DON'T EAT YOUR HEART OUT COOKBOOK

P9-DFA-521

by Joseph C. Piscatella
Recipes by Bernie Piscatella

WORKMAN PUBLISHING, NEW YORK

Library of Congress Cataloging in Publication Data

Piscatella, Joseph C.
Don't eat your heart out.

Bibliography: p.
Includes index.
1. Heart—Diseases—Diet therapy—Recipes.
I. Piscatella, Bernie.   II. Title.
RC684.D5P57   1983   641.5'6311   83-14810

ISBN 0-89480-488-X
Book Designed by Vlahovich Design Associates

Workman Publishing Company, Inc.

708 Broadway

New York, NY 10003

Manufactured in the United States

First printing September 1983
Second printing January 1984
Third printing April 1984
Fourth printing July 1984
Fifth printing November 1984
Sixth printing June 1985
Seventh printing November 1985
Eighth printing March 1986
Ninth printing July 1986
Tenth printing October 1986
Eleventh printing March 1987
Twelfth printing March 1987
Thirteenth printing July 1987

Revised edition: first printing October 1987

30 29 28 27 26 25 24 23 22 21

Originally published under the title
Don't Eat Your Heart Out.

At age 32, I underwent coronary bypass surgery. It forced me to come to grips with the fact that heart disease is an American epidemic; it doesn't just happen to "the other guy." It also forced me to recognize that certain aspects of my lifestyle, particularly my diet, were greatly responsible for my condition.

After the surgery, I found myself facing a very difficult problem: how to eat healthfully and still be a part of the modern American lifestyle. The standard "heart-healthy" diets were tasteless and unrealistic. In addition, none of them paid attention to permanent dietary change. They just said, "Don't eat that!" about every food I liked.

To overcome this problem, I had to develop an appealing, real-life diet. The result is this book. *Don't Eat Your Heart Out* presents a diet with healthy, appetizing foods—a hassle-free approach to eating for cardiac patients and others concerned about the health of their heart. Complete with recipes, menus and meal plans, it explains the practical application of low-fat, low-salt, low-sugar and low-cholesterol principles to the contemporary American diet. It is a blueprint for permanently changing a diet pattern.

Don't Eat Your Heart Out has become the standard for a heart-healthy diet in over 4500 hospitals and is used in both cardiac rehabilitation and prevention programs. Its sensible, practical approach has made it a favorite of medical professionals and patients alike. This revised edition contains current information on diet, including research on the effects of olive oil and fish oil on cholesterol. While much of the information is new, the premise of the book has not changed: eating well and eating healthfully can be the same thing.

Joseph C. Piscatella

ACKNOWLEDGEMENTS

No one person produces a book such as this by himself. *Don't Eat Your Heart Out* would not exist were it not for the support and help of many people. In particular, I am grateful to Dr. John Nagle, Dr. James Early, Dr. Gail Strait, Dr. Denton Cooley, Dr. J. Ward Kennedy, Dr. Jack Copeland, Diane Gallagher (R.N.), Carole Gentry (R.N.), and Jean Macy (R.D.), all of whom gave generously of their time and expertise, providing valuable appraisals of the manuscript. In addition, Bonnie Nelson, Joan Imhof, Mary Piscatella, Em Stern and Pam Andrew furnished helpful editorial comment and suggestions for change. For their able and efficient secretarial support, my thanks to Flor Covey and Denise Johnson. A special note of thanks to John Vlahovich and Jim Gibson for balancing incredible patience with strong guidance in developing the graphic design of the book. And finally, my overwhelming thanks to my wife, Bernie, my most vocal critic and best friend, for her original contributions and for her untiring dedication to making this book become a reality.

CONTENTS

FOREWORD 9

PREFACE 13

INTRODUCTION 17

1. THE HEART AND THE CORONARY
    ARTERIES 37
    The Heart 37
    How the Heart Works. 40
    The Coronary Arteries 42

2. CORONARY HEART DISEASE 47
    Who Gets Coronary Heart Disease? 48
    The Development of Coronary Heart
        Disease 50
    The Results of Coronary Heart Disease 53
    Focusing on the Real Problem 57

3. THE AMERICAN DIET IS A CARDIAC
    RISK FACTOR. 59
    Fat and Cholesterol .61
    Salt. 72
    Sugar 77
    Myths of the American Diet 82
    A Last Word 89
    The Reversibility of Atherosclerosis. 90

4. THE POSITIVE DIET. 93
    The Basic Principles. 96
    The Basic Tools 98
    Applying the Basic Principles and the Basic
        Tools 103

5. IMPLEMENTING THE POSITIVE DIET .105
   Reducing Fat and Cholesterol............105
   Reducing Butterfat......................124
   Summing Up Fat and Cholesterol........130
   Reducing Salt...........................131
   Summing Up Salt.......................137
   Reducing Sugar.........................140
   Summing Up Sugar....................144

6. THE SECRET TO SUCCESS: TIMING ...151

7. WEIGHT CONTROL 159
   Obesity Is a Cardiac Risk Factor..........160
   Quick Weight Loss.....................163
   The Positive Diet Approach to
      Weight Loss.........................164

8. HOW TO HANDLE EATING IN A
      RESTAURANT......................171

COOKBOOK

9. COMMENTS FROM THE COOK........181

10. MEAL PLANNING 195

11. APPETIZERS AND BEVERAGES.......235

12. BREADS AND BREAKFASTS..........265

13. SOUPS AND SANDWICHES 293

14. SALADS AND SALAD DRESSINGS 329

15. VEGETABLES........................367

16. SEAFOOD 413

17. POULTRY...........................445

18. RED MEATS 475

19. DESSERTS...........................499

SOURCE NOTES........................529

BIBLIOGRAPHY 531

GENERAL INDEX.......................537

INDEX TO RECIPES 544

FOREWORD

At last the lay public has become seriously concerned about the growing problem of heart disease in contemporary society, and many self-designated authorities on preventive medicine give convincing advice, often based, however, upon meager scientific knowledge. While some risk factors are beyond our control, such as heredity and genetics and gender, others are subject to deliberate and meaningful change. Diet and nutrition are obviously conducive to planned alteration and control, and we, as potential victims of death or disability from heart disease, should accept the obligation to improve our eating habits. Abuses are equally present for both the type and the quality of the food we consume.

First, the problem of obesity in our modern society should be addressed. More than a century ago, Sir Richard Burton (1821-1890), a person whom I have often found quotable said, "Gluttony is the source of all our infirmities and the fountain of all our diseases. As a lamp is choked by a superabundance of oil, and a fire extinguished by excess of fuel, so is the natural health of the body destroyed by intemperate diet." Gluttony is an inborn sin or vice, and most healthy humans are already guilty at birth. Self control must, therefore, be developed in an opulent environment where foodstuffs abound.

Starvation and famine, which still confront some geographic regions, are problems seldom confronting western societies. In past generations, parents overfed their children believing that this would provide a good "start" in life with healthy bones, teeth, and full growth. Poor eating habits, mostly from dietary excesses, which were instilled at an early age often prevailed in young minds and continued throughout life. Everyone can recall the "fatty" in grade school whom other children ridiculed. The fault was not his or hers, but their parents who were ill-informed about sound nutrition.

During adulthood, overeating leads not only to obesity which causes cardiovascular hardship, but also to deposits of excess, unused nutritional elements, not the least of which are cholesterol and triglycerides. Obese individuals consistently claim that they eat sparingly or "like a bird," but in truth that bird must be more like a bald eagle than an English sparrow.

The second alterable dietary factor is the quality or type of nutrients we ingest. Scientific knowledge has accumulated which incriminates fats (particularly the saturated animal fats), refined sugar, salt, and cholesterol. Taken in excess, these substances affect the cardiovascular system, and when all of these dietary abuses are supported by cigarettes, alcohol, and stress, the consequences may be disastrous. Thus, attention to diet is mandatory to good health.

But in addition to diet, a well-balanced life including time for work, recreation, and rest must be developed. In a modern society such as ours with a strong work ethic, intelligent individuals fail to appreciate the need for all three. One's work should be recognized as a privilege which provides the necessities of a comfortable environment. Recreation is vital to relieve stress by providing diversion. Healthful exercise habits should be developed to maintain muscular tone and general physical and mental fitness. But one should not overlook the physiologic importance and need for rest and sleep.

The author of this book, Joseph C. Piscatella, when confronted with coronary arteriosclerosis and cardiac surgery at just 32 years of age, responded dramatically to an obvious need to change his lifestyle. This book, which describes his experience with heart disease and outlines a plan for a positive diet, reveals a true fighting spirit coupled with an inquisitive and determined mind and should help others to prevent similar problems and still others to cope better with the realization that they have heart disease and need surgical treatment. *Don't Eat Your Heart Out* should be available not only to sufferers from heart disease, but also to all young adults before the devastation of arteriosclerosis becomes critical.

Denton A. Cooley, M.D.
Surgeon-in-Chief
Texas Heart Institute

PREFACE

As a cardiac surgeon performing coronary artery bypass operations on a daily basis, I have been surprised over the last ten years at the safety and efficacy of the operation which represents the first surgical intervention in a line of many previous failures which actually helps people with coronary artery disease. Ninety-five percent of patients are relieved of angina and the mortality rate is 1% to 3% in the hands of adequately trained cardiothoracic surgeons. It would be wonderful if these results persisted over the postoperative years. Unfortunately, when one critically reviews the long-term results, this is not true.

Even though coronary artery bypass surgery relieves pain and in certain anatomic configurations of coronary obstructive lesions, such as left main coronary or triple vessel disease, prolongs life beyond that expected with medical therapy, the operation must be placed in the category of those procedures called palliative. Simply placing a venous or arterial conduit such that it bypasses a coronary obstruction providing increased blood flow to the heart does nothing about the underlying process, arteriosclerosis. And in all coronary bypass patients we can expect that the underlying disease will continue.

We know from late follow-up studies that six years after coronary artery bypass only 40% to 50% of patients will be free of symptoms compared to the 95% figure for the early postoperative period. Admittedly, some of the poor postoperative results may be due to bypass graft closure in the first 3 postoperative months (15%), but even with a 15% graft closure rate, most patients remain asymptomatic. I believe that the arteriosclerotic process accounts for most of the late problems.

We have seen in numerous patients returning for second, third, and even fourth bypass operations, evidence of more arteriosclerotic disease of their own coronary arteries and in their saphenous vein bypass grafts. Therefore, I view the coronary bypass operation as a temporary improvement in blood supply to the heart. It is not a curative procedure. It does not make the patient any more or less susceptible to arteriosclerois than he was before the surgery. And, unless some drastic measures are taken, particularly in younger patients, the "window" of symptom-free, infarction-free time provided by coronary artery bypass may be measured in just a few years to a decade.

All of my coronary artery bypass patients are considered for a multiphasic rehabilitation program involving dietary modifications, stress control, a carefully monitored program of progressively increasing exercise and a long-term medical follow-up including lipid analysis and treadmill exercise testing. I firmly believe that reduction of risk factors tailored to the individual patient in the long run may be as important as doing an excellent bypass operation. Obviously, not all patients are able to participate in all phases of the program, but they all must eat and therefore may change their diets.

The "American diet" is, I believe, a major reason for the high incidence of coronary artery disease in our society. Mr. Piscatella's book attacks this diet, and also provides abundant examples of a less atherogenic alternative. I believe this information should be available to every American male, his mother, and his mate if we are to decrease the dietary risk factors contributing to the epidemic of coronary artery disease in the United States. I intend to recommend *Don't Eat Your Heart Out* to all of my coronary bypass patients and to make it an often used resource in my own home.

Jack G. Copeland, M.D.
Professor & Chief
Section of Cardiothoracic Surgery
University of Arizona Health Sciences Center

INTRODUCTION

It was a hot July afternoon, and for the second time in a week, I was seated in the office of Dr. John Nagle, a prominent cardiologist in Tacoma, Washington. I was bewildered as to why I was there.

Five days earlier I had been in to see my internist, Dr. James Early, about what I thought was a lung problem. For about a month I had been experiencing some pain in my chest while I warmed up to play tennis. By the end of the warmup, the pain would usually disappear. But the day before I saw Dr. Early, the pain had remained with me through six hours of tennis. It was then that I decided to call Dr. Early. He asked me to come in the following morning.

He was concerned about the pain, more concerned than I was at the time, and he advised that an electrocardiogram, called an EKG, be taken. An EKG measures the electrical impulses of the heart and is used as a standard indicator of cardiac health. A previous EKG had been taken just four months earlier during my annual physical exam and the results then had been normal. The results now, however, were drastically different.

"Joe, the EKG indicates a heart abnormality, perhaps indicative of a very serious heart problem," said Dr. Early. "I want you to see a cardiologist immediately."

So, three hours after my "routine" exam with

Dr. Early, instead of meeting a business associate for lunch as planned, I found myself in Dr. Nagle's office undergoing a thorough cardiac examination. Jim Early is a respected and competent physician. I did not take his sending me to a cardiologist lightly. But I did not believe that there was anything seriously wrong either; I was sure that it was a mistake.

The result of Dr. Nagle's examination was the same: a heart problem existed. But he could not tell how serious the problem was. There was only one way to determine its extent, and that was to undergo a coronary arteriogram, a surgical procedure in which the heart and the coronary arteries are X-rayed. Two days later I underwent this procedure. Now Dr. Nagle was ready to review the results with me.

"Joe," he said, "you have a severely blocked coronary artery, about a 95 percent obstruction from what we can tell, which is causing the chest pain, called angina. This condition is identified as 'coronary heart disease.' The blockage is a buildup of fat and cholesterol on the artery wall. It is badly located, being in the coronary artery which supplies the main pumping chamber of the heart. The smallest blood clot could stop the flow of blood completely and trigger a heart attack. The result of such an attack could be fatal.

" We could put you on certain drugs to try to keep the artery open, but I don't think they would be very effective in the long run. I would recommend open-heart surgery be done immediately. . . I mean within the next few days. At this moment you are a heart attack statistic just waiting to happen."

I was 32 years old.

The shock of his words hit me like a slap in the face. This couldn't happen to me! I was not prepared to hear what he had to say; I had difficulty understanding his words. He was speaking about a heart problem — my heart problem! — that psychologically I could not accept. Several thoughts of escape filled my mind. "Just get up and leave," I told myself. "It's all a mistake. You're not supposed to be here." Once safely back in my world, I reasoned, I would surely awaken from this horrible nightmare.

As I continued to listen numbly to Dr. Nagle, I was confused. Like most people, I knew something about the workings of the heart, but the information was principally of the Biology 101 variety. It had been a number of years since I had cause to study the human body, so the details concerning the heart were nebulous at best. About the coronary arteries, those tiny channels which supply blood to the heart; about the blockage, the result of coronary heart disease; and about the potential result, the heart attack, I knew nothing.

It wasn't that information about the heart and coronary heart disease was not available, for it was. The American Heart Association, among others, had produced and disseminated a tremendous amount of such information. But, quite frankly, it had been of remote interest to me. The information, indeed the entire subject matter itself, was simply not relevant to my life.

What did blocked arteries or heart attacks have to do with me? After all, I was just 32 years old and in the prime of my life. There was plenty of time, I thought, to read all those Heart Association pamphlets while I was rocking in retirement. There were many other things in my life which were of more immediate importance to me.

Unknowingly I had succumbed to the "what I don't know won't hurt me" syndrome. But in reality what I didn't know could not only hurt me, it

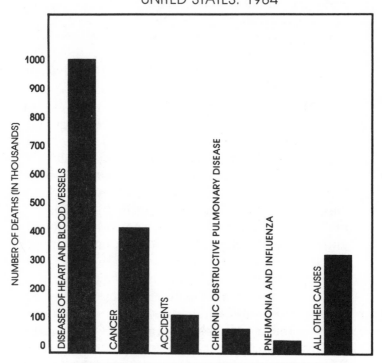

LEADING CAUSES OF DEATH
UNITED STATES: 1984

SOURCE: NATIONAL CENTER FOR HEALTH STATISTICS, U.S. PUBLIC HEALTH SERVICE, DHEW

could kill me.

What I didn't know was that coronary heart disease develops silently, insidiously over a long period of time, generally 20 to 40 years. Once it surfaces, however, the results — angina, stroke and heart attack — are often rapidly devastating.

What I didn't know was that over 5.5 million Americans have coronary heart disease and that every year some 1.5 million are struck by heart attacks, causing an estimated 600,000 to 800,000 fatalities annually

What I didn't know was that two people die every 60 seconds in the United States from some form of heart disease.

What I didn't know was that heart disease causes 51% of all the deaths in the United States each year — more than cancer, auto accidents, floods and airplane disasters combined.

What I didn't know was that for 50% of all heart attack victims, their initial heart attack resulted in sudden death.

And what I didn't know was that lifestyle — the way in which we live — could increase or decrease the risk of coronary heart disease and that my dietary lifestyle had resulted in a culturally induced heart problem.

Information such as this was simply outside the realm of my everyday life. But it all changed on that hot July day. Listening to Dr. Nagle, I became intensely interested. I thought of El Cordobés, the famous Spanish matador, who once said that his interest in the bullfight increased in direct ratio to the closeness of the bull's horns. Confused, but "close to the horns," I struggled to understand the nature of the problem.

My second reaction was one of irritation and anger, the typical "Why me?" response. As I saw it, I was young, physically active, in the midst of building a career, raising a family, and contributing to my community. I took care of my health and had no physical problems. Moreover, I didn't beat my wife, steal from the poor or kick the family dog.

What could have caused such a thing as coronary heart disease to strike me and to imperil my life? It wasn't fair. There was no logic in the selection process. It was like being seated with 100,000 others in the Rose Bowl and having your ticket number announced as the winner in a lottery for a firing squad. Why me?

Then I remembered a comment made by President Kennedy at the beginning of the Viet Nam war on the fact that life was unfair, that unfairness was a part of its nature. There were no guarantees. The randomness of death existed for everyone. All at once I understood. Why not me?

I was gripped by pure stomach-churning fear. Dr. Nagle wanted the surgery performed "immediately . . . in the next few days." He would not consider any delay because of the high potential for a fatal heart attack. I was, in his words, a heart attack waiting to happen. The prospect of death, of leaving my wife, Bernie, and our children, Anne, then 6, and Joey, then 4, was crushing.

I had never carried that weight before. At 32, I had felt a kind of immortality that only the young experience. The concept of death had been a remote one for me. I pictured it at the end of a long life, after years of accomplishment, fulfillment and joy. Old age was something that I looked forward to sharing with Bernie. For death to take me in my prime had never been contemplated.

On that July day the alarm clock of reality rang. I realized that not only could death happen now, but that it probably would happen now, the result of a time bomb located inside of my chest.

As we talked that afternoon, Dr. Nagle calmly and deliberately explained the many facets of the problem and the options. We talked about the physiology of the heart and the coronary arteries, and of the impact of heart disease. We talked about some of the reasons that could cause the disease to develop, the so-called risk factors. We talked about why the surgery was necessary ("At this stage we don't know if drugs could keep the artery open; it's too severely blocked."); about how it was performed ("We can't clean out the existing artery, so we'll create a new one for you."); about what the potential problems were ("The operation is a serious one. Any time you are on the heart-lung machine, there is a risk of stroke and cardiac arrest, which could be fatal."); and about what the long term risks were ("The procedure is relatively new and about 10% of all bypasses close up in the first year. Statistically we do not know the long term results.").

Soon the late afternoon shadows began to grow and I knew that the day was almost done. Like the day itself, I was also out of time. A decision was needed. Treat the problem with drugs and be satisfied with the half-life of a cardiac cripple? Or undergo cardiac surgery, a risky procedure which was less than 10 years old and could promise no long term success?

I chose the surgery.

Less than a week after meeting with Dr. Nagle, Dr. Kari Vitikainen, a gifted surgeon practicing in Tacoma, conducted a 5-hour coronary surgery at Tacoma General Hospital in which he took a piece of vein from my left leg and used it to create a new arterial channel to the heart. The new channel would allow the blood in the coronary artery to flow freely around the blockage. It literally "by-passed" the blockage, from whence the operation gained its name. The procedure was not without problems and I had to return to surgery two days later due to complications. Ultimately, however, it was a success. Life-sustaining blood was once again flowing freely to my heart.

Ten days after surgery I was recovering at home. Initially I felt terrible and was in considerable pain and discomfort. I was weak and had neither strength nor stamina; I felt as though I had been hit by a train. In this physical condition my mental faculties were taxed to the limit with simple decisions. Comprehension and reasoning were difficult. It was a time of physical and mental anguish, but I was elated to be alive.

As I began to mend physically, I slowly began to comprehend what had taken place. I began to think about what was ahead of me. Despite the sheer joy of survival, I was very concerned about the unknowns in my future. Surgery had circumvented the disease, but it had not stopped it. I asked a number of questions: How did I get coronary heart disease? What had caused its development? Would new blockages develop in the future? What had to be done to retard or abate the disease?

Reflecting upon my experience, I concluded that there were many things about coronary heart disease that I did not know. But there were some things that I did know. I knew that I did not want the disease to reoccur in me. I knew that I did not want to die a premature death from a heart attack. I knew that I did not want to live the half-life of a coronary cripple. And I knew that I did not want to undergo a second coronary surgery.

I was seriously concerned about how I was going to live the rest of my life. I would do whatever was within my power to prevent future heart problems. I understood how lucky I had been.

Coronary heart disease could have killed me, but it did not. Instead I was alive and recuperating. The surgery was in the past; I was interested in the future.

It was a turning point in my life: I could slip back into my comfortable old lifestyle, or I could develop a different, more healthful lifestyle.

Since my old lifestyle had contributed to the coronary problem, returning to it was not a viable alternative. It was only prudent for the sake of my heart to adopt a new lifestyle.

I wanted to do something positive to enhance my cardiac health, and with it, the quality and the longevity of my life, but I was immobilized by a lack of clear direction. What should I do? How should I do it? What was it in my lifestyle that was harmful to my health, and why was it so? It became obvious that no serious change could be accomplished based upon my current fragments of information. I needed to better understand the causes of coronary heart disease before I could determine how to alleviate those causes. Again I turned to Dr. Nagle.

"I'm glad you are interested in cardiac risk factors," he said. "In my opinion the identification and the control of these risk factors will be the key to the future health of your heart.

"During the past ten to fifteen years, a number of major developments have taken place concerning coronary heart disease. You have already benefited from some of those developments, Joe, such as the arteriogram, the heart-lung machine, and the by-pass surgery technique itself. As important as those developments are, they may prove to be less significant in the long run than the discovery that certain aspects of our lifestyle can increase the risk of coronary heart disease.

"The way a person lives may dictate how healthy his heart will be. Because many relevant aspects of lifestyle can be controlled or modified, a person has some ability to influence his cardiovascular health. Unlike the other developments which deal in correction, the discovery of cardiac risk factors provides us with a means to deal with prevention.

"The discovery of cardiac risk factors is not a new one," he continued. "In fact it's about 25 years old. And during those years enormous amounts of time, energy, and money have been expended in medical and scientific research to identify exactly how the risk factors work to produce coronary heart disease. Despite all this effort, we still do not have many definitive answers. But we do know two things: one, certain aspects of lifestyle foster the development of coronary heart disease, and two, most of these lifestyle aspects occur in Americans. Our particular way of life contains a multitude of cardiac risk factors, enough to have made heart attacks in the United States a culturally-induced epidemic."

I could understand in general what Dr. Nagle was explaining, but I was not certain what a cardiac risk factor was. "The most common risk factors," he explained, "are genetics; gender; diets high in fat, sugar, salt and cholesterol; obesity; lack of physical exercise; high blood pressure; cigarette smoking; and stress.

"Obviously two of these risk factors — genetics and gender — are beyond our control. Should either one of them be the primary cause for coronary heart disease, there is not much that can be done to prevent the disease from occuring. But the rest of the risk factors are controllable.

"To a certain extent, the development of coronary heart disease is also controllable. How you eat, whether or not you exercise, whether or not you smoke; how you manage your stress — those are aspects of lifestyle over which you have control. Since we know that these aspects can increase the risk of heart attack, their control does provide a person with some say about the destiny of his or her cardiac health.

"In your case, Joe, your diet pattern, which is a manifestation of your lifestyle, is a primary risk factor. Your diet is the contemporary American diet: rich in cholesterol, fats, salt, sugar and total calories. Our 'go-go' society has developed fast foods, snack foods, convenience foods, canned foods, frozen foods, and junk foods. The result of this diet pattern for you has been a high level of cholesterol and fat in your blood, a condition that raises the risk for the development of coronary heart disease. And you are not alone. The American diet pattern may be the single largest contributing factor to the high incidence of coronary heart disease and heart attack in this country."

"Does anyone else know about this?" I interjected. "Why isn't this publicized? I never knew our national diet constituted a health problem."

Dr. Nagle smiled. "Yes, Joe, many people are aware of it. But it never ceases to amaze me that people have not been educated about the proper role of diet. The American Heart Association has been working for a change in our diet pattern since 1961. The U.S. Senate's Select Committee on Nutrition has established dietary goals that are at odds with the contemporary American diet pattern. Indeed, many organizations today are concerned about the level of non-nutritive food in the American diet.

"While Americans consume great quantities of food, they simultaneously suffer from malnutri-

27

tion that may be as damaging to the nation's health as were the widespread contagious diseases of the early part of the century. Our national diet is a nutritional travesty, and we are paying for it with increasing numbers of degenerative diseases, including coronary heart disease. McDonald's has spent over $230 million, Coca Cola over $197 million, and Mars candy over $40 million annually to promote products which are high in fat, salt, and sugar. How does a message about diet as a cardiac risk factor overcome those advertising dollars?

"Let me make an additional point," he continued. "It is a common misconception that the American diet pattern is a healthy one as evidenced by the longevity of life in the United States. American longevity is a myth. Life expectancy today has increased statistically by some 20 years since 1900, but much of that statistical increase is due to a decrease in the infant mortality rate. In 1900 more babies died, so the life expectancy averages were lower. Today fewer babies die, so the averages are not significantly altered by infant mortalities. For a 50-year old man, the increase in life expectancy today over 1900 is only 2.2 years — despite our modern medicine, drugs and technology. A good part of the reason is our national diet.

"Coronary heart disease is a modern disease. Pathologists report that less than 50 years ago arterial blockages were infrequent and not a cause for concern. Today these blockages are present in virtually all adult Americans and in many children as well. They are responsible for 1 out of every 2 Americans dying from heart attack or stroke. I think one of the most important things which you can do for yourself, Joe, is to institute a more healthful way of eating."

As he was speaking, I realized the extent of my ignorance. I knew very little about my diet or my nutritional needs and absolutely nothing about diet as a cardiac risk factor. While I suspected that not all the food on my diet was highly nutritional, I had no inkling that this diet could produce such a negative impact upon the health of my heart. I was encouraged by his words, however, for I believed that we had identified an aspect of my health problem about which I could take some action.

All that was needed, I thought, was for Dr. Nagle to fill in the blanks — to explain clearly the relationship of my particular diet pattern to my cardiac health, to design a new diet for me, and to instruct me as to how that new diet should be instituted. Naively I thought that just because he was a physician, all this information would be at his finger-tips. He would tell me what to do and how to do it, and it would easily be accomplished.

Unfortunately, we were dealing with realism. "Much as I would like to do the whole thing for you," he said, "the fact is that few physicians can offer much more than general advice and direction in the reorientation of diet. We can be helpful, but we can't make it happen. Only you can do that. The starting point is, of course, understanding the role of diet in coronary health and identifying the problems of our diet pattern in general. I can certainly help you in that regard. I can tell you about tested principles (such as a diet rich in saturated fat will elevate blood cholesterol levels), and I can direct you to research and clinical studies which can provide more indepth information.

"Once you understand the problems with your diet, you have only solved one-third of the equation. The other two-thirds are the really difficult tasks: *1. designing a new diet pattern;* and *2. implementing it.* Unfortunately, in these areas I can help you very little. Medicine can provide you with general principles and a sense of direction, but it can't do the work for you. You are the only person who can restructure your own diet.

"Much information has been published by the American Heart Association and others concerning heart-healthy diets. My recommendation is that you investigate the available information and use it to construct a new diet which will fit both the needs of your personal lifestyle and the needs of your heart. Once you have done that, it will be a matter of making the diet permanent. No one else can do that for you."

I wasn't happy about what Dr. Nagle had to say. I was looking for an easy answer — a pill or a prescription. Instead he gave me straightforward information: the task would not be easy, and the responsibility was mine. It was my heart; it was my life; it had to be my effort.

The next six months were spent in study and investigation, trying to understand the many facets of diet and cardiac health. I struggled with medical texts about the heart and the coronary arteries, about cholesterol, and about coronary heart disease. Books, papers and articles were read and re-read. I attended seminars, lectures and clinics from coast to coast, and interviewed a number of physicians, nutritionists and chemical biologists. I digested every cookbook, pamphlet, and article published by the American Heart Association. And I continued to visit with Dr. Nagle. Finally, after much work, I was able to complete the first one-third of the equation: I understood the mechanics of my coronary problem, how my diet had contributed to that problem, and what had to be done to change my diet and to reduce the risk of future coronary problems.

The process of collecting and evaluating information was not an easy one. As a layman, my background and experience were not suited for medical reasearch, and often my limitations were reached. At the same time, however, I knew that there had to be a way for a layman to more clearly understand the nature of coronary heart disease and the role of diet in the disease process.

It was not my role, as I saw it, to discover something new; I merely wished to synthesize and to evaluate current information, and arrive at a rational conclusion as to what was the best, most healthful diet pattern for me. My research led me to certain conclusions:

1. *Diet Pattern Is A Cardiac Risk Factor.* The evidence linking diet to coronary heart disease comes from various epidemiologic studies, such as the Framingham Study, where the incidence and potential causes of disease in different populations have been surveyed. Studies of populations since World War II have illustrated a strong correlation between dietary fat, blood cholesterol and coronary heart disease. While diet may not be the only factor in the development of the disease, clearly it is a factor.

2. *The Contemporary American Diet Significantly Increases The Potential For Coronary Heart Disease.* Americans eat well by world standards, but our national diet is a major factor in the high number of coronary fatalities in the United States. While much of the world suffers from nutrient deficiency diseases, Americans suffer from chronic diseases caused by nutrient excesses. Too much dietary fat, cholesterol, salt, sugar and total calories have contributed to elevated levels of obesity, high blood

31

pressure, stroke and heart attack. With a diet consisting of 42% fat, 24% sugar and 5% alcohol, many nutritionists consider Americans to be the most overfed and undernourished people in the world. The American Heart Association, the U.S. Surgeon General, the Department of Agriculture, the Department of Health and Human Services, the United States Senate Select Committee on Nutrition, and 17 other major health organizations consider the American diet to be a significant coronary risk factor.

3. *Diet Pattern Can Be Controlled And Cardiac Risk Can Be Diminished.* Laboratory tests and field studies have illustrated that dietary change can produce a lowering of blood cholesterol. During World War II, Scandinavians were denied their typically high-fat diet. Consequently, the incidence of heart attack diminished. After the war their high-fat diet was resumed and the incidence of heart attack also increased. More recently, clinical tests on Rhesus monkeys have indicated that a reversal of coronary artery blockage buildup may be possible through a low-fat, low-cholesterol diet.

4. *The Responsibility For Dietary Change Rests With The Individual.* Help is available from family, friends, physicians and organizations. But they cannot make the change happen. Only the individual can do that. One physician stated it succinctly: "We doctors are trained in disease. That is why coronary problems can be diagnosed and corrected. But what you are talking about — the control of diet in order to reduce coronary risk — is not disease. It is health. And health, strangely enough, is not our field. Health is the responsibility of each person."

So, armed with basic knowledge about diet and coronary health, and motivated by an intense desire to reduce my cardiac risk, I began to translate what I had learned into a specific and practical program of dietary change. This was neither an easy nor a quick effort; progress was slow and was measured in small increments. Trial and error ruled. Some meals were disasters; others were very good. Some new cooking techniques worked well; others did not and had to be abandoned. Some days I could easily stay on a diet; other days I experienced cravings for pizza, pastrami sandwiches, or chocolate bars. There was much frustration in designing a new diet plan. But there were also many resources to call upon. A diet for me might not have existed, but after combing many cookbooks and experimenting in the kitchen, I knew that such a diet was possible.

It was then that I ran into the second problem: how to specifically institute and maintain such a diet. The cookbooks and other resources could tell me how to prepare a recipe, but not a single one told me how to institute permanent dietary change. I found that I was building the proverbial bicycle as I was riding it. Many times I came close to giving up the struggle, but I knew that the alternative — returning to my old diet — was not the answer. Finally, the progress started to take root and a totally new dietary program began to take shape. The new diet that evolved was realistic, practical and workable, and it had a positive impact upon my coronary health. For that reason, I called it "The Positive Diet."

After a year on the Positive Diet, I returned to see Dr. Nagle for a checkup. He was well pleased with my condition. My cholesterol count had gone from a high of 360 to a low of 208. My weight went from 185 pounds to 165 pounds. He remarked that all of his cardiac patients should follow such a diet.

"Why don't they?" I asked.

"For a variety of reasons," he replied. "Many of them aren't as young as you are, and most wouldn't be able to put in the effort to design and implement such a diet. Nevertheless, they need it as much as you do."

It was then that I first thought of writing this book. *Don't Eat Your Heart Out* is a personal statement of how one person altered his dietary lifestyle in order to enhance cardiac health. It was developed not as an academic exercise, but as a program of survival to control my dietary destiny.

The book includes information about healthful and harmful foods, menus, recipes and cooking tips.

However, it is not simply a compilation of dietary information. It is a "how-to" book, a step-by-step outline of how to achieve a permanent change in dietary pattern. It is dedicated to the premise that no one — least of all a cardiac patient — should suffer a heart attack as the result of inadequate or insufficient information.

Will the Positive Diet be of help to cardiac patients and others interested in heart health? I believe it will. Obviously, no cardiac patient should institute dietary change without first consulting his or her physician. However, the individual should understand that all of us are ultimately responsible for our own cardiac health. For those who want to institute a heart-healthy diet, this book is a tool. If it helps even one person, it will have been worth the effort.

A friend of mine recently asked, "Why did you write the book? It took a long time and it must have been painful to recall unpleasant memories." I was reminded of the story of the chicken and the pig which I related to him as an explanation.

The chicken and pig were walking down the main street of town and they came to a restaurant with a sign in the window, "Ham and eggs, $2.00." The chicken beamed and pointed to the sign. "See that," she said, "I'm an integral part of the process. I'm involved." The pig studied the sign for a long moment, then turned to the chicken. "For you, it's involvement," he answered. "For me, it's total commitment."

For me, also, it's total commitment.

Joseph C. Piscatella
Tacoma, Washington

CHAPTER ONE

THE HEART AND THE CORONARY ARTERIES

Until the time of my coronary surgery, I had felt no need to understand the function and the operation of the heart. Its health, much like freedom, was taken for granted. With the shock of surgery, however, came the desire to understand more about the heart. Suddenly, I was hungry for information about its functions, about the role of the coronary arteries, and about the complex arrangement of blood vessels in the circulatory system. I knew that the heart had to first be understood before an appreciation of the role of coronary heart disease could be gained.

THE HEART

The word "heart" is one of the most frequently used words in the English language. It is a word with many meanings which has been used throughout the ages in history, music and literature to describe love and affection, "to win her heart"; courage or spirit, "lion-hearted"; the core or vital part, "the heart of the matter"; a capacity for sympathy, "a heart of gold"; and as an expression of affection, "dear heart." These, along with ace of hearts, heart crops, the game of hearts, heartache. . . are all secondary meanings of the word.

One would think that with the number and the richness of the secondary meanings, the prime definition of "the heart" would be spectacular. Alas, it is not. Webster defines "the heart" simply as a "hollow muscular organ which by rhythmic contractions and relaxations keeps the blood in circulation." This is certainly an adequate, if vastly understated, definition, but it does not truly capture the nature of this wonderful organ.

The heart is what the heart does: it is a pump. Pure and simple, pumping is what the heart is all about. Certainly there are many physiological complexities concerning the heart, such as celluar structure, electronic impulses, oxygen sensitivity and so forth. But when these complexities are removed, the essential nature of the heart remains. . . it is a pump. To describe the heart merely as "a pump," however, is akin to describing Mt. Everest merely as "a mountain" or the Amazon simply as "a river."

The heart is not just "a pump" — it is *THE PUMP!* Every day this unbelievable organ pumps 2100 gallons of blood continuously at the rate of over one gallon a minute through some 60,000 miles of blood vessels to reach over 300 trillion body cells. In order to accomplish this monumental task, the heart must beat over 100,000 times a day. At this rate, in an average lifetime the heart will pump over 135 million gallons of blood in more than 2½ billion heartbeats, and that is just when it is resting. It can pump six times its resting volume during exercise!

This pumping is such an amazing feat that its magnitude is often difficult to comprehend. Two and one-half billion heartbeats. . . It's like talking about the national debt. The figures are too large to be realistic. Perhaps that is why the heart is taken for granted by most people and often is not appreciated until a problem occurs.

Many misconceptions abound about the heart. Upon learning of the awesome amount of work that is required of it, I assumed that the heart would be rather large. It is, in fact, quite small, about the size of a clenched fist, and usually weighs between seven and twelve ounces, depending upon the size of the person. By comparison, the heart of a bull elephant can weigh over 50 pounds.

A second misconception concerns the location of the heart. Most people believe, as I did, that the heart is located in the left breast. But in actuality the heart is located in the center of the chest directly behind the protective breastbone. Before my coronary surgery, I gave no thought to the location of the heart; but now, smug in my newly acquired anatomical knowledge, I smile inwardly each time I stand in Seattle's Kingdome and see 60,000 people sing the national anthem with a hand over their left lung.

A third misconception generally held concerns the shape of the heart. The heart is simply not "heart-shaped." It does not remotely resemble the classic valentine heart. While it may come as a shock to romantics and candy manufacturers alike, the heart is really shaped like. . . an eggplant! Suspended in its protective sac, the pericardium, the heart looks exactly like a grocery store eggplant in a plastic bag. Can you imagine Valentine's Day with chocolate eggplants and eggplant-shaped boxes of candy? For some people, myself included, this might take "truth in advertising" one step too far.

HOW THE HEART WORKS

The human body is made up of over 300 trillion individual cells. Each of these cells is a life unto itself, and each has a metabolic need for oxygen and nutrients in order to produce energy and new cellular material. Each cell also has a need to expel waste products and carbon dioxide. In this respect, the life of each cell parallels the life of the body as a whole.

The process of "in with the good, out with the bad" must occur continuously if the cells are to remain healthy. Any disruption in the process — too little oxygen and nutrients going in or too little waste and carbon dioxide coming out — will negatively impact their good health. Of critical importance to each cell is an uninterrupted supply of oxygen, for no cell can live more than 30 minutes without oxygen. Some cells, notably those in the brain and in the heart, live for a considerably shorter time when deprived of oxygen.

For this reason blood is constantly being circulated throughout the thousands of miles of arteries, arterioles, capillaries, veins and venules which make up the blood vessel system. The blood vessels are the vehicle by which oxygen and nutrients are delivered to the cells and by which waste and carbon dioxide are removed from them. It is much like an enormous freeway system which is connected to a city. On the incoming roads are found a flow of food trucks going into the city; on the outgoing roads are found garbage trucks hauling refuse from the city. The life of the city depends upon the constant movement of the trucks on the freeway. Any slowing or stopping of this traffic could result in famine or disease. It is the same for the body. Blood must circulate constantly throughout the blood vessel system. But it can only do so as a result of the pumping action of the heart.

While the heart is considered a single organ, biologically it is two separate pumps which work together: the right heart and the left heart. The two pumps are completely separated from each other by a wall of muscle. Each heart has two chambers, the atrium, or holding chamber; and the ventricle, or pumping chamber. The right heart receives the blood containing waste products and carbon dioxide in the right atrium. This blood, called "poor blood" is low in oxygen. (Contrary to social myths concerning the blue-blooded rich, "poor blood" is characteristically blue; "rich blood," blood high in oxygen, is characteristically red).

After the right atrium is filled, the poor blood is sent to the right ventricle, which in turn pumps it to the lungs. This is a fairly easy activity for the heart due to the low pressure maintained in the lungs. Only an easy pumping action is required, and that fact is reflected by the relatively thin walls of the right ventricle.

Once the poor blood is in the lungs, it is cleansed of carbon dioxide, takes on oxygen and is transformed into rich blood. The rich blood then moves from the lungs into the left heart, where it is received and stored in the left atrium and is subsequently passed to the left ventricle. The left ventricle is the powerhouse pump of the heart. It is the chamber which will pump the blood to distant parts of the body, under high pressure and against much resistance, through arteries and capillaries which may be only 1/2500 of an inch wide.

Resistance to blood flow is a product of the diameter of the blood vessel. The smaller the blood vessel, the higher the resistance. This pumping takes tremendous power. As such, the

41

left ventricle is a heavily muscular chamber with thick walls measuring one-half inch in width. The pressure necessary to drive the blood out of the left ventricle is so great that if the aorta were opened in the neck, a column of blood would spurt out to a height of five or six feet. Intense pressure is essential in order to keep the blood circulating.

Even from this simplistic description of the purpose and the function of the heart, it is easy to understand the importance of cardiac health. When the heart is healthy, it can pump needed oxygen and nutrients to the farthermost cells and can promote good health for the body. When the heart is not healthy, its pumping ability is diminished, and ill health can result. The heart — this small, misshapen, and wonderfully powerful organ — is essential to life. Its health cannot be taken for granted.

THE CORONARY ARTERIES

While the heart is often viewed as the key element in the delivery system — the pump which keeps the oxygenated blood circulating — its own dependence on oxygen and nutrients is often overlooked. The heart is a super-organ in terms of its capacity for work and its efficiency. However, like all other organs and body tissue, it also needs a constant supply of oxygen and nutrients; it cannot operate without fuel. The cardiac muscle has a need to be served, and that need is met by blood which flows through the coronary arteries.

I had assumed that the heart was somehow nourished by the thousands of gallons of blood which pass through its chambers. This is not the case. In spite of the large volume of blood which the heart processes, it must, like the rest of the body, be served by arteries. Only the blood which reaches the heart through the coronary arteries can provide nourishment.

The two main coronary arteries which originate from the aorta are the right and the left coronary arteries. They lie on the surface of the heart and divide into smaller branches so that every portion of the heart has a blood supply. The right coronary artery nourishes the right side of the heart and has branches which extend to the back of the heart. The left coronary artery has two main branches: the left anterior descending branch which nourishes the front of the heart, and the left circumflex branch which carries blood to the back of the heart. These arteries surround the heart and actually curl around its surface like a crown. It is this crown-like characteristic that gives the arteries their name. In Latin crown is "corona."

In establishing the coronary arteries as the supply line for the heart, nature has developed an efficient delivery system. Each time the heart pumps rich blood through the aorta to the body, a portion of that blood is syphoned from the aorta through the coronary arteries back to the heart itself. It's like a commission that the heart pays itself for the work performed. Of the rich blood that is pumped into the aorta, 95% is supplied to the body and 5% finds its way back to the heart. Every time the heart pumps, it works to nourish itself. The fact that only 5% of the rich blood is sufficient to meet the needs of the heart is due to the ability of the heart to extract more oxygen per milliliter of blood than any other organ of the body.

Although the location of the coronary arteries and the 5% commission system are designed in

THE CORONARY ARTERIES

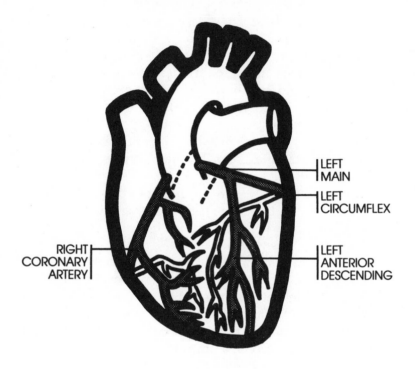

combination to provide all areas of the heart with an adequate blood supply, that design is fraught with potential problems. The arteries themselves are extremely small, about the size of cooked spaghetti. Thus, any blockage or obstruction can easily reduce the blood supply to the heart.

In addition, unlike other arteries in the body which are protected by muscle tissue, the coronary arteries are located on the surface of the heart. They are afforded no protection by the heart itself.

The coronary arteries are forced to move, stretch and kink as the heart muscle contracts and relaxes. This constant movement can cause much wear and tear, expecially at the points where the arteries bend, and can make them susceptible to small tears on the inside wall of the artery. These tears often become important in the development of artery blockages. The fact that the arteries are not protected and can easily tear is a major reason why a blockage can develop. And the fact that coronary arteries are very small is a major reason why such a blockage can impede the blood flow and cause a heart attack. These arteries, the weak link in the circulatory chain, are the real Achilles' heel of man.

CHAPTER TWO

CORONARY HEART DISEASE

Coronary heart disease is found in epidemic proportions in the United States today. It is estimated that over 5.5 million Americans are afflicted with the disease, which contributes to over 1.5 million heart attacks and 600,000 to 800,000 deaths each year.

Basically, coronary heart disease is a condition in which the blood flow to the heart is restricted due to the buildup of blockages on the inner walls of the coronary arteries. This condition is the product of a disease called atherosclerosis, which is derived from the Greek *athere,* meaning "mush," and *skeros,* meaning "hard." Literally translated as "hard mush," it is an apt description of the fact that an arterial blockage begins as a soft, mushy accumulation of fat and cholesterol and ends as a deposit of hard, encrusted material.

Atherosclerosis progresses silently, often without any outward manifestation of its debilitating effects. As it does so, blockages begin to form and the arterial walls begin to thicken. The channel through which the blood flows becomes more and more narrow. In addition, the arteries themselves lose their ability to expand. The resulting impediment to blood flow can seriously impair cardiac performance. Should the blood flow be completely stopped, a heart attack will take place.

WHO GETS CORONARY HEART DISEASE?

Coronary heart disease is mostly identified with middle-aged and elderly people. While this is the age when the disease is made manifest, many young people also carry arterial blockages. In some infants the disease is detectable at birth, and studies have illustrated that coronary artery blockages may even be present in a fetus. Dr. Forest H. Adams of the Pediatric Atherosclerosis Clinic at UCLA has demonstrated that traces of the disease are common in American children by the time the tenth birthday is reached. Dr. Charles J. Guleck of the University of Cincinnati has found that elevated cholesterol levels — a prime indicator of the disease — can be found in children as young as eight years old. In addition, research involving autopsies performed on children killed in auto accidents have confirmed that coronary artery blockages exist even in young children.

Significant studies were also conducted during the Korean and Viet Nam wars involving young adults. These confirmed that youth offers no immunity to coronary heart disease. The young men studied, whose average age was 22, were in excellent health until the time of their battlefield death. Their autopsies revealed that despite their young age, many cases of severe coronary heart disease existed. It was concluded that some 35% of these young men were well on their way to a heart attack.

It is often thought that females are generally immune to coronary heart disease, but statistics illustrate that sex provides no ultimate immunity either. Males between the ages of 30 and 49 are 6.5 times as likely to develop the disease as females of the same age. This is probably due to the female production of estrogen, a sex hormone which seems to protect against coronary blockages. As the female ages, however, her risk of developing coronary heart disease increases rapidly. Shortly after menopause her odds become equal to those of the male.

No one is immune to coronary heart disease. The insidious aspect is its silent progression, its ability to remain undetected until it has reached an advanced stage. It is only when the blockage seriously restricts the blood flow to the heart that the disease becomes noticeable. Often it is too late. While a heart attack may be described as "sudden," the blockages which produce the attack do not "suddenly" grow, but develop silently over a period of years. Although blood cholesterol measurement may indicate the probability of the disease in a person, there exists no practical, fool-proof early detection device.

Like most people, I had relied on an annual physical examination to disclose any potential heart problems. This exam always included a resting electrocardiogram. Unfortunately, a resting EKG will generally not disclose a blockage in a coronary artery until that blockage obstructs some 90% or more of the channel opening. Since an EKG is taken at "rest" when the heart is not under a heavy workload demand, the results may be "normal" whether the channel is 100% clear or 20% clear, as long as the heart is getting enough oxygen to sustain its resting beating pattern. It is only when the artery is obstructed more than 90% and the blood flow is impeded to the point where the heart has difficulty in sustaining a normal resting beating pattern that the EKG will show an abnormality. Four months prior to my coronary surgery I had received a resting EKG as a part of my annual physical. It showed no abnormalities.

Either my 95% blockage had totally developed within a 4-month period, which would have been highly unlikely, or it had developed over a period of time but had not as yet been large enough to show up on my resting EKG exam. Obviously, the latter is what occured. So, while my physical examination indicated that all was well, in reality atherosclerosis was in an advanced stage in my coronary arteries. This same situation has occured with other people as well. Not too long ago a prominent mayor of Chicago died of a heart attack as he was leaving his cardiologist's office after an examination in which his resting EKG was normal!

THE DEVELOPMENT OF
CORONARY HEART DISEASE

The coronary arteries are the only channel through which oxygenated blood is supplied to the heart. The exact sequence of events leading to the formation of blockages in those arteries is unknown. However, it is known that at birth the artery channel is smooth and that blood flows through it unimpeded, much as water will flow through a new pipe.

The coronary artery is lined with a smooth tissue, the intima, which by its nature helps the blood to move freely. Soon after birth, minute cracks begin to develop in the intima, the result of the constant movement of the coronary arteries as they twist and flex each time the heart contracts and relaxes. And with the heart beating some 100,000 times in a single day, it is not surprising that the wear and tear on the coronary arteries would produce such a result. When a crack does occur, blood cells and clotting material are rushed to the wound in order to repair it. As happens with external cuts or scrapes, a "patch" of new cells covers the wound and soon a protective scar is formed. Coronary artery cracks are common, and consequently each of us carries many coronary artery scars. Few of these scars pose a significant health hazard for the heart.

But a hazard does arise when the blood contains a high level of fat and cholesterol. The bloodstream then not only deposits blood cells and clotting material for repair purposes, but fat and cholesterol as well. The latter are quickly absorbed by the cells which surround the crack. As more and more fat and cholesterol are deposited and absorbed, the surrounding cells are forced to multiply rapidly in order to maintain the absorption rate. The result can be a wild, cancerlike growth of new cells which soon become swollen to the bursting point. The accumulation of these new cholesterol-filled cells is called a fatty streak, a protuberance which thickens the artery wall much as accumulated rust and corrosion can thicken the inside of an old water pipe.

The cells which constitute the fatty streak sometimes become stable and cease growing. In such a case they may not cause significant disruption of blood flow to the heart. But should the cells continue to absorb fat and cholesterol, the fatty streak can grow from the artery wall like a cancerous tumor and can constitute a dangerous impediment to the blood flow. This impediment is called a blockage or a plaque. It is estimated that well over 50% of all adult males in the United States today harbor one or more of such coronary artery blockages.

The natural consequence of coronary disease is a heart attack. In the situation where a blockage is large, or where a series of blockages exist, the

THE DEVELOPMENT OF ATHEROSCLEROSIS

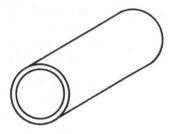

No Atherosclerosis.

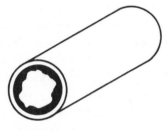

Only Moderate Atherosclerosis.

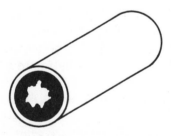

Severe Atherosclerosis.

blood supply to the heart can be curtailed to the point where the heart can no longer function normally and a heart attack results. Often even moderate sized blockages can be responsible for a heart attack.

If the blockage itself develops a crack in its hard exterior which allows the blood cells to come in direct contact with the fat and cholesterol, a clotting action will take place and frequently an enormous blood clot will be formed. The blood clot can act as an extension of the blockage, and the combination of clot and blockage may be of such size as to completely obstruct the artery channel and stop all blood to the heart. When this happens, a heart attack can result. In some instances the blood clot will break free to float in the blood stream. Should this floating clot become lodged with another artery blockage to stop blood flow, a heart attack can again be the result.

THE RESULTS OF CORONARY HEART DISEASE

Coronary heart disease commonly causes four cardiac conditions. The first is angina, or angina pectoris, which in Latin means a "pain in the chest," and is the result of the heart muscle receiving insufficient oxygen to maintain its workload. It is estimated that over two million American adults suffer angina. For many people, angina is a sharp pain in the chest, jaw, neck, arm or shoulder. For others, it is a discomforting sensation of tightening in the chest or heavy pressure behind the breastbone. It was described to me by one cardiac patient as "like having an elephant sit on my chest." Frequently angina is misinterpreted as a gas pain or an indigestion that will not go away.

In my case, it was a burning sensation in the area of my lungs.

Whatever its manifestation, the pain of angina is generally sufficient to force a person to curtail his physical activity. For many people angina dictates a lifestyle moderation which precludes physical activities. In jogging, tennis, or for some people just walking up a hill, the heart is called upon to pump blood at an increased rate to those muscles which require oxygen. A jogger's legs, for example, may demand six times the amount of blood when running as when at rest. This increased demand in workload usually poses no problem for the heart. But when coronary artery blockages prevent the heart from receiving sufficient oxygen to maintain its high workload, angina becomes the warning sign to the body that the heart is in trouble.

Usually a person experiencing angina will be required by the pain to stop the activity, and the heart is allowed to return to its slower beating pattern. With the workload reduced, the oxygen requirement is dimished and the angina generally disappears. Sometimes drugs are needed to produce relief from the pain. Angina is a principal indication that coronary artery blockages exist and are of sufficient size to warrant concern about a heart attack.

The most common result of coronary artery blockages is the heart attack, also referred to as a myocardial infarction or MI. A heart attack takes place when the blood supply to the heart is completely stopped and an area of the heart muscle is without oxygen for too long a period of time. When this happens, the area affected suffocates and dies. The dead area can be large or small; however, once it dies, it remains dead. There is no healing or rejuvenating process which will restore

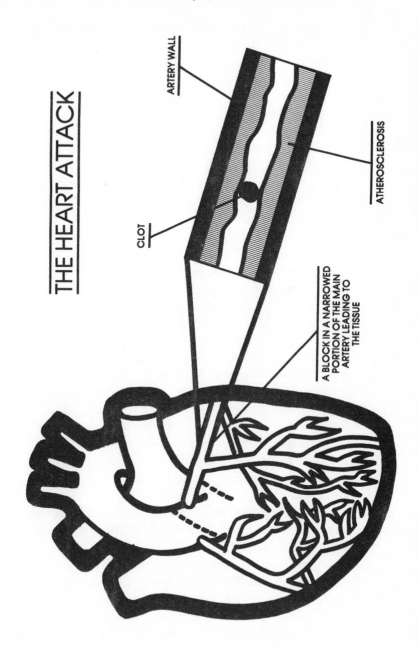

THE HEART ATTACK

ARTERY WALL

CLOT

ATHEROSCLEROSIS

A BLOCK IN A NARROWED PORTION OF THE MAIN ARTERY LEADING TO THE TISSUE

the original muscle. Scar tissue replaces muscle tissue. Unfortunately, scar tissue does not have the ability to contract, and it is useless in the pumping activity of the heart. The scarred area consequently causes the heart to lose some of its effectiveness as a pump.

The odds of having a heart attack are 1 out of 158 for every American over 15 years of age. In about 50% of the persons experiencing first heart attacks, the result is sudden death. Of those that survive the attack, some 8% to 13% die in the first year following the attack. If the area of heart muscle death is great, the first year death rate can be in the 25% to 33% range.

Congestive heart failure can occur when a heart attack has reduced the pumping power of the heart so that blood in the veins leading to the heart becomes backed up. A heart attack often causes significant scar tissue to form in the area of the left ventricle, the principle pumping chamber. When this happens the left ventricle may no longer have the ability to pump vigorously. But if the right ventricle is without scar tissue, it will continue to pump blood into the lungs at a rapid rate. The difference in pumping abilities of the two chambers may cause blood to back up in the lungs and in the veins, disrupting the normal circulatory flow and causing distension of the tissues and a leaking of fluid into the abdomen and the extremities. The swelling due to abnormally large amounts of fluid in the body tissue is called pulmonary edema. The liver and the kidneys are susceptible to damage when edema takes place, and a painful death can occur.

After an area of the heart muscle dies and scarring takes place, the muscle area which borders the scar is often in a half-alive state. It is injured, yet alive and receiving a supply of blood, but that supply is so inconsistent that the muscle area is always on the verge of death. It very much resembles a drowning man who is gasping for breath. Often in this situation the muscle will panic.

Instead of following the master electric rhythm sent out by the heart to establish the heartbeat rate, the affected muscle area begins to generate its own electrical rhythms in an attempt to increase the heartbeat rate and to gain more blood flow for itself. The new rhythms may be strong enough to override the master rhythm, which is usually about 72 beats per minute, and the heart can race wildly to 150 or 250 beats per minute. This condition is called tachycardia. Where the heart enters completely into undisciplined, uncoordinated contractions in excess of 250 beats per minute, the condition is called fibrillation. In either case, the heart muscle can be seriously damaged and death can result.

FOCUSING ON THE REAL PROBLEM

The consequences of coronary heart disease are serious and often fatal. Much effort and money have gone into the medical research involving angina, heart attack, congestive heart failure and fibrillation. Much media attention has been given to the tragic impact of these coronary problems on the lives of millions of Americans. And many physicians have spent countless hours helping their cardiac patients to cope with coronary heart disease.

While the consequences of the disease rightly demand our attention, it is imperative not to lose sight of the real problem: atherosclerosis, the cause of coronary heart disease. If we are to have

57

any control over coronary heart disease and its consequences, we must first exercise control over the development of atherosclerosis itself.

This can be achieved only if individuals take action to reduce their risk of atherosclerosis before the disease becomes evident. The beginnings of the disease are found in the small tears in the intima which are a product of the human condition. About that we can do nothing. But its festering development is the product of elevated fat and cholesterol levels in the bloodstream, a situation in part caused by our national diet pattern. About this we can do much.

Without preventive measures, the disease is allowed to develop slowly, almost imperceptibly, over a period of time. It is like the progressive pinching of the fuel line until, no more fuel being available, the auto engine suddenly dies. It is the same for the heart when its fuel line, the coronary arteries, become blocked. It too, suddenly dies.

CHAPTER THREE

THE AMERICAN DIET IS A
CARDIAC RISK FACTOR

The German poet Goethe once wrote that "Man is what he eats." This statement made no sense to me until my coronary problem forced me into a better understanding of the relationship between diet pattern and cardiac disease. It was only then that Goethe's insight could be fully appreciated.

Many health professionals today consider the contemporary American diet to be the single most important factor in the development of coronary heart disease. They view our national diet as influencing a number of other life-threatening diseases prevalent in the United States, such as cancer, high blood pressure, diabetes and stroke.

The problem is that what we eat bears little resemblance to what we need to eat for good health. Dietary decisions are based upon impulse, convenience, economics, status, taste . . . on a number of influences other than nutritional value. The American diet consists of too much fat and cholesterol, too much sugar and alcohol, too much salt and too many calories. One nutritionist categorized it to me as consisting basically of "sweet and salty fat." The ramifications of our national diet have not been good for coronary health. As Dr. John W. Farquhar, Director of the Stanford Heart Disease Prevention Program has stated, "The American diet may be hazardous to your health."

The relationship between diet and cardiac health has long been recognized by the American Heart Association. Since 1961 that organization has been clamoring for a change in the way Americans eat. More recently a comprehensive study was concluded by the United States Senate's Select Committee on Nutrition and Human Needs which resulted in the establishment of national dietary goals. These goals are intended to, among other things, reduce the high incidence of coronary heart disease and heart attacks in Americans.

The Committee has called for a reduction in the amount of unhealthy elements consumed by Americans, notably fat, cholesterol, salt, sugar, alcohol and total calories, and for an increase in the consumption of fresh fruits, vegetables, and whole grains. The recommendations specifically include:

>A reduction in fat from 42% to 30% of total calories.

>A reduction in saturated fat from 16% to 10% of total calories.

>A reduction in cholesterol from 600 milligrams to 300 milligrams per day.

>A reduction in refined sugar from 18% to 10% of total calories.

>A reduction in salt from 8,000 milligrams to 3,300 milligrams per day.

The Committee also recommended a diet with less red meat and whole milk; fewer processed foods; and fewer non-nutritive foods, such as candy, soft drinks and alcoholic beverages. Dr. Mark Hegsted, Director of the Human Nutrition Center of the Department of Agriculture, has stated:

"The diet of the American people has become increasingly rich — rich in meat, other sources of saturated

fat and cholesterol and in sugar . . . The diet we eat today was not planned or developed for any particular purpose. It is a happenstance related to our farmers and the activities of our food industry. The risks associated with eating this diet are demonstrably large. The question to be asked, therefore is not why we should change our diet, but why not? . . ."

FAT AND CHOLESTEROL

A diet rich in saturated fat and cholesterol has been identified as a major risk factor for coronary heart disease. As Dr. Nagle succinctly summarized the problem for me, "If you remember nothing else about the relationship of diet pattern to your cardiac health, remember these things:
>A diet pattern which is high in saturated fat will raise the cholesterol level of the blood.
>Where blood cholesterol levels are high, so is the risk of coronary heart disease and heart attack."

The Clinical Evidence

Much of the very early research concerning the impact of dietary fat and cholesterol upon the development of coronary heart disease was conducted on rabbits, dogs and cats. It illustrated that a high-fat diet caused both elevated levels of blood cholesterol and fatty artery deposits to occur in these animals. Diet pattern was found to be the principal factor in the elevation of blood cholesterol.

A certain amount of difficulty existed in assessing the importance of the test results due to the fact that the basic metabolism of the animals used differed so greatly from that found in humans. Some researchers said the results were significant; others said that they had little meaning. It was subsequently decided to conduct these same tests using the Rhesus monkey, an animal with a basic metabolism quite similar to that of humans. In the test a monkey was fed a high-fat diet which was similar in fat and cholesterol content to the modern American diet.

After being on this diet for 2½ years, the monkey suffered a massive heart attack and died. During the autopsy it was discovered that he had developed multiple coronary artery blockages. His heart closely resembled that of a human with severe atherosclerosis.

The notable point was that under normal circumstances the Rhesus monkey would not have been susceptible either to coronary heart disease or to heart attack, for neither are part of the natural animal condition. But this monkey did suffer a heart attack, one which the researchers concluded was induced by diet. The test findings clearly illustrated that the high-fat diet produced elevated cholesterol levels, which in turn contributed to the production of coronary artery blockages.

A number of studies and field tests involving humans have been conducted since World War II. One of the first studies was initiated in 1947 by Dr. Ancel Keys, a pioneer in cardiac research, at the University of Minnesota. In this test 281 businessmen in their 40's and 50's were studied over a 15-year period. During that time, some of the businessmen had heart attacks; some did not.

It was found that the men who had heart attacks had a significantly higher amount of cholesterol and fat in their blood than did those who did not suffer any heart attacks. Dr. Keys concluded that a direct relationship existed between a high level of cholesterol in the blood and a high incidence of heart attack. A person with a high blood cholesterol level, it seemed, was much more likely to have a heart attack than a person with a low blood cholesterol level. This was the first time that cholesterol was linked to coronary heart disease in humans; however, the study did not concern itself with diet pattern.

Other research projects followed. Among the most famous was the Framingham Study, started in 1948 by the Public Health Service. In this project, conducted over a 12-year period, some 5,000 adults were studied. The conclusion drawn was similar to that of Dr. Keys findings: the cholesterol level of the blood was the most significant factor in determining the risk of a heart attack.

Many other tests and studies were conducted which indicated again and again that a relationship existed between elevated blood cholesterol and heart attack. The results of a series of studies involving over 4,000 men concluded that a man with a cholesterol level of 260 had four times as much risk of a heart attack as a man with a cholesterol level of under 200. The consensus from these many tests was clear: the higher the cholesterol level, the greater the risk of heart attack.

It was not until the early 1950's before the role of diet as a risk factor was seriously examined. Again it was Dr. Keys who played an instrumental role. He developed a study of three groups of Japanese, each of whom were living in a different environment. Differences in heredity and physiology, which were evident in his prior studies, were set aside in this study, allowing Dr. Keys to concentrate on the differences in the diet patterns and in the cholesterol levels of the three groups.

The first group consisted of Japanese who lived in Japan. They ate a traditional low-fat Asian diet. This group had a low blood cholesterol level and a low incidence of heart attack. The second group were Japanese who lived in Hawaii. Their diet was a mixture of the low-fat Asian diet and the contemporary American high-fat diet. The second group had higher levels of blood cholesterol and a higher incidence of heart attack. The third group were Japanese who lived in Los Angeles. They consumed the American diet exclusively. Their blood cholesterol levels and their incidence of heart attack were much higher than the second group, and were significantly higher than the first group.

Dr. Keys concluded that the blood cholesterol level was influenced directly by diet pattern. This conclusion, coupled with his previous finding that elevated blood cholesterol is linked to an increased incidence of heart attack, opened the door to the modern medical approach to diet as a risk factor for coronary heart disease.

Another notable research test, the Seven Country study, was one in which diet, cholesterol levels, and frequency of heart attack were measured in communities in Finland, Greece, Italy, Japan, the Netherlands, the United States and Yugoslavia. In all, some 12,000 men in the age range of 40-49 years old were tested and observed. The study illustrated that cultures in which fat made up a significant percentage of total caloric intake were also cultures which demonstrated a high incidence of coronary heart disease. Thus, the Netherlands, where 40% of the diet was fat, had a far greater incidence of coronary heart disease than did Japan, where the diet was only 9% fat.

A further study done in Europe divided that continent into two distinct geographic areas based upon dietary patterns. High-fat Europe, with a diet similar to that of the United States, consisted of the British Isles, Germany, Holland, Scandinavia, Belgium, Northern France and Northern Switzerland. This group was categorized as a "beer and butter" culture, and their diet pattern, while differing in national foods, was uniformly rich in fat. Low-fat Europe, on the other hand, exhibited a diet pattern which was lower in fats. This group, categorized as a "wine and oil" culture, consisted of Spain, Italy, Southern France, Southern Switzerland, and Greece. The study illustrated that a high level of blood cholesterol and a frequency of heart attack existed in high-fat Europe, while just the opposite existed in low-fat Europe. It concluded that blood cholesterol levels and incidence of coronary heart disease cut across geographic and ethnic boundaries where similarities in diet patterns did the same.

One additional study deserves comment. During the Korean and Viet Nam Wars, autopsies were performed on American and Asian servicemen. All of these servicemen were young, about age 22, were fit and were without health problems. The American servicemen autopsied showed consistent evidence of coronary artery blockages already in evidence, while the Asian servicemen had relatively few blockages. The salient difference between these two groups was their respective diet patterns. The Americans ate a high-fat diet; the Asians, a low-fat diet. The evidence from this study corroborated the conclusions of the many other studies: diet pattern does have an impact, positively or negatively, on the development of coronary heart disease.

The Role of Cholesterol

Cholesterol has frequently been identified as the principal culprit in the development of coronary heart disease mainly because it is the chief component of artery blockages. The result is that cholesterol has received exclusively "bad press" and is perceived by the general public as a dangerous substance.

In truth, the role of cholesterol is not totally negative. Indeed, cholesterol is necessary to the normal chemical process of the body. Produced primarily in the liver, cholesterol is utilized in cell wall construction. It also serves as an insulator between cells that are receiving electronic signals from the brain, thereby preventing an electrical short. No cell could survive without cholesterol.

The liver is not the only source of cholesterol. It also enters the body through foods that are eaten. This is dietary cholesterol, and it is found in foods of animal origin such as beef, pork, lamb, shrimp, organ meats and egg yolks. Many of these foods also contain saturated fat, a type of animal fat that causes the body to increase cholesterol production. Thus, a diet rich in animal fats (and therefore rich in dietary cholesterol and saturated fat) can cause blood cholesterol levels to rise. The more cholesterol in the blood, the greater the risk for coronary heart disease.

Cholesterol Levels

Blood cholesterol level is a key indicator of cardiac risk potential. The amount of cholesterol in the blood is determined by a blood test and is expressed as a number. This represents the number of milligrams (mg) of cholesterol in one deciliter (dl) of blood. For example, a person who has 275 milligrams of cholesterol in a deciliter of blood would have a cholesterol level of 275.

The higher the blood cholesterol level, the greater the potential risk for coronary heart disease and heart attack. According to the Framingham Study, a person with a cholesterol level of 260 has four times the risk of heart attack as a person with a level of 200. The opposite is also true: the lower the cholesterol level, the lower the risk. Indeed, a study by the National Institutes of Health has shown that a 1% reduction in blood cholesterol level results in a 2% reduction in heart attack risk.

A relative scale has been established to define the relationship of cholesterol level to cardiac risk. Historically, a level of 300 and above constituted a high risk, while 200 and below represented a low risk. The normal or acceptable range used in the United States has been 225 to 275, with a mean of about 250. Today, however, many physicians no longer consider this to be a true indicator of risk potential because of the wide range involved. In addition, they've concluded that what Americans define as "normal" is considered excessively high in other parts of the world. In Third World nations where many people are vegetarians, the normal cholesterol range is 100 to 140. In the Mediterranean, Latin America and the Orient, normal is a range of 150 to 180. The normal mean level for Americans is 250. But in Italy it is 175, in Japan it is 163, in India it is 146, and in Peru it is just 137.

Because the fat- and cholesterol-rich American diet has produced elevated blood cholesterol levels in the United States, the normalcy range for Americans has been adjusted upward. Americans are not biologically different from other people in the world, yet the mean level of the normal range is 100 milligrams higher. Americans may feel better hearing that their cholesterol level is "normal," but this façade of normalcy cracks and breaks under the staggering weight of the number of heart attacks suffered every year in the United States.

A more accurate view of cholesterol risk, according to the National Institutes of Health, is the following:

Age	Recommended Level	Moderate Risk	High Risk
2–19	Less than 170	170–185	Greater than 185
20–29	Less than 200	200–220	Greater than 220
30–39	Less than 220	220–240	Greater than 240
40 +	Less than 240	240–260	Greater than 260

Types of Cholesterol

In addition to the total amount of cholesterol in the blood, attention must be paid to the types of cholesterol that make up that total. There are two main types: one is harmful and considered "bad" cholesterol; the other is healthful and considered "good" cholesterol.

The chief distinction between good and bad cholesterol involves their chemical packaging. All cholesterol is insoluble in water, so it cannot be transported in a pure state via the bloodstream. It must first be combined with fat and protein molecules in order to become soluble. This combination, or chemical package, is called a lipoprotein.

One type is called a high-density lipoprotein, or HDL, and is described as "good" cholesterol. An HDL, which is primarily protein and contains very little fat, is very stable from a chemical viewpoint and will not come apart easily. Thus, should an HDL escape the bloodstream and penetrate an artery wall, the package will remain intact and the cholesterol will have very little chance to come in direct contact with the artery. In such an instance, the HDL will generally return to the bloodstream without causing damage. A high level of HDL's in the blood enhances cardiac health. The best way to improve HDL level is through a regular program of aerobic exercise.

A low-density lipoprotein, or LDL, on the other hand, is predominantly fat and contains very little protein. Unlike an HDL, an LDL is not a stable chemical package and comes apart quite easily. For this reason, it is described as "bad" cholesterol. Should an LDL penetrate an artery wall, the cholesterol could be released and become embedded. When this happens, the start of an arterial blockage could occur. LDL is what lines the artery walls and forms blockages. The higher the LDL level in the blood, the greater the risk for arterial buildup. Because of this, many physicians believe that its measurement is important in predicting the potential for future heart attacks. LDL's are very sensitive to diet and are increased by foods rich in saturated fat and cholesterol.

While it is an oversimplification to state that HDL is "good" cholesterol and LDL is "bad," this relationship is basically correct. HDL works to minimize the harmful effects of LDL by causing the body to excrete LDL. In fact, HDL helps to prevent the arterial buildups that LDL can cause. At birth, a person has equal amounts of HDL and LDL. But as a result of a diet that is rich in saturated fat and dietary cholesterol, most Americans have four times as much LDL as HDL. And this is an important reason why coronary heart disease is of major consequence in the United States today.

The Role of Fat

The amount of dietary cholesterol a person consumes does have some bearing on his or her blood cholesterol level. Indeed, the American Heart Association guidelines specify an intake of no more than 300 milligrams of cholesterol per day. While dietary cholesterol is important, dietary fat provides a more significant problem for most people.

Fat is one of the main classes of food essential to the body (the others are protein and carbohydrate) and has an important role to play in good health. Because it is a more efficient fuel than either protein or carbohydrate, it is a concentrated source of energy. The body stores fat as an energy reserve and draws upon it when extra fuel is needed. In addition, fat insulates the body against heat loss and cushions many organs against injury. Indeed, fat has a legitimately important role to play in the healthful functioning of the body.

The problem with fat on the American diet involves the amount and type consumed. We eat a lot of fat because it is a basic component of our foods. We like it because it provides flavor and texture to what we eat. Because it is digested slowly, fat also helps to satisfy our appetites. Foods with high fat values include red meats such as beef, pork and lamb; processed meats such as luncheon meats, frankfurters and sausage; dairy products such as milk, butter and cheese; margarine; cooking oils; commercially baked goods such as pies, cookies and doughnuts; fast food fried in fat, such as hamburgers, chicken and French fries; and convenience foods such as canned pork and beans, chili con carne and cream soups.

The result is that 42% of all calories consumed by Americans are in the form of fat. Most health professionals believe fat should constitute no more than 30% of total calories consumed. Too much dietary fat contributes to obesity, a condition that can cause blood cholesterol levels to go up.

More significant, however, is the type of fat consumed on the American diet. Basically there are three types: saturated, polyunsaturated and monounsaturated. Saturated fat is found in animal foods, such as the visible fat on a steak, bacon drippings, lard and butter. An estimated 44% of all fat on the American diet is saturated. What makes this fat a cardiac risk factor is that it tends to raise LDL cholesterol in the blood, thus contributing to the development of coronary artery blockages.

Conversely, polyunsaturated fat has a lowering effect on LDL blood cholesterol. The drawback is that it lowers not only bad LDL cholesterol but good HDL cholesterol as well. Examples of polyunsaturated fat are safflower oil, sunflower oil, corn oil, cottonseed oil and soybean oil. (Two vegetable oils to avoid are palm oil and coconut oil—both contain more saturated fat than lard.) Another good source of polyunsaturated fat is fish. Omega-3, an ingredient of fish oil, has been shown to protect against coronary heart disease. According to the *New England Journal of Medicine*, eating "as little as two fish dishes a week may cut the risk of dying from heart attack in half." Fish with high fat content include salmon, mackerel, herring, fresh tuna, whitefish and lake trout.

Olive oil is the best example of a monounsaturated fat. Once seen as neutral, neither helpful nor harmful to cardiac health, it has been shown to lower LDL levels but not HDL levels. Thus, more and more healthy diets include olive oil in moderate amounts.

The amount and the type of fat consumed do impact blood cholesterol levels. When the total quantity consumed is too high, and when the total quality is too saturated, then dietary fat can constitute a risk for coronary heart disease. Unfortunately, such is the condition of the American diet. It is the prime reason why 5.5 million Americans are victims of coronary heart disease.

71

SALT

It is dinnertime, and throughout the United States people sit with family and friends to enjoy a meal together. Somewhere between the grace and the first forkful of food comes the inevitable hallmark phrase of American table conversation: "Please pass the salt!"

For most Americans, salt constitutes a basic dietary element. But recently many people have begun to question the amount of salt consumed on the typical American diet. The reason? Excessive salt intake has been linked to high blood pressure (hypertension), stroke, kidney and thyroid disease, and edema. Indeed, both the U.S. Surgeon General and the U.S. Senate's Select Committee on Nutrition have concluded studies and have issued separate reports advising Americans to restrict their salt consumption. Noted food columnist Craig Clairborne, himself a victim of high blood pressure, has stated that, "They should label salt, just as they do cigarettes, saying that it is injurious to your health."

What Is the Problem?

The warnings issued about salt are very serious. In order to understand the health risks associated with excessive salt consumption, it is first necessary to distinguish sodium from salt. Salt, or sodium chloride, is a combination of two minerals: sodium, a metal; and chlorine, a gas. Approximately 40% of salt is sodium. Thus, a diet which is high in salt is also a diet which is high in sodium. It is the sodium content of foods on the American diet which constitutes a health issue.

Sodium, which is essential to life, displays both positive and negative characteristics. On the positive side, it is the chief regulator of the fluid balance of the body. The tissues in the human body must constantly be bathed in a saline solution. The correct ratio of sodium-to-water in this body fluid is critical to proper metabolic functioning.

Sodium regulates that balance by triggering a thirst sensation when body fluid is too low or sodium content is too high. For example, when a person loses fluid by sweating, the ratio of sodium-to-water is increased, causing that person to become thirsty. By drinking liquids to satisfy his thirst, he is also replacing the fluid necessary to restore the proper fluid balance. This relationship of excess sodium to thirst has long been understood by bartenders who offer free salted peanuts or popcorn to their patrons.

When the concentration of sodium in the body is constantly high, as it often is as a result of the high-salt American diet, the fluid balance mechanism can be perverted to produce negative health results. A characteristic of sodium is that it holds water. When the body contains too much sodium and consequently too much water, the excess is eliminated through the kidneys.

Should this happen occasionally, it generally poses no health problem. But when the kidneys are required to work constantly over a long period of time to eliminate excessive sodium and water, they become overworked and are placed under great strain. Many times they simply become unable to perform at the required level of elimination, and kidney damage or failure results.

Excessive amounts of sodium and water in the blood vessels also tax the heart by increasing the volume of blood to be circulated. When this happens, the heart is required to pump harder and to create more pressure in order to move the

73

additional pounds of fluid in the bloodsteam. At the same time sodium causes the small blood vessels to constrict, thereby increasing resistance to blood flow. The heart is forced to respond by further increasing blood pressure, which is a significant strain on the heart muscle.

Hypertension, or high blood pressure, is the most serious health consequence of excessive sodium intake. Over 35 million Americans (one out of every six) are afflicted with the disease, and 100,000 deaths result each year. Like atheroscleroisis, the disease makes a silent progression. Blood pressure may be increased year after year with no overt symptoms of any health problem. Then quite suddenly, usually in middle age, the disease appears. But by this time it is usually too late to repair the damage done to the heart, blood vessels and kidneys. Chronic illness and death often occur. According to the National Heart, Lung and Blood Institute, about 50% of Americans with hypertension do not know that they have the disease.

The causes of hypertension are not fully understood. Many factors, such as weight, age, stress, genetics and diet, are thought to contribute to it. Although it is difficult to prove a direct cause and effect relationship between salt and hypertension, numerous studies have established that a clear link does exist between a high-salt diet and the incidence of hypertension. These studies have shown that in low-salt cultures, such as New Guinea and parts of Brazil, high blood pressure is virtually non-existent and blood pressure does not rise steadily with age. In high-salt cultures, such as Japan and the United States, high blood pressure is rampant.

In a study conducted in the Solomon Islands by Dr. Lot Page of Harvard, six primitive tribes

74

were studied. All six exhibited a common lifestyle with one notable exception: three tribes ate a high-salt diet. It was only in the tribes which ate such a diet that incidence of high blood pressure could be found. In Japan, where salt consumption is three to six times that of the West, areas can be found where over 40% of the adult population suffers from serious high blood pressure. It is that country's leading cause of death.

Not everyone with an excessive sodium intake is susceptible to the disease. In many people the excess is promptly excreted no matter how high the intake. But in 10%-30% of all Americans there exists a genetic predisposition to hypertension. For these people a diet high in salt, and consequently high in sodium, can increase the risk of hypertension and of heart disease. No procedure exists which identifies with certainty those Americans who have the genetic weak-link. Consequently, a person with a sodium-rich diet is playing Russian roulette with his health.

Salt Is Found Everywhere

Salt is the major source of sodium for most Americans. The National Research Council has stated that an "adequate and safe" level of sodium intake is between 1100 and 3300 milligrams daily. This is about one teaspoon of salt. Many physicians feel that these figures are still too high and that a much lower daily requirement — about 220 milligrams, or one-tenth of a teaspoon of salt — could be established. The average American consumes two to four teaspoons of salt daily, which translates into 4000-8000 milligrams of sodium. It is the salt-rich American diet, producing a per capita consumption rate of 15 pounds of salt annually, which has caused sodium intake to go well beyond the "adequate and safe" levels.

Where does all the salt on our diet come from? About 15% comes from natural sources such as meat, fish, dairy products, vegetables and drinking water. Another 35% is the result of table salt used as a condiment and a cooking spice. But the remaining 50%, the largest source, comes from processed foods found on the American diet.

Salt and other sodium products are used by food manufacturers as a curative for fish and meats; as a brine agent for pickles, olives and sauerkraut; as a levening agent in bread and crackers; and as a fermentation control agent in cheese. The result has been to make foods which are low in sodium in a natural state into high-sodium foods in a processed state. A 5.5 ounce potato, for example, contains just 5 milligrams of sodium. But processed as potato chips, it contains 1562 milligrams. A tomato contains 14 milligrams of sodium. But processed into tomato sauce, one cup contains 1498. One-half a chicken breast has 69 milligrams of sodium; a fast food chicken dinner contains 2243.

Why do processed foods contain so much salt and sodium? There are many answers beyond food preservation. One is found in economics. Salt is an inexpensive filler which adds weight and substance to processed foods. In addition, because food processing often removes the natural flavor of the food, salt is added as a flavoring substance to provide the product with some semblance of recognizable taste, thereby masking the blandness of the product. It is this salty taste which the American consumer has been conditioned to accept. And finally, the fact that salt can be addictive has not been lost on food processors.

There is no natural affinity for the taste of salt.

We are not born with such a craving. The preference for a salty taste is an acquired one. The more salt eaten, the more impervious the taste buds become, and the more salt is necessary to produce a "too salty" taste. By maintaining a high level of salt in their products, many food processors have insured that their foods will be purchased not for reasons of nutrition, but for reasons of taste. From a profit standpoint, the heavy use of salt as a food additive can be justified. From a health standpoint, it cannot.

SUGAR

Excessive sugar intake has been characterized as one of the major health hazards of the American diet. It is a contributing factor to tooth decay, obesity and diabetes. And according to many cardiac experts such as Dr. John W. Farquhar, excessive sugar constitutes a risk for coronary heart disease as well. Despite evidence of its detrimental effect upon good health, Americans continue their love affair with sweet taste. It is estimated that the average American consumes about 128 pounds of sugar annually, or more than one-third of a pound (600 calories) each day. Sugar constitutes better than 24% of all calories consumed by American adults; the figure is even higher for children and adolescents.

Much of this sugar is consumed in the form of sweets and soft drinks. The average American eats 15 pounds of candy and drinks 40 gallons of pop annually — and that constitutes a lot of sugar. But the main source of sugar is processed foods: canned fruits, soups, gravies, cereals, salad dressings and catsup are some of the foods in which sugar is a hidden principal ingredient.

Dr. John Yudkin of London University, long a critic of sugar as a food additive, states that "if only a fraction of what is already known about the effects of sugar were to be revealed in relation to any other material used as a food additive, that material would promptly be banned."

Two Types of Sugar

An appreciation of the potential health problems associated with excessive sugar intake requires an understanding of the two types of sugar consumed. The first type is the sugar contained in fruits, berries, dairy products, grains, vegetables and other unprocessed foods. It is called "natural sugar" since it is an inherent part of the food itself. The second type of sugar is that which is added to processed foods, such as canned fruits, or that which is used as a condiment, such as table sugar sprinkled on breakfast cereal. This sugar is called "concentrated sugar." It is manufactured to produce a super-sweetness not found in natural sugar. Concentrated sugars include granulated table sugar (sucrose), brown sugar, powdered sugar, unrefined sugar, turbinado, and invert sugar.

Both types of sugar produce energy at the rate of 4 calories per gram. In this respect it can be said that "sugar is sugar." But very significant differences appear when nutrition and caloric density of the two sugars are considered. Nutritionally, foods which contain natural sugar also contain protein, vitamins, minerals and fiber. When strawberries are consumed for their sweet taste, vital nutrients in the fruit are also supplied to the body.

Foods high in concentrated sugar, on the other hand, are often totally devoid of nutritional value. When a piece of chocolate cake is eaten for its sweet taste, it produces nothing but pure calories for the body. For this reason, foods which contain natural sugar are preferable to foods which contain concentrated sugar as an additive.

The second difference concerns caloric density, the amount of calories supplied in ratio to the bulk of the food. A food with high bulk and low calories, such as cantaloupe, has low caloric density. A food with low bulk and high calories, such as a brownie, has high caloric density.

The caloric density of foods is important because the body requires a balance between calories consumed and calories burned. When more calories are consumed than burned, the excess calories are converted into fat and stored. It does not matter what is the source of the calories — fat, protein or carbohydrate. As long as more calories are consumed than are used up, body fat will be produced.

Foods containing natural sugar generally demonstrate a low caloric density. A great many strawberries at 55 calories per cup, for example, would have to be consumed before excess body fat would be created. The chances are that because of the bulk of the food, a person would feel full before consuming too many calories.

It is not the same with foods containing concentrated sugar. These foods are generally high in caloric density. A 4-ounce milk chocolate candy bar, for example, contains 600 calories. Because this food lacks bulk, several candy bars, representing hundreds of calories, could be consumed before a person felt full. Foods containing concentrated sugar often allow a person to simultaneously occupy two opposing dietary extremes: to be overfed and to be hungry.

What Is the Problem?

A diet high in sugar represents many dangers for the heart. The first is obesity, the storage of excessive amounts of body fat, a condition that places tremendous strain upon the heart and the circulatory system. Obesity can cause the heart to be overworked in its attempt to circulate blood to the excess fat, and can promote elevated blood cholesterol. Permanent damage to the cardiac muscle can result. A recent study by the National Center for Health Statistics cites that 33% of all Americans are overweight. This statistic does not bode well for our national cardiac health.

The second danger is that foods rich in concentrated sugar can displace more nutritionally valuable foods in the diet. What is often perceived as a craving for sugar may simply be a hunger pang. But instead of appeasing the hunger with nutritional foods, many people satisfy their hunger with foods containing concentrated sugar — a cookie, a doughnut, or a piece of pie. While these foods may satisfy, they are a poor substitute for a balanced meal. In this situation the heart is robbed of needed nutrients.

Finally, sugar has been shown to raise triglycerides. Clinical studies in Yemen, South Africa, Japan, East Africa and the United States have concluded that concentrated sugar acts to increase triglycerides in certain people and can increase their risk of coronary heart disease.

The Sweet Tooth Syndrome

Why do we eat sweet foods? The fact is that man genuinely has a "sweet tooth." A preference for sweet taste has been demonstrated throughout history. Even the Bible described the Promised Land as "flowing with milk and honey." No other animal (with the possible exception of cats) demonstrates such an inclination. But the craving in man is sufficiently strong to affect his dietary decisions.

Foods containing natural sugar had been used to satisfy the sweet craving until the time of the Industrial Revolution. Fruits and berries not only were sweet, they were also important nutritionally to a proper diet. With the advent of the sugar refining process around 1800, man began to gravitate toward foods which contained concentrated sugar. Industrialization produced a more civilized lifestyle for many people, including dietary changes which called for sweeter and richer foods as a symbol of affluence and status. Cream, butter and refined sugar became popular. Fruits and berries were replaced by pastry, cakes and candies.

Very little concentrated sugar was consumed in the early 1800's — only about two pounds per person annually. Refined sugar was an expensive commodity and not everyone could afford it. But a more important reason was one of taste. The sweet tooth of 1800 could be satisfied on only two pounds of sugar a year.

Advances in technology reduced the cost of producing refined sugar and by the late 1800's it was available to the entire population. By 1875, the average American consumed 40 pounds of concentrated sugar annually; by 1910, it was 70 pounds. As people continued to increase sugar consumption, the amount of sugar needed to satisfy the sweet tooth also increased. The more sugar eaten, the more sugar desired.

It took thirty-five times the amount of sugar in 1910 than it did in 1800 to meet the sweet craving.

The development of the processed food and beverage industry in the 20th century has caused the consumption of refined sugar and other sugar concentrates to skyrocket. Sugar has replaced salt as the most popular food additive. The average American now consumes 128 pounds of refined sugar and other sugar concentrates, such as corn syrup, each year.

Even these statistics, high as they are, may be misleading as they are only averages. Some Americans do not consume concentrated sugar at all for reasons of health and weight. This means that those who do consume sugar probably eat more than the statistical average. In a test conducted on children in Washington State, Dr. Alexander G. Schauss found that the average consumption of the test group was 12.02 ounces of sugar per day — or 274 pounds a year!

According to Dr. John Yudkin and other experts, sugar is addictive. The more of it contained in the diet, the more of it that is needed to satisfy the sweet tooth craving. The result is a diet which contains more sugar intake in a single week than our forefathers consumed in an entire year. The health consequences for Americans have been disastrous.

MYTHS OF THE AMERICAN DIET

During the research process I became convinced of two things: 1. *that diet pattern does have an impact upon cardiac health,* and 2. *that my diet pattern — the contemporary American diet — was too full of fat, cholesterol, salt, sugar and total calories.* The need to change the way I ate was evident.

Nevertheless, to do so still was a cultural shock. For 32 years I had eaten the classic American "meat and milk" diet, based on the premise that the more of these products consumed, the better for you. So my Mother dutifully prepared meals rich in red meat and dairy products, and I dutifully consumed them. After all, we thought, fortified with quantities of protein and calcium, I would grow straight and strong, have sparkling teeth, and leap tall buildings in a single bound.

Nothing was ever said about coronary heart disease. Somehow the information linking diet to atherosclerosis fell through the cracks. As a result, it was not until my coronary surgery that I came to understand many of the shortcomings of the American diet. A number of these have become solidified in our culture as myths.

Myth Number 1: Eat Lots of Red Meat.

A TV commercial fades into a football player. "Hi," he says. "I'm Lance Superjock, and I'm here to tell you that the protein in beef is what makes me so terrific. I eat beef at every meal. Remember how we were losing the Super Bowl?

"Well, at halftime I ate two steaks, three hamburgers and part of a rib roast, and only then was I able to throw those six touchdown passes."

Facetious as this is, it is an example of the advertising which has perpetrated this myth. There is no argument that red meat is an important source of protein. That is an undisputable fact. The fallacy concerns the amount of protein needed for good health. And the amount of saturated fat consumed with the protein.

The recommended quantity for an adult is no more than 0.8 grams of protein per 2.2 pounds of body weight, or about 56 grams for an average man and 46 grams for an average woman. This amount is adequate to maintain good health, provide for growth, and insure proper tissue repair. Large quantities of red meat can provide more protein than is needed each day for good health. The body cannot always utilize excessive protein and in some instances it may even cause health problems.

The most significant problem, however, is that making animal food the principal source of protein overloads the diet with saturated fat. When red meat is consumed for protein, fat is consumed as well. Generally, the fat content of red meat is many times more than the protein content. In truth, red meat consumption can be diminished drastically without neglecting protein needs.

Myth Number 2: Eat and Drink Lots of Dairy Products.

Whole milk dairy products also constituted a large percentage of my pre-surgery diet. I drank 2-4 glasses of milk each day, and ate butter, cheese, and ice cream. These foods provided me with calcium for the development and maintenance of strong bones and teeth. But the same problem existed here as with red meat: the consumption level of dairy products far outstripped the needs of my body for calcium, resulting in a high intake of saturated butterfat as well.

It was not the nutrition of the food which was in question. It was the quantity of the food seen as necessary to provide calcium benefit. Many nutritionists believe that a calcium intake of 0.8 grams per day is sufficient for an adult. This can be provided by just 3½ ounces of low-fat cheese or three cups of skim milk. A number of vegetables, notably spinach, also are rich in calcium. The great amount of dairy products on my diet not only produced excess calcium but also were a significant source of saturated fat.

Myth Number 3: Start Each Day with a High-Protein Breakfast.

How many times had I heard this message in the course of my life? Each time the pitch would advocate the classic American high-protein breakfast: eggs, ham, bacon and sausage; toast with butter; cereal with whole milk or half-and-half; juice; and coffee. It is undeniable that this breakfast is a high-protein meal. But it constitutes a high-fat meal as well. The promotion of the protein content exclusively is a little like saying that Pill "X" will clear your sinuses without revealing a side effect that will cause your nose to fall off!

Let's examine this high-protein breakfast. The juice is wholesome, as may be the cereal (unless it is sugared). But the milk used on the cereal and in the coffee and the butter on the toast are high in saturated butterfat. The eggs are rich in cholesterol, especially when cooked in butter or fat. And the breakfast meats could easily be over 75% in fat content.

This might be a high-protein breakfast, but it is also a breakfast that is too rich in saturated fat to be healthful. It took coronary surgery for me to appreciate this fact.

Myth Number 4: Fast Foods Are Nutritious and
Healthful.

My guess was that this was dependent upon who
was defining "nutritious." By my post-surgery
standards, I find this claim to be pure bunk, aimed
at unaware children and guilt-ridden parents.

It cannot be argued that fast foods and convenience foods are not tasty, for they are. No one
enjoyed the taste of hamburgers, tacos, milk
shakes, pizza and doughnuts more than I did.
And I was not alone. It takes millions of people to
spend $25 billion annually on fast foods and
$10 billion on snacks — and that does not count
the money spent in grocery stores for convenience
foods such as frozen dinners. We are attracted to
these foods because they are fast, filling, inexpensive and attractive to youngsters, and because we
have learned to like the taste.

But nutritious? That is quite another thing.
The amount of fat, sugar and calories — not to
mention fillers, preservatives and chemicals — in
these foods may overshadow any nutritional content. A McDonald's Big Mac has 570 calories and
is 55% fat; Burger King's Whopper has 626 calories
and is also 55% fat; the seafood platter at Long
John Silver's has 976 calories and is 58% fat; and a
Kentucky Fried Chicken Extra Crispy Thigh contains 343 calories and is 64% fat. These foods can
be too high in saturated fat to be healthy.

Fast food processing has changed the nutritional benefit of many foods. Potatoes in the raw
state, for example, can supply a large percentage of
daily requirements for protein, vitamins and minerals. They are low in calories and fats, and high
in desirable complex carbohydrates. But when
processed as a French fry or a chip, the raw potato

is fried in deep fat and its original nutritional benefit is decreased. It then becomes a high-fat, high-calorie, high-salt food.

The fast food industry, I concluded, might talk about nutrition and food composition, but in reality they were really concerned with predictability, cleanliness and efficiency. It was name recognition, not nutrition, which was the paramount goal. As a fast food aficionado, I knew that they were tasty. But as a cardiac patient, I know that they may be neither nutritious nor healthful.

Myth Number 5: Processed Foods Are As Nutritious As Natural Foods.

The same argument holds here as with fast foods. Certainly canned, frozen, and dehydrated foods offer some nutritional value. Some offer considerably more than others. But the additives in many of these foods are of sufficient quantity to offset most nutritional value. Salt and refined sugar are the two most popular food additives. An excess of salt in the diet can lead to high blood pressure; an excess of sugar can lead to elevated blood fats and obesity. In addition, many processed foods use saturated fat in the form of butter or lard as a flavor enhancer.

Salt, sugar, fat . . . these are dietary elements which in excess can lead to coronary heart disease. Not all processed foods are bad. But enough of them contain additives that no one can simply assume that processed foods are nutritious and healthy.

Myth Number 6: Refined Sugar Is an Energy Food.

Every day millions of Americans reach for a candy bar or soft drink for quick energy. They have been convinced by the sugar industry's advertising that refined sugar is an energy food. This is simply not the case.

Confusion over the word "sugar" is what has provided the advertisers with the literary license to produce the energy myth. The term "sugar" can be applied to natural sugar, such as that found in fruit, as well as to concentrated refined sugar, which is found in candy.

The most important of the natural sugars is glucose. Food is converted into glucose, which in turn is burned by the tissues for energy. As such, glucose is always in the bloodstream, available to the tissues when needed. It is referred to as "blood sugar."

But "blood sugar" has nothing to do with refined sugar. When it is said that sugar is an energy food, what is meant is that glucose is an energy food. The sugar industry, however, has created the impression that refined sugar is what the body uses as fuel. This myth has contributed to a diet pattern in which the average American consumes 128 pounds of refined sugar annually.

Myth Number 7: Salt Is a Needed Preservative.

Almost any canned, prepackaged, dried or frozen food available in the supermarket today contains salt or sodium derivatives, such as sodium benzoate, sodium nitrate or sodium glutamate, as a "necessary preservative." In fact, salt does act as a preservative; but that is not the chief reason for its addition to many processed foods. The main reason lies in the fact that many processed foods are tasteless. They are often refined to the point where no taste is left in them. So, the food processors needed to create an artificial taste that people would like. Salt creates that taste.

Salt is often referred to as a "flavor enhancer" or as a "natural seasoning." In reality, it is neither. It is a means to capitalize on the American addiction to salty taste in order to sell more processed foods. This myth has contributed to a diet pattern which supplies about twenty times more salt than is needed each day.

Myth Number 8: It Is Natural and Acceptable To Put On Weight As You Get Older.

The average American gains one or two pounds a year after age 20. This has made us a nation of overweight people. Many adults who are 20 or 30 pounds overweight consider themselves to be normal and healthy, their weight a natural occurrence of aging.

It is not "normal" to gain weight as you get older. Weight gain is not a natural occurrence. Instead, it is a product of overconsumption of calories and under-activity in physical exercise. In many less developed, less sedentary countries, adults lose weight as they age, a product of the normal loss of heavier lean muscle mass that comes with growing older. Americans are fatter at 50 than at 20 not because age and fatness go together naturally, but because the American diet encourages us to eat too much, eat too often, and eat too many high caloric foods.

A LAST WORD

St. Thomas Aquinas, a most intelligent and scholarly person, subscribed to the thesis that all things should be done in moderation. This was for him the key to both physical and spiritual health. Fortunately for him, St. Thomas never had the opportunity to meet an American and to be confronted with a lifestyle which often reflects extremes.

One of the most significant extremes of the American lifestyle is our diet pattern. There is so much available to our affluent society that we eat without any sense of what we are doing or why we are doing it. By eating excessive amounts of cholesterol, saturated fat, sugar, salt and total calories, we have contributed to our own demise. The epidemic proportions of coronary heart disease, obesity, high blood pressure and heart attacks in the United States today are culturally induced, in part by a diet which is too extreme to be healthful.

THE REVERSIBILITY OF ATHEROSCLEROSIS

Not all the news concerning diet is bad. Recent medical research has indicated that atherosclerosis may be reversible, that coronary artery blockages could be reduced in number and size, as the result of dietary changes. This research illustrates not only that a high-fat diet is a risk factor for developing coronary heart disease, but conversely, that a low-fat diet could minimize the risks of that disease. It means that by controlling his diet, an individual could exercise some control over his cardiac future.

Among the most significant of the studies made in this area were those conducted by Dr. M.L. Armstrong. Over a 5-year period he tested a group of 30 Rhesus monkeys. All the monkeys were fed a high-fat/high-cholesterol diet during the first two years in order to determine the effect of the disease. (Neither the diet pattern nor the disease was common to the Rhesus monkey.) At the end of that time, 10 animals were examined and found to have severe atherosclerosis. Their coronary artery blockages were numerous and of significant size. This information became the baseline for further testing.

The remaining animals, whose arteries were presumed by Dr. Armstrong to be equally atherosclerotic, were divided into two equal groups. Group 1 was placed on a low-fat/low-cholesterol diet, while Group 2 was placed on a medium-fat/low-cholesterol diet. At the end of three years, the animals were examined. The Group 1 animals were found to have arterial blockages which were 75% smaller than those found in the baseline group. The blockages in Group 2 were 35% smaller than the original group.

A significant reduction in blockages had taken place in this test as a result of dietary change. Dr. Armstrong concluded that a diet low in fat and cholesterol could be effective in reversing the buildup of coronary artery blockages.

A great deal of research is still to be done in this area for the evidence is much less conclusive in humans than in test animals. However, the initial results indicate that diet pattern may be a two-edged sword: it can work for you as well as against you. And that means that if properly managed, diet need not constitute a cardiac risk factor.

CHAPTER FOUR

THE POSITIVE DIET

"Lifestyle" is a very contemporary word. It has unique shades of meaning for different individuals, but for all of us it says much about the way in which we live and about what is important to us. How we live often dictates how we eat. Diet pattern is frequently a product of custom, habit, convenience, economics and social standing. Some families enjoy a certain special meal on Sundays or on holidays. Modern wives often utilize convenience foods to save time. Young people congregate at fast food restaurants. Those who can afford it dine on haute cuisine. And children, often responding to television advertising, beg for certain breakfast cerals.

The body, however, has no concept of lifestyle. It is a machine which needs to be fueled in order to perform. The food which is eaten provides that fuel. The body does not care about the appeasement of psychological, social and culinary appetites. It is concerned exclusively with the nutritional value of what is consumed. It is like an automobile which needs gasoline to run. It cares not whether the pump is in Beverly Hills or Tortilla Flats, just so long as it produces usable fuel.

I had not understood this in the past and consequently the food choices on my diet had been made for other than nutritive reasons. After my surgery, I began to realize that the decisions concerning food choices had to be based upon the results generated, rather than upon taste, preparation time or the endorsement of a superjock.

Along with this realization came an understanding of the word "diet." In my pre-surgery lifestyle, diet had a singular connotation. It was a weight reduction program, a means of shedding excess pounds rapidly by controlling the intake of calories. Only fat people were concerned with diet. Periodically they went on and off a diet, much like Toynbee's cyclical theory of history, until either the on, or more likely the off, would eventually dominate. In this context, there was no relationship between diet and health.

After researching diet as a risk factor, I understood that *a diet could be a long-term manner of eating* and *a diet pattern could generate negative or positive results.* In analyzing my diet, it was obvious that it was a "negative diet," that indeed it had produced a negative impact upon my cardiac health. What was needed, I reasoned, was a "positive diet," a diet which would be a permanent program of healthful eating.

Using the knowledge gained, I determined the important elements of such a "Positive Diet":
>It must be in tune with the contemporary American lifestyle.
>In order to be achievable, it must be realistic.
>It must meet psychological needs as well as physical needs.
>It must be motivated by an understanding of the importance of healthful eating.
>It must maximize the heart-healthy foods and minimize the harmful foods.

It was easy to understand and to accept the "why" of the Positive Diet. Much information testified to the fact that such a diet could be instrumental in the prevention and perhaps the reversal of coronary heart disease. The difficulty as Dr. Nagle had indicated, would be in the "how."

When I left the hospital after surgery, I was issued a standard low-cholesterol diet, really nothing more than a listing of good and bad foods. It was based on the premise that some foods were healthful and should be eaten, while others were harmful and should be avoided.

The missing link was that the standard diet did not explain how to apply the premise, how to change the eating habits of a lifetime, or how to make it work. It just said, "You better do it!" Granted, with the surgery fresh in my mind, my motivation to stay on a new diet was great. But how long, I asked myself, could I survive on carrot sticks — the Peter Rabbit approach to cardiac health — before saying, "The hell with it!" and reverting to my tasty, old, comfortable diet? Without the "how," the new diet was meaningless.

"We can only make general dietary recommendations for you," Dr. Nagle had said to me. "We can't design a diet to specifically suit your needs and your tastes, and we can't make it work for you. Many of my patients have had a strong motivation to modify their diet. Yet, the vast majority have been unable to do so with any degree of success. A number have returned to their original diet — the same diet which had contributed to their cardiac problem in the first place. Why? Because without a realistic, step-by-step program to follow, the patient never understands how a new diet can be accomplished. Generally, after a few months of trying, the cardiac patient gives up in frustration."

As I experimented over the months to develop a new diet, his words became even more meaningful to me. Frustration plagued me. Progress was elusive. Without a tested plan to follow, I was never quite sure whether or not my new diet was working. The author Graham Greene had once said that there was no black and white but only shades of gray. And that was how the Positive Diet initially appeared to me: in ellusive, chiaroscura form.

Gradually, however, it emerged from the gray and took on clarity in the light. After more than a year of work, it existed not just in theory, but in reality, and in the process it became an integral, permanent part of my lifestyle. I finally understood not only why I had made the dietary change, but how I made it as well.

The Positive Diet

Before the Positive Diet can be successful, one needs to understand its basic principles and tools. He also needs to recognize the underlying premise for the practice of the diet:

>That each individual is responsible for his own health.
>That a decision to eat "positively" must include an understanding of diet as a cardiac risk factor.
>That a firm commitment must be made to make the Positive Diet a permanent diet pattern.

THE BASIC PRINCIPLES

The fundamental cardiac risk involved with the contemporary American diet concerns excesses. While dietary deficiencies are still the major problem in many other areas of the world, in the United States the biggest problem is the inordinate amount of fat, cholesterol, sugar, salt and total calories consumed. Recognizing this fact, the basic principles of the Positive Diet are designed to reduce or to eliminate certain harmful foods. The four basic principles are as follows:

1. Reduce the intake of animal fat and cholesterol. As has been illustrated in numerous medical studies and field tests, a direct and causal relationship exists between the intake of animal fat and cholesterol, the elevation of blood cholesterol levels, and the development of coronary heart disease. While a diet high in fat and cholesterol may only be one of a number of factors which ultimately cause the disease, it clearly is a factor.

2. Reduce the intake of butterfat. Butterfat, which is a saturated fat, contributes to cardiac problems in the same way as does animal fat by promoting high blood cholesterol.

3. Reduce the intake of salt. Salt consumption in the United States has risen over 600% since the turn of the century, today averaging about 15 pounds annually per person. Excess salt in the diet contributes to the development of hypertension, hardening of the arteries, and coronary heart disease.

4. Reduce the intake of refined sugar. The annual average per capita consumption of refined sugar by Americans is 128 pounds, or about one-third pound a day. Not only has sugar displaced needed nutritive foods in the diet, but it has contributed to obesity and to high blood fat levels, both of which constitute significant risks for coronary heart disease.

THE BASIC TOOLS

The four basic principles, concerned with reduction, must be combined with meal planning and creative substitution for permanent change to take place. Meal planning and creative substitution — called the basic tools of the Positive Diet — allow for the creation of new healthful meals. They are dedicated to the belief that if satisfaction can be found in the foods which should be eaten, then there will not be the inclination for the foods which should not be eaten.

Meal Planning

The meal plan is the first step to success and is critical to the practice of the Positive Diet. In a number of ways, the meal plan is like the game plan in football. It provides advance direction for what to do to be successful. In football, the quarterback relies heavily on the game plan. Although he may have a strong arm and sturdy legs, without a game plan his physical talent can be wasted and the team effort can be dissipated.

It is the game plan which defines for the quarterback how he can best move his team against the opposition; it is the game plan which allows him to know in advance what plays he must run. Without such a game plan, even an All-Pro quarterback could find himself approaching the line of scrimmage only to ask, "What do I do now?"

It is the same in establishing the Positive Diet. Instead of a game plan, a meal plan defines in advance how to successfully stay on the diet. The Positive Diet meal plan is the selection of which foods to eat over a designated period of time, usually one to three weeks. By listing the foods for each meal ahead of time, the meal plan can insure the inclusion of nutritious foods and the exclusion of harmful foods. The meal plan minimizes the meals which are left to chance. As with the quarterback, it prevents an individual from approaching a mealtime only to ask himself, "What do I do now?"

Meal planning was essential to my success with the Positive Diet. I began the planning process by dividing the week into 21 meals. Using the basic principles as a guide, I began to plan a meal schedule which either reduced or eliminated harmful foods. On my pre-surgery diet, for example, I frequently ate red meat. To insure that the fat and cholesterol content of my meals would be drastically reduced, I charted a meal plan for the Positive Diet that reduced red meat to just four meals per week.

Another advantage to using a meal plan is that it allows for certain favorite, but not-so-healthy foods to be phased out gradually, rather than eliminated abruptly. Abrupt elimination can cause a feeling of being unjustly deprived and result in resentment.

For example, abruptly giving up a daily breakfast of bacon and eggs could be very discouraging. All of the fat and cholesterol arguments in the world might not work. With meal planning, however, one could begin to practice the Positive Diet by reducing the number of times bacon and eggs were eaten for breakfast. Further reductions and possible elimination could come in future meal plans. The result not only would be an immediate reduction in fat and cholesterol, but also a more ready acceptance of the Positive Diet as a permanent diet pattern.

An additional reason for using a meal plan is to involve all members of the family in the act of planning. Eating is a family affair, and good cardiac health is the business of the entire family. When everyone in the family understands why the Positive Diet is necessary and provides input as to what should be eaten, there generally is more cooperation.

In our family, we decided together what meals to eat during the coming week. Even our youngest child had his say. Total family participation reduced the number of surprises at meals and led to a firmer commitment by each person to practice the Positive Diet. It resulted in a sharing of responsibility, pride and support which helped to keep everyone eating healthfully. Even the children could understand that we were eating right not just for Daddy's heart, but for their own hearts as well.

Meal planning does take some work to be successful. In the beginning I found our meal plans to be restrictive and repetitive. This was to be expected — after all, I was attempting to change the dietary habits of a lifetime. After a while we developed a larger selection of tested menus and recipes, which gave me more culinary choices.

Today, with the Positive Diet an integral part of our family lifestyle, meal planning has become more a guideline and less a rigid plan. It has become second nature to the extent that a formal meal plan is no longer necessary. However, had meal planning not been used at the beginning of the diet, I do not believe that success would have been possible.

There are sample meal plans provided in this book. It is not necessary to use my meal plans to practice the Positive Diet successfully; but it is necessary to use a meal plan.

Creative Substitution

Creative substitution is the process of substituting healthful foods and ingredients for harmful ones while still preserving the appeal and the taste of the food. It is one thing to remove harmful foods from the diet. It is quite another to fill the void with alternative foods which are nutritive, tasty, easily prepared, and acceptable to the American palate.

The long term challenge is to produce satisfying meals made up of healthful foods, so that harmful foods will not be missed. Creative substitution is a necessary tool to effect permanent dietary change. Fortunately, it is easily done. It is an art, and like any other art it can be perfected over time.

I knew when I began the Positive Diet that creative substitution would be essential to its success. While there was a legitimate place in my diet for raw carrots and unmilled grain, without the creative use of these foods in acceptable recipes such a diet was doomed. For that reason, I spent time during the development period talking with physicians, nutritionists and, most importantly, other cardiac patients about the problem of permanent acceptability of a heart-healthy diet.

Their comments coincided with my own experience and led to this conclusion: in order for a healthy diet to become permanent, it must offer foods which are acceptable to the American palate. This meant that "American-type" meals had to be made more healthy, rather than eliminated. And it meant that creative substitution was of extreme importance in accomplishing such a change.

For example, saturated animal fats, often used in American cooking, are unhealthy. Fish oil is a healthy alternative, but is not familiar to American tastes. For that reason, it is an unrealistic sub-stitution despite its healthful qualities. Safflower oil would be a more acceptable substitute. Thus, in creating the menus and the recipes for the Positive Diet we paid as much attention to American taste as to healthfulness.

The process of creative substitution took two forms. The first was a simple "one-for-one" ex-change of heart-healthy food for less healthful food. Barbecued or broiled salmon, for example, replaced beefsteak. Since salmon is lower in fat and cholesterol, it is a good one-for-one substitution. Many other harmful foods were easy to re-place: skim milk for whole milk; egg substitute for whole eggs; chicken sandwiches for pastrami sandwiches; unsalted peanuts for salted peanuts; and fruit juice for soft drinks. Even for those new to the Positive Diet, this form of creative substitution is an easy one to learn, especially when used in conjunction with a meal plan.

The second form of creative substitution was more difficult to master, but was also fundamental to the success of the diet. This form involves the substitution of healthful ingredients for harmful items in a recipe. It allows a meal normally unac-ceptable to a heart-healthy diet to become accept-able by removing the harmful ingredients and substituting more healthful ingredients. For example, in beef stroganoff, fat-rich sour cream and commercially prepared cream of chicken soup were replaced by non-fat yogurt and homemade chicken broth. In effect, the form and the taste of the American diet pattern can be preserved, while the quality can be drastically changed for the bet-ter.

Another form of creative substitution is to alter the cooking method. For example, commer-cially prepared, fat-laden French fries are artery blockers. But heart-healthy French fries can be made by substituting unsaturated liquid vegetable oil for animal fat and by using oven-baking in place of deep fat frying. And chocolate cake can include safflower oil in place of butter and shortening and cocoa powder in place of baking chocolate.

Creative substitution with ingredients takes time and practice to develop, but with proficiency comes an increasing ability to turn negative diet meals into Positive Diet meals. When that happens, the best of both worlds is gained.

APPLYING THE BASIC PRINCIPLES AND THE BASIC TOOLS

After I understood why adherence to the Positive Diet was critical for me, I began to deal with the real question: how to make it work? Could I produce meals which were tasty and healthful? Would too much time be spent in cooking? Would the meals be expensive? Was the Positive Diet a practical one?

My decision was to disregard the "woulds" and the "shoulds," and to direct my attention to just getting started, but to do so in an orderly fashion. I did not believe that even with an understanding of diet and motivation to change, I could totally reverse a 32-year-old behavior pattern instantly.

Instead of attempting complete dietary control by simultaneously adopting all four basic principles, I decided to work with one at a time. Start with the first basic principle, I reasoned, get it firmly established in my diet pattern, then move on to the second. When that one was in place, go to the third, and so on. By taking the time to concentrate on specific pieces of the program, I could make steady progress. This method would be far preferable to the quick, but potentially short-lived adoption of all the basic principles simultaneously.

And so I began.

CHAPTER FIVE

IMPLEMENTING THE POSITIVE DIET

The practical application of the Positive Diet involves two steps. The first is to analyze diet pattern and identify the sources of fat, cholesterol, salt and sugar. The second is to design and implement specific actions to reduce these unhealthy elements.

REDUCING FAT AND CHOLESTEROL

The first basic principle, the reduction of fat and cholesterol, is one of the most important. Remember that the average American consumes a diet which is 42% fat, and of this amount, almost one-half is saturated. In addition, average daily cholesterol consumption is estimated at 600 milligrams.

Guidelines established by the American Heart Association and the United States Senate's Select Committee on Nutrition prescribe a daily diet not in excess of 30% fat, with one-third or less being saturated, and no more than 300 milligrams of cholesterol. Some dietary experts think that even these guidelines are too liberal. They believe that fat should constitute no more than 15% of total calories and cholesterol no more than 200 milligrams per day. I subscribed to the American Heart Association guidelines as my initial goal. Over time, I am trying to better that goal.

Step Number 1: Identification of Fat and Cholesterol Sources

Red meat was the largest single source of fat and cholesterol on my pre-surgery diet. I ate ham, sausage or bacon for breakfast; bologna sandwiches, salami sandwiches, hot dogs, or fast food hamburgers for lunch; steaks, chops, roasts, or meat loaf for dinner. As indicated by the following composition analysis based upon information compiled by the U.S. Department of Agriculture, fat often constitutes 50% of the total calories from red meat products.

Food	% of Calories from Fat
Pork Sausage	87%
Bacon	82%
Frankfurter	81%
Rib Roast	80%
Spareribs	79%
Sirloin Steak	76%
Salami	76%
Lamb Chop	74%
Pork Chop	73%
Rump Roast	71%
Ham	69%
Leg of Lamb	61%

A review of this information also highlights the high-protein myth of the American diet. If every 100 calories from sirloin steak produces 76 calories of fat and just 24 calories of protein, there is no reasonable way this food can be classified as "high-protein" without also being classified as "high-fat." The same holds true for other meat products.

Fats and oils were also a major source of fat on my diet. Hydrogenated margarine, even when made from unsaturated vegetable oil, is about 99% fat. I used it on toast, rolls, and bread. It was also used in sauces, baking and frying. Salad dressings, such as Blue Cheese, Thousand Island and Roquefort, are about 75% fat. Palm oil and coconut oil, both of which are rich in saturated fat, are included in most crackers, convenience foods and non-dairy substitutes.

The list did not stop there. Gravies and sauces made from meat drippings were high in saturated fat, as were fast foods. Ten French fries, about 2 ounces, contain 156 calories. That in itself is frightening. But over 40% of those calories are derived from fat. And most canned, pre-mixed, frozen or dehydrated convenience foods use animal fat. Of the fat contained in pork and beans, for example, 40% is saturated; of that in a frozen meat loaf dinner, 35% is saturated; and of that in a chocolate cake mix, 37% is saturated.

The sources of cholesterol were the next aspect of my diet to be analyzed. Any food which comes from an animal contains cholesterol. However, certain foods contain more than others, and these cholesterol-rich foods had to be identified and restricted or eliminated if I were to reduce my intake to below 300 mg. a day.

The red meats on my diet, already damned for being high in saturated fat, contained much cholesterol. Just 12 ounces of beef, pork, lamb or veal could put me over the 300 mg. level. Two average frankfurters could constitute almost one-fifth of that level, and a single salami sandwich could comprise over one-third. Organ meats, such as liver, kidney or sweetbreads, also had too much cholesterol to remain on my diet. A 4-oz. portion of liver, for example, contains 500 mg. of cholesterol.

Animal fats used in cooking also contributed to my cholesterol level, as did eggs. One large egg (1.8 oz.) contains 251 mg. of cholesterol. With two eggs for breakfast, I could almost double the daily recommended guideline. According to the U.S. Census Bureau, the average American consumes 273 eggs per year, not only eaten as poached, scrambled and fried, but also as a component of other foods such as pancakes, baked goods and packaged cake mixes. When I ate these foods, I ate eggs. And when I ate eggs, I consumed cholesterol.

Step Number 2: Reduction of Fat and Cholesterol

Dinner was the starting point for the practice of the Positive Diet. It was selected because it was the most easily controlled meal in our family schedule, it was regularly eaten at home, a variety of foods were heart-healthy as dinner fare, and normally more preparation time was available than for other meals. My pre-surgery diet had included red meat at five or six dinners in the course of a week. My initial action was to develop a meal plan which would limit red meat dinners to no more than three per week, or about a 50% reduction from my old diet. The following is an example of a two week meal plan:

Week 1	Red Meat Dinners
Sunday	Chili Con Carne
Monday	
Tuesday	
Wednesday	Beef-Barley Soup
Thursday	
Friday	Roast Beef
Saturday	

Week 2	Red Meat Dinners
Sunday	Spaghetti With Meatballs
Monday	
Tuesday	
Wednesday	French Dip Sandwiches
Thursday	
Friday	
Saturday	Hamburgers

Further steps were also taken with these red meat dinners to reduce the amount of fat and cholesterol consumed. They were as follows:

▶Reduce meat portions in size and increase complex carbohydrates (vegetables, fruit, grains and legumes).

▶Use only lean-grade meat and trim it of all visible fat before cooking.

▶Broil, roast, bake or barbecue meats as these methods allow the fat to drip away during cooking.

▶Cook meat to medium or to well-done to maximize the fat loss during cooking.

▶Avoid frying foods in hydrogenated margarine or animal fats; instead use chicken or beef broth, wine, water, flavored vinegars, or use a non-stick pan.

▶Always de-fat meat drippings and broths by refrigeration (the fat coagulates and can be skimmed and discarded) before using in gravies or sauces.

▶Avoid packaged, canned or frozen meat dishes as their fat content cannot be controlled.

▶Be careful of restaurant foods, especially fast foods, as their fat content cannot be controlled.

For three nights I could eat red meat which, with the exception of portion size and cooking method, was close to those meals on my old diet. But what about the other four nights?

The answer was found in simple one-for-one substitutions using poultry and seafood. Skinless, white poultry is only about 20% fat. Only 19% of the calories in trout are fat, and only 6% of those in water-packed tuna are fat. In addition, poultry and seafood, with the exception of shrimp, are generally lower in cholesterol than is red meat. (Although shrimp is high in cholesterol, many medical professionals now feel that the healthful benefits of fish oil allow shrimp to be eaten on a moderate basis.) A 3½ oz. serving of cooked trout, halibut or chicken, for example, yields cholesterol values respectively of 55 mg., 60 mg., and 79 mg. Four ounces of cod contain just 57 mg. and 3 oz. of tuna just 54 mg. of cholesterol. Four ounces of sirloin steak, by comparison, contain 107 mg. of cholesterol.

One-for-one substitutions were effective in limiting fat and cholesterol. We also took other steps to insure that the substitutions would be as low-fat and low-cholesterol as possible. These steps were:

▶Reduce poultry and seafood portions in size. Although lower in cholesterol than red meat, poultry and seafood are still sources of cholesterol.

▶Always cook poultry without the skin so that the fat in the skin does not drip into the meat.

▶Select the white meat of the chicken or turkey,

rather than the dark meat, as the white is lower in cholesterol.

▶Broil, roast, bake, steam, poach or barbecue poultry and seafood as these methods allow the fat to drip away during cooking.

▶Use wine, herbs, lemon juice or flavored vinegars, rather than margarine, oils and sauces, to flavor poultry and seafood dishes.

▶Use shellfish that are high in cholesterol (such as shrimp) moderately.

▶Avoid packaged, canned or frozen poultry and seafood dishes.

▶When ordering seafood and poultry in restaurants, avoid any sauces and gravies, and select only heart-healthy cooking methods.

The one-for-one substitutions were easily made. Soon barbecued chicken replaced barbecued steak, baked salmon replaced roast beef, a tuna sandwich replaced a hamburger. Before long, I was ready to substitute ingredients.

Our goal was to preserve the taste of my old diet while stripping the dishes of their not-so-healthy elements. Chili made with ground round, for example, had always been a favorite of mine. But it was also a high-fat meal. So, I began to make it using chicken rather than beef. The result? A delicious, heart-healthy chili. The same was true of cioppino. By substituting liquid safflower oil or olive oil for butter or margarine in the recipe, cioppino could be adapted to the Positive Diet. Through creative substitution, it was possible to make low-fat food taste good.

Soon the two-week dinner meal plan was complete.

Week 1	Meal Plan
Sunday	Chili Con Carne
Monday	Roast Chicken
Tuesday	Salad Niçoise
Wednesday	Beef-Barley Soup
Thursday	Stuffed Fillet of Sole
Friday	Roast Beef
Saturday	Vegetable Stir-fry

Week 2	Meal Plan
Sunday	Spaghetti With Meatballs
Monday	Steamed Clams
Tuesday	Roast Breast of Turkey
Wednesday	French Dip Sandwiches
Thursday	Cioppino
Friday	Chicken Soup
Saturday	Hamburgers

The red meat substitutes on this plan were not the tasteless meals of a bland diet. They easily kept me from craving red meat or feeling deprived. I was too busy eating savory, wholesome foods to be concerned with those foods no longer on my diet.

In addition, the meal plan was economical. Monday's roast chicken produced the stock for Friday's soup. Roast beef yielded French dip sandwiches. The vegetable stir-fry used vegetables left over from earlier meals. And the cioppino was a product of the sole and clam dinners.

After a few months I began to prefer this dinner pattern to that of my old meat-rich diet. Soon I was able to adjust red meat dinners downward to 2 per week without any problem. I was eating better and was more satisfied, yet the saturated fat and cholesterol were reduced. Thanks to meal planning and creative substitution, I had the best of both worlds.

Other refinements were made to further reduce fat and cholesterol. They were as follows:

▶Use fresh vegetables whenever possible. If it is necessary to use canned or frozen, read the label to insure that the product does not contain saturated fat, such as lard, bacon fat, palm oil or coconut oil. If a label lists "vegetable fat" without revealing the specific source, assume that it is palm oil or coconut oil and do not purchase the product.

▶Use only those salad dressings made from olive oil or from an unsaturated vegetable oil (safflower, corn, cottonseed, sesame, soybean and sunflower). Use homemade rather than commercial salad dressings for maximum control over the oil, salt, sugar and preservatives. Avoid dressings made with cheese. Serve dressings on the side as only 1 tablespoon can be 75 to 100 calories.

▶Use soft tub-type margarine made from an unsaturated liquid vegetable oil in place of hydrogenated stick margarine. Again, label reading is the key. To be acceptable, the label must list liquid vegetable oil as the first ingredient and show that the product contains twice the amount of unsaturated as saturated fat.

▶Reduce the amount of margarine used on breads. Even tub margarine made from an unsaturated vegetable oil is 99% fat and contains 95 calories per tablespoon. Eliminate margarine as a sauce for vegetables, rice and potatoes; instead use herbs, spices, wine, lemon juice or flavored vinegars.

▶Avoid commercial bakery products and desserts that are high in saturated fat and calories.

113

►Increase the amount of complex carbohydrates (such as rice, beans, pasta) to satisfy in a low-fat manner and reduce the portion size of the entrée.

Lunch. After practicing the Positive Diet for about two months, dinner was under control. Meal planning and creative substitution were being utilized regularly; fat and cholesterol were being reduced; and I was satisfied physically and psychologically with my meals. I then began to apply the first basic principle at lunch.

Lunch had always posed a fat and cholesterol problem. This was especially true during the weekdays, when time often dictated a fast food lunch. But I had not realized how much fat was consumed in these lunches. Research by the Center for Science in the Public Interest educated me to the fact that many fast foods were over 50% fat:

Fat Content of Fast Foods		% of Calories
Fast Food	Calories	from Fat
HAMBURGERS & CHEESEBURGERS:		
Wendy's Triple Cheeseburger	1040	68%
Burger King Double Beef Whopper with Cheese	970	59%
Carl's Jr. Super Star	780	58%
McDonald's McD.L.T.	680	58%
Wendy's Double Cheeseburger	630	57%
Burger King Whopper	626	55%
McDonald's Big Mac	570	55%
Jack in the Box Ham & Swiss Burger	638	54%
CHICKEN:		
Kentucky Fried Chicken, Extra Crispy Thigh	343	64%
Kentucky Fried Chicken, Extra Crispy Side Breast	354	60%
McDonald's Chicken McNuggets	323	56%
Dairy Queen Chicken Sandwich, fried	670	55%
Burger King Specialty Chicken Sandwich	688	52%

Fat Content of Fast Foods

Fast Food	Calories	% of Calories from Fat
FISH:		
Long John Silver's Seafood Platter	976	58%
McDonald's Filet-O-Fish	435	53%
Burger King Whaler Sandwich with Cheese	530	51%
Jack in the Box Moby Jack	444	50%
ROAST BEEF:		
Arby's Roast Beef Deluxe	486	43%
Roy Rogers Roast Beef with Cheese, large	467	40%
Arby's Super Roast Beef	501	40%
FRENCH FRIES:		
Burger King French Fries, regular	227	52%
Hardee's French Fries, large	406	49%
McDonald's Fries, regular	220	47%
Roy Rogers French Fries, large	357	46%
Wendy's French Fries, regular	280	45%
Kentucky Fried Chicken Kentucky Fries	268	43%
SHAKES:		
Burger King Vanilla Shake (10 oz.)	321	28%
Burger King Chocolate Shake (10 oz.)	374	26%
Dairy Queen Chocolate Shake (20 oz.)	990	24%
McDonald's Strawberry Shake (10.2 oz.)	362	22%

Source: Center for Science in the Public Interest.

It became obvious that fast foods, as well as fatty luncheon meats such as salami or bologna, had to be eliminated. This was not easy. In fact, I found the institution of the Positive Diet at lunch to be more difficult than it had been at dinner. There was no intelligent alternative but to make it work; but eating, I soon found out, was not always a matter of intellect. It was more often a matter of emotion.

Strawmen arguments were raised in my mind about why eating Positive Diet lunches were impossible: "I was in a hurry"; "I was with friends and they chose the restaurant"; "It would have been embarassing to complain about the buttersauce"; or my favorite, "I work hard and I deserve a salami sandwich!" Lunch became a battleground as to which would control my diet, intellect or emotion.

Finally, after much tribulation, common sense won. Sticking to the diet was not only a matter of rational choice, it was also a matter of having the will and the determination to do what I knew was right. I had to control my diet, not let it control me, if I were to have any say in my cardiac destiny.

I accepted the necessity of having to pack a lunch, but I did not like it. I had never taken my lunch to work in the past. I told myself that was because I liked to eat out. But the real problem was not my affinity for restaurant lunches . . . it was my ego. I was really concerned with whether or not I would continue to be viewed as a "successful executive" by my business peers if I carried a brown bag lunch. What would people say?

Ridiculous as this seems in retrospect, at the time the problem was real for me. After awhile, I concluded that my identity problem was secondary to my coronary problem. At this early state of the Positive Diet, restaurant lunches meant no control, and no control meant no diet. Bringing my lunch from home was the only viable alternative.

Since salads were somewhat cumbersome, the meal plan was designed around sandwiches, fresh fruit and crisp raw vegetables. I knew what I should not have: fast foods and fatty luncheon meats. I also decided to eat sandwiches containing red meat no more than once a week.

I used creative substitution to plan lunches for the remaining four days. Many of these lunches were a product of previous dinners. Roast turkey breast for a Monday dinner yielded sliced turkey sandwiches for a Wednesday lunch. Chicken dinner leftovers became a chicken sandwich for lunch. I also rediscovered two old favorites: water-packed tuna and natural peanut butter.

Breads became very important. They needed to be tasty and filling, and to provide variety, as well as to meet the low-fat standards of the diet. Reading labels helped me find many acceptable choices such as certain brands of sourdough, rye, French, pumpernickel, Armenian, whole wheat, bran wheat and whole grain. Lettuce, tomatoes, onions, sprouts, almonds and water chestnuts were great garnishes and provided me with needed raw vegetables. Safflower mayonnaise, either commercial or homemade, was an acceptable spread. And I always packed fresh fruit for dessert. Soon my two-week meal plan was complete.

Week 1   Lunches

Monday	Water-packed tuna with lettuce, tomato, onion, sprouts and water-chestnuts on whole wheat bread; Granny Smith apple.
Tuesday	Sliced roast turkey with lettuce, tomato and sprouts on thick crust French bread; fresh or frozen grapes.
Wednesday	Sliced cold roast beef with tomato and onion on sourdough roll; tangerine.
Thursday	Thinly sliced low-fat cheese with lettuce and tomato on light Bohemian rye bread; delicious apple.
Friday	Chicken salad in Armenian pocket bread with sliced green peppers; celery sticks; fresh pineapple spears.

Week 2   Lunches

Monday	Thinly sliced extra-lean ham and low-fat mozzarella cheese with lettuce and tomato on thick crust French bread; fresh or frozen raspberries.
Tuesday	Water-packed tuna with lettuce, tomato, onion and sprouts on dark rye bread; orange.
Wednesday	Sliced chicken with tomato and sprouts on sourdough bread; fresh or frozen berries.
Thursday	Natural peanut butter on whole grain bread; celery and carrot sticks; sliced green pepper; banana.
Friday	Turkey with tomato, lettuce, sprouts and sliced mushrooms on whole wheat bread; pear.

These low-fat lunches actually provided more variety than did my pre-surgery meals. I soon enjoyed the new lunches more than the old. After about four months, I felt secure in my practice of the Positive Diet at lunch, and I decided to reward myself with a salami sandwich. As I walked into the deli, I was overwhelmed by the heady aroma of luncheon meats. I could almost taste how delicious the sandwich would be.

What a disappointment!

It was not delicious at all. The salami tasted greasy; it did not even look appealing. The sandwich had not changed. It was made the same as always. But I had changed, or, more specifically, my taste buds had changed. The Positive Diet had oriented them away from fatty foods. It was then that I knew that my lunch diet pattern had changed fundamentally and permanently. By following a few simple rules, I could keep my lunches under control. These rules were as follows:

▶At the start of the diet, avoid all restaurant food, especially fast food.
▶Reduce red meat lunches to no more than one per week; use poultry, fish and low-fat cheese instead.
▶Avoid fatty luncheon meats such as bologna and frankfurters. Check the fat content of the so-called "low-fat" luncheon meats such as turkey bologna and "95% fat-free" sandwich ham. Many of these products are over 50% fat.
▶Use safflower or corn oil mayonnaise and soft tub-style margarine as sandwich spreads.
▶Use different breads and rolls for maximum sandwich variety.
▶Take advantage of seasonal fresh fruits and vegetables.

Breakfast. On my old diet, breakfast had been a meal of extremes. On weekends I might eat a logger's meal of hash browns, bacon and eggs. On weekdays, I would eat no breakfast at all or I might have a cup of coffee and a roll. I decided to treat each type of breakfast separately.

Weekday breakfasts needed changing for two reasons. The first was to reduce whatever fat and cholesterol existed in the meal. This was done by using soft margarine on toast and by excluding commercially baked goods such as doughnuts, Danish pastry and sugar-coated buns. The second reason was to introduce additional healthful foods into my diet.

For example, research by Dr. James Anderson at the University of Kentucky has shown that oat bran, available as a hot breakfast cereal, can lower blood cholesterol. For that reason, I began to eat oat bran on a regular basis for breakfast. In addition, no breakfast or a poor breakfast could make me so ravenous by lunchtime that a Positive Diet lunch might not be sufficient. This could open opportunities for pastry at a coffee break or a bag of potato chips at lunch. However, if the breakfast fare could keep me satisfied until lunch, not only would I benefit nutritionally, but the chances for lunch success would be enhanced.

My new weekday breakfasts were planned around low-fat protein, whole grains and fresh fruits. The protein was in the form of natural peanut butter, low-fat cheeses, egg substitute, non-fat yogurt and skim milk; the whole grains were in the form of cereals, particularly oat bran, toast, bagels, English muffins or bran muffins and the fruits were eaten in their natural state or squeezed into juice. A typical weekday meal plan would be as follows:

Week 1   Breakfasts

Monday	½ grapefruit; low-fat mozza-rella cheese and fresh tomato slices broiled on a whole grain English muffin.
Tuesday	Non-fat yogurt with fresh raspberries; crumpet with a dab of honey; skim milk.
Wednesday	Sliced banana; toasted bagel with natural peanut butter; skim milk.
Thursday	Chilled fresh melon; hot oatmeal or oat bran cereal; skim milk.
Friday	Fresh strawberries; scrambled eggs (egg substitute) with salsa; bran or English muffin.

Week 2   Breakfasts

Monday	Freshly squeezed grapefruit juice; hot or cold cereal with skim milk; bran wheat toast.
Tuesday	Freshly squeezed orange juice; homemade oat bran muffin; skim milk.
Wednesday	Chilled orange slices; non-fat frozen yogurt; toasted English muffin; skim milk.
Thursday	Baked apple; hot oatmeal or oat bran cereal with skim milk; whole wheat toast.
Friday	Chilled grapefruit; French toast made with crusty French bread; skim milk.

These breakfasts met my needs extremely well because:

>They did not take great forethought in planning.

>They did not take a great deal of time either to prepare or to eat.

>They offered sufficient variety.

>They were low in fat and in cholesterol.

>They kept me satisfied for the entire morning.

Weekend breakfasts were a different matter. On my old diet these frequently had been brunches, often including fresh fruit, sausage, ham, bacon, eggs, hashbrowns, pancakes, waffles or French toast. The fat and cholesterol in these meals were astronomical. The meats were fat, the eggs were high in cholesterol and almost everything except the fruit was fried in animal fat. I had two choices: I could either eliminate these breakfasts altogether or I could modify their content.

The first element to be examined was eggs. A single large chicken egg contains 251 mg. of cholesterol, or almost the entire maximum recommended daily allowance. The white of the egg contains 60% of the protein and only 1% of the cholesterol, while the yolk contains 40% of the protein and 99% of the cholesterol. For this reason, egg whites did not have to be removed from my diet, but only egg yolks.

Consequently, egg substitute (made from egg whites and unsaturated oil) was very important to the preservation of my weekend breakfasts. Egg substitute, available in the supermarket or made at home, allows breakfasts to include such foods as scrambled eggs, omelets, huevos rancheros, pancakes, French toast, waffles and crepes. By using egg substitute rather than whole eggs in these dishes, cholesterol was either reduced or eliminated, yet the taste and the appearance remained virtually unchanged. To further reduce cholesterol, these dishes were cooked on a non-stick teflon griddle or in a non-stick teflon frying pan, thus eliminating the need for fat or oil as a lubricant.

My last move was to eliminate breakfast meats. Pork sausage is 87% fat, bacon 82% fat, and ham 69% fat. These meats are also rich in cholesterol. One ounce (one link) of pork sausage contains 30 milligrams and 4 ounces of ham contains over 100 milligrams. It was only prudent to eliminate these foods from my diet.

REDUCING BUTTERFAT

The second basic principle, the reduction of butterfat, is concerned with the fat in whole milk and whole milk foods, such as cheese, cream and ice cream. Because butterfat is a saturated fat, it has the same negative impact upon the health of the heart and the blood vessels as does the saturated fat in red meat. Initially, it was difficult to relate dairy products to harmful saturated fat. These foods meant calcium and protein to me, essential elements for good health. A study of the U.S. Department of Agriculture Composition of Food Analysis altered this concept.

Food	% of Calories from Fat
Butter	99%
Heavy Cream	96%
Light Cream	88%
Sour Cream	88%
Cream Cheese	84%
Half and Half	82%
Roquefort Cheese	74%
American Cheese	74%
Cheddar Cheese	74%
Blue Cheese	73%
Parmesan Cheese	60%
Ice Cream	55%
Whole Milk	51%
Creamed Cottage Cheese	34%
2% Milk	34%

Whole milk products are an important source of calcium and protein. But many also contain over 50% fat and are high in cholesterol as well. About one-third (100 mg.) of the recommended maximum daily cholesterol allowance can be reached by consuming any one of the following:
>3 cups of whole milk
>4 tablespoons of butter
>4 ounces of American cheese
>3 ounces of cream cheese
>²⁄₃ cup of sour cream
>1 cup of ice cream

Once whole milk products were placed in their proper perspective, there was no alternative but to reduce their use.

Step Number 1: Identification of Butterfat Sources

Whole milk foods were consumed at virtually every meal on my old diet — whole or 2% milk at breakfast, lunch and dinner; cheese in sand-wiches and in casseroles; butter on bread and in cooking; cream in cheese, snacks, and desserts; and ice cream in cones, milkshakes and floats.

Step Number 2: Reduction of Butterfat

I began by applying the second basic principle to whole milk. My first move was to eliminate it in favor of 2% milk. Touted as "low-fat" by the dairy industry, I assumed that this milk contained only 2% butterfat. As such, it would be extremely low in saturated fat. Unfortunately, this is not the case. The term 2% is very misleading; it applies only to the weight of the butterfat in the milk. As a per-centage of calories, butterfat constitutes about 34% of the milk (whole milk is about 51% fat). It is hardly possible to call a product which is over one-third fat a "low-fat" food. Certainly this term is a misnomer. This milk may be lower in fat than whole milk, but it is not a "low-fat" product. As far as the heart and blood vessels are concerned, 2% milk is "high-fat."

The only genuine low-fat alternative is skim milk, a product which has only 2% of its calories derived from butterfat, yet has all the benefits of whole milk (calcium, protein) and none of the drawbacks (high butterfat). In addition, skim milk has a much lower cholesterol value than whole milk.

It took about a month to get used to the taste of skim milk. Initially, I found that adding ⅓ cup of powdered non-fat milk to each quart of skim milk produced a creamier taste. After awhile, I began to prefer the lighter taste of skim milk to the creamier taste of 2% or whole milk, and I no longer needed to add the non-fat milk powder.

There was another benefit to the change: my

total milk consumption decreased. At first I did not care for the taste of skim milk; and by the time I came to like it, I was already used to drinking less milk.

Butter was another source of fat. I used it on toast, pancakes, waffles or French toast; on rolls, bread or in sandwiches; on potatoes, rice or vegetables; and in snacks, such as pies, cakes, cookies or popcorn. Not only is butter almost 100% fat, but over half of its fat content is saturated. In addition, butter is high in cholesterol; a single tablespoon contains 35 mg.

I eliminated butter in favor of soft tub-style margarine. I always made sure that the prime ingredient was liquid safflower oil or corn oil and the amount of unsaturated fat was at least double the amount of saturated fat. Once again label reading was very important. Tub-style margarine does not need to hold its shape and is less hydrogenated than is stick margarine, which contains saturated fat because of the hardening process.

The change to soft tub-style margarine minimized the amount of saturated fat consumed. The change did not, however, reduce the total amount of fat consumed. In order to do that, I followed these steps:

▶Reduce by ½ the amount of margarine used on rolls, toast, pancakes . . . After a time, reduce this amount again by ¼.

▶Avoid commercially baked goods, such as rolls, pastries, pies, cakes and doughnuts.

▶Avoid the use of buttersauce on potatoes, rice, vegetables and main dishes; instead use herbs, spices, flavored vinegar or lemon juice. Dip shellfish, such as crab, clams, mussels and lobster in fresh lemon juice, rather than butter.

▶Avoid foods fried or sautéed in butter or margarine. For home cooking use a non-stick teflon pan or use lemon juice, flavored vinegar, vermouth, wine, broth or water.

▶Beware of restaurant foods. Generally, they are rich in butter and/or margarine. Ask how the food is prepared. If it's fried in butter, do not order it. Do not assume anything — ask questions! A broiled or barbecued salmon fillet may automatically be served with a butter sauce.

Cheese was another dairy food that called for modification. Most cheese is over 50% fat and is rich in cholesterol (generally one ounce of cheese contains about 28 mg. of cholesterol or about 10% of the maximum recommended daily intake). As much as I loved cheeseburgers, and Swiss or Cheddar cheese on sandwiches, it was only prudent to remove this fat source from my diet. I did this by substituting non-fat and low-fat cheese for that made with cream and whole milk.

Many types of low-fat cheese are available. Pot cheese is quite low-fat and is suitable as a spread on crackers and vegetables and as a dip. Hoop cheese and part-skim-milk Mozzarella can be sliced and are suitable for sandwiches. Other types of low-fat cheese include Ricotta, Edam, Somerset, Danbo, Cheddar and Jack. Remember, however, that all low-fat cheese is still relatively high in fat and should be eaten judiciously.

Since much of this cheese is produced in a high-fat as well as a low-fat variety, label reading becomes very important. The low-fat varieties are generally made from skim or partially skim milk. Some cheese may be labeled "low-fat," but the fat content may still be over 50%. Kraft's Philadelphia Brand Cream Cheese, for example, is 90% fat. Kraft's Neufchatel Cheese, promoted as a low-fat alternative, is 79% fat.

In my opinion, a true low-fat cheese should have a fat content of 20% or less. If the label does not reveal the fat content, do not hesitate to ask the dairyman in your supermarket. A trip to a specialty cheese store can be very rewarding if the salesperson is knowledgeable. These stores usually carry the newest varieties of low-fat cheese and the salespeople generally know the fat content of each cheese as well.

Other dairy products, such as cottage cheese and yogurt, are available in low-fat versions. However, the fat content often is considered low only when contrasted with that of its whole milk counterpart. Low-fat yogurt, for example, can be over 50% fat. For that reason, I avoid the low-fat variety in favor of non-fat yogurt, either purchased or produced at home with the aid of an inexpensive, simple-to-use yogurt maker. In the case of cottage cheese, dry cottage cheese is the best bet for a truly low-fat alternative.

Sweet cream, ice cream and whipped cream made from whole milk are too rich in saturated fat to be acceptable on a heart-healthy diet. But with creative substitution, homemade recipes for these foods exist, allowing low-fat variations to be enjoyed periodically. Refer to the cookbook for our recipes.

SUMMING UP FAT AND CHOLESTEROL

The Positive Diet is not totally free of foods that contain fat, butterfat and cholesterol. However, these elements can be drastically reduced using a few simple guidelines:

▶Make use of meal planning and creative substitution.

▶Avoid high-cholesterol foods such as liver, kidneys and other organ meats.

▶Reduce whole egg consumption; use egg substitute or egg whites.

▶Avoid red meats rich in saturated fat such as sausage, bacon and luncheon meats; use more poultry and fish.

▶When red meat is eaten, reduce the portion size; use a lean grade trimmed of all visible fat; broil, roast, bake or barbecue, but never fry; cook to medium or well-done.

▶De-fat meat drippings and broths before using.

▶Always cook poultry without the skin; choose white meat over dark.

▶Sauté in wine, broth, water, vermouth or flavored vinegar or use a non-stick pan; never sauté in hydrogenated margarine, lard, butter or shortening.

▶Oils of choice include olive, safflower and corn. Avoid butter and stick margarine; instead, use soft tub-type margarine made from liquid vegetable oil; reduce the amount of margarine used.

▶Avoid whole milk and whole milk products; use skim milk and low-fat cheese.

▶Learn to read labels.

▶Avoid convenience foods and commercially baked goods; beware of restaurant food, especially fast food.

▶Increase complex carbohydrates (vegetables, fruit, grains and legumes).

REDUCING SALT

The third basic principle of the Positive Diet addresses the reduction of salt and sodium. I had eaten salt-rich foods, such as pickles, bacon, and potato chips. I used salt in cooking and at the table and I used processed foods, such as soups, pork and beans, chili and frozen hashbrown potatoes. It was time to re-educate my taste buds.

Step Number 1: Identifying Salt Sources

The sources of salt on my pre-surgery diet could be divided into two categories: obvious and hidden. Obvious sources are those in which salt is expected to be found, such as potato chips or pickles. Hidden sources are those in which salt is a surprise ingredient, such as certain brands of peanut butter or dehydrated chicken noodle or onion soup.

The obvious sources included:
>table salt used as a condiment
>table salt used in cooking as a seasoning
>table salt used in alcoholic drinks, such as in Bloody Marys
>salty condiments, such as seasoning salt, soy sauce and bouillon cubes
>salty foods, such as pickles, olives, anchovies, salted herring, sauerkraut, potato chips, pretzels, popcorn and salted nuts.

The hidden sources included:
>processed luncheon meats, such as bologna, salami, and frankfurters
>ham, bacon, sausage and cured pork
>canned tuna or salmon packed in oil
>cheese and cheese spreads
>vegetable juice and tomato juice
>canned tomato sauce, paste and puree

>commercial salad dressings
>condiments such as catsup, relish, chili sauce, steak sauce and mustard
>fast food hamburgers, French fries, chicken, tacos and pizza
>commercially baked bread, crackers, rolls, breadsticks, pastry and desserts
>cereals and pancake mixes
>salted butter and margarine
>baking soda and powder
>canned, frozen and dehydrated processed foods such as chili, macaroni and cheese, TV dinners, and canned vegetables

Step Number 2: Salt Reduction

The Obvious Sources. I used table salt regularly on my old diet. I salted all food even before it was tasted. This was an automatic, knee-jerk reaction. In order to curtail salting, I had to remove the salt from the table. So I threw the salt shaker away!

In the beginning this proved to be a problem. Saltless food tasted bland and I longed to spice up meals with a dash of salt. I resisted this temptation by reminding myself of the importance of salt reduction to cardiac health and by handling the reduction one day at a time. "Certainly you can last one day without your salt shaker," I told myself each morning.

Soon a month had elapsed and I noticed a subtle change taking place in my taste buds. I began to enjoy the natural flavor of the saltless foods. A tossed green salad with fresh vegetables, for example, contained a myriad of pleasing tastes. In the past it had existed merely as a vehicle for carrying salt. Now, with my taste buds no longer dulled, I could taste the many distinct flavors. I also began to appreciate other sources of seasonings — black pepper, garlic powder, parsley, tarragon, chili powder and lemon juice. Meals could be spiced up I learned, without using my salt shaker.

After about two months of eating in this manner, I decided to test my taste buds. I made a large salad and salted it just as I had on my old diet. The taste of the salad was not like I had remembered. It was too salty to be enjoyable; there was no taste to the food itself. I might as well have been eating cardboard. It was then that I knew that my desire for salt could be diminished permanently and that I could live and eat well without my salt shaker.

The next step was to reduce the amount of salt used in cooking by 25%. If a recipe called for 1 teaspoon of salt, I used only ¾ teaspoon. Much to my delight, I found there was very little change in the taste of the food. After a few months, I made a second reduction of 25%, again without adverse results. And finally, I made a third reduction of 25%. I further reduced the amount of salt when cooking with processed foods such as canned tomatoes, tomato sauce, tomato paste or chicken broth, as these foods are already high in sodium. To bring out the natural flavors of foods, I relied on lemon juice, flavored vinegars and herbs and spices which were low in sodium. Black pepper or sage, for example, each contain less than 1 milligram of sodium per teaspoon; the same amount of salt contains 2300 milligrams of sodium.

Finally, I restricted or eliminated those foods which were obviously too salty to be on a heart-healthy diet. Such foods were easy to identify, for to taste them was to know they were rich in salt. Keeping in mind that an "adequate and safe" sodium level is no more than 3300 milligrams daily, it was easy to see how such foods could cause that level to be exceeded.

Food	Milligrams of Sodium
Salted Popcorn—2 oz.	1100
Salted Potato Chips—2 oz.	568
Salted Nuts—2 oz.	680
Sauerkraut—1 cup	1755
Dill Pickle—1 large	1940

In some instances low- or no-salt versions were available, such as unsalted peanuts or potato chips. But for foods such as pickles, sauerkraut or salted herring, where no viable substitute existed, drastic reduction or total elimination was the only answer.

The Hidden Sources. With the obvious sources of salt under control, I turned my attention to the more difficult problem of controlling the hidden sources. The solution lay in totally revising my dependance upon processed foods.

In researching hidden salt, I was shocked at the number of canned, frozen and dehydrated foods in which salt and other sodium products are main ingredients. The same was true for fast foods. A U.S.D.A. listing of the sodium content of sampled foods illustrates the degree to which sodium is used as an additive:

Food	Milligrams of Sodium
Chef-Boy-Ar-Dee Beef Stroganoff — 6⅔ oz.	1067
Heinz Beef Stew — 8½ oz.	1272
Kraft Macaroni and Cheese — 12½ oz.	1593
Swanson Meat Loaf Dinner — 16½ oz.	1915
Snow's New England Clam Chowder — 8 oz.	1368
Lipton's Cup-A-Soup (Chicken) — ⅓ oz.	931
Heinz Baked Beans — 8 oz.	1307
Shake 'N Bake Chicken Coating — 2⅜ oz.	2557
Prince Spaghetti Sauce — 4 oz.	1030
Chicken of the Sea Tuna (oil packed) — 6 oz.	1196
Morton Turkey Dinner — 12 oz.	1397
Campbell Cream of Celery Soup — 8 oz.	930
Del Monte Carrots — 4 oz.	1852
Green Giant Broccoli Spears — 3⅓ oz.	444
Hormel Genoa Salami — 1 oz.	454
Oscar Meyer Bologna — 1⅓ oz.	342
Oscar Meyer Frankfurters — 1⅔ oz.	364
Pepperidge Farms Herb Stuffing — 8 oz.	3931
Betty Crocker Bisquick — 8 oz.	1475
Wonder Bread — 1 slice	148
General Mills Cheerios — 1 oz.	320
McDonald's Big Mac — 1	962
Kentucky Fried Chicken 3-piece dinner	2285
McDonald's Egg McMuffin — 1	914
Dairy Queen Hot Dog	868
Nabisco Saltines — 1 oz.	430
McDonald's Chocolate Shake — 8 oz.	329

The amount of salt and sodium included in processed foods is incredible, especially when contrasted with the sodium content of these same foods in their natural state. Peas, for example, contain just .9 milligrams of sodium per serving; the same amount of canned peas contains 230 mg. An ear of corn contains about 1 mg. of sodium, a cup of canned corn about 384 mg. Three ounces of steak contain 55 mg., a frozen meat loaf dinner about 1304 mg. Three ounces of pork contain 59 mg., the same amount of canned ham about 1114 mg. Processed foods, a mainstay of the heat and serve American diet pattern, guarantee Americans a sodium intake high enough to be a health hazard.

Not all processed foods contain the same level of sodium. A 6-ounce can of Del Monte's tomato paste, for example, contains 90 milligrams of sodium, while the same size can of Hunt's has 620. Unfortunately, sodium content information is not universally listed on food labels. In fact, only 13% of all foods regulated by the Food and Drug Administration are presently labeled for salt or sodium content. Under the present laws, the FDA "permits" but does not "require" sodium content to be identified on food labels. Food processors face relatively few restrictions in the use of salt or other sodium additives such as sodium benzoate, sodium nitrate, monosodium glutamate, sodium bicarbonate or sodium phosphate, as far as their use as food additives. As long as the processor does not use salt to "exceed the amount reasonably required to accomplish its intended physical, nutritional or other technical effect in food," he is free to do what he wants. And that is the way most food processors want it. Congressman Albert Gore, in a *Time* interview, stated, "There is an enormous competitive advantage to loading food with salt and not telling people about it."

With no requirement existing for food proces-sors to display specific sodium information, even the most prudent shopper is at a disadvantage when purchasing processed foods. This situation may change in the future as more and more or-ganizations demand such information. In fact, legislation requiring sodium labeling has been in-troduced in Congress a number of times, but as of this writing no new law has been passed.

Under the present circumstances, consumers can take two actions to protect themselves. One is to consult a good sodium dictionary, such as Bar-bara Kraus' *Sodium, Fats, and Cholesterol.* Such books list the sodium content of foods by brand name. They can be extremely helpful in product selection. Second, adopt a simple rule not to pur-chase any processed food that lists salt or sodium as one of the first three ingredients on the label. While this rule provides less than a precise mea-surement, it does provide an acceptable standard against which processed foods can be measured.

The only true solution to the high-salt prob-lem is to incorporate more natural foods into the diet. These foods are fresher, taste better, and are significantly lower in salt, sodium and other addi-tives than are processed foods. They are the key to a successful low-sodium diet.

SUMMING UP SALT

The Positive Diet is not salt-free. However, it is designed to restrict excessive salt and sodium con-sumption through the use of a few guidelines:
▶Avoid using salt as a condiment; remove the salt shaker from the table.

▶Reduce the salt called for in recipes by 25% initially, by 75% ultimately; never add salt to processed foods.

▶Avoid using sodium-rich seasonings, seasoning salt, and soy sauce; use low-sodium alternatives such as garlic, onion, lemon juice, flavored vinegars, fresh herbs and spices.

▶Avoid obviously salty foods such as pickles, salted nuts, salted potato chips and sauerkraut.

▶Avoid fast foods; they specialize in high-salt.

▶Avoid processed foods as much as possible. When using them, read food labels carefully. If sodium content is high (one of the first three ingredients), avoid the food. For best results, consult a sodium dictionary.

▶Use more natural foods. Take advantage of fresh raw fruits, berries and vegetables in season.

Sodium Content of Common Spices

Food	Milligrams of Sodium Per Teaspoon
Allspice	1.4
Basil Leaves	0.4
Bay Leaves	0.3
Caraway Seed	0.4
Cardamon Seed	0.2
Celery Seed	4.1
Cinnamon	0.2
Cloves	4.2
Coriander Seed	0.3
Cumin Seed	2.6
Curry Powder	1.0
Dill Seed	0.2
Fennel Seed	1.9
Garlic Powder	0.1
Ginger	0.5
Mace	1.3
Marjoram	1.3
Mustard Powder	0.1
Nutmeg	0.2
Onion Powder	0.8
Oregano	0.3
Paprika	0.4
Parsley Flakes	5.9
Pepper, Black	0.2
Pepper, Chili	0.2
Pepper, Red	0.2
Pepper, White	0.2
Poppy Seed	0.2
Rosemary Leaves	0.5
Salt	2300.0
Sage	0.1
Savory	0.3
Sesame Seed	0.6
Tarragon	1.0
Thyme	1.2
Turmeric	0.2

Source: American Spice Trade Association

REDUCING SUGAR

The fourth basic principle of the Positive Diet calls for a reduction of sugar. I had not considered my old diet to be rich in sugar, but a close examination revealed multiple sources. Refined sugar was used in cooking and baking, sometimes as a condiment on fruits or berries, and as an ingredient in ice cream, soft drinks, cookies, canned fruit, and even processed spaghetti sauce and canned soup.

Step Number 1: Identification of Concentrated Sugar Sources

As with salt, the sugar sources could be classified as obvious and hidden. The obvious sources constituted about 36% of the concentrated sugar intake; and the hidden sources about 64%.

The obvious sources included:
>granulated sugar, powdered sugar, and brown sugar used on cereal, fruit, berries, and in coffee
>granulated sugar, powdered sugar and brown sugar used as an ingredient in cooking and baking
>granulated sugar used in drinks, such as iced tea, Kool-Aid, and lemonade

The hidden sources include the following:
>candy and sugary snacks, such as gum drops, mints, and chocolate bars
>soft drinks, such as soda pop and cocoa mixes
>ice cream, milk shakes, flavored milk
>commercially baked pastry and desserts, such as doughnuts, pies, cakes, cupcakes; frostings
>commercially baked bread, crackers, rolls, biscuits and breadsticks
>jams, jellies, marmalades
>sugared breakfast cereals

>canned fruits
>cured meats
>salad dressings, ketchup and other such condiments.
>peanut butter
>processed convenience foods such as baked beans, tomato sauce, soups

Step Number 2: Sugar Reduction

The Obvious Sources centered around refined table sugar. My first action was to remove the sugar bowl from the table. Initially, the sugarless food often tasted bland. Again, the one-day-at-a-time method was employed. By never looking forward more than 24 hours, the reduction of sugar became a short-term problem. Within six weeks, my taste buds became acclimated to the natural taste of foods. I began to relish new flavors and textures. A bowl of blueberries could now be appreciated for its natural sweetness; to add sugar was to gild the lily. The natural flavor of fruit, cereal and other foods more than compensated for the loss of the super-sweet table sugar.

The second area where concentrated sugar posed a problem was with baked goods and candy. A 4-ounce piece of iced chocolate cake contains 10 teaspoons of sugar; a 1-ounce square of fudge contains 4½ teaspoons. There was no way to reconcile this amount of concentrated sugar with a healthy diet pattern.

Fortunately, by the time I began to work on the sugar problem, a break away from many of these foods had already been made due to their high fat content. In their place I substituted fresh fruit. A ripe peach became as satisfying to my sweet tooth as a milkshake or a candy bar. I also used nuts and sunflower seeds to replace sugary snacks. As my need for sugar gradually decreased, so did my desire.

There were certain occasions when cakes or pies were appropriate, such as a birthday or Thanksgiving. For these special times, I used low-fat ingredients and reduced the sugar and the salt as much as possible. It is important to keep these special occasions to a minimum so as not to negatively impact cardiac health.

The most difficult area to control was the hidden sugar used as an additive in processed foods and beverages. Sugar is often a surprise ingredient in such foods as frozen chicken dinners, baked beans and non-dairy creamers. It can even be found as an ingredient in certain pipe tobacco! A number of nutritionists have identified processed foods as the chief contributor to the 30-teaspoon-a-day habit of Americans.

Many food processors routinely add concentrated sugar during processing for sweetening, moisture control, and spoilage control. For that reason, label reading is essential. Food processors are required to list on the label all ingredients in the food product in decreasing order according to weight. Only by identifying the position of sugar on the ingredient list can the sugar content of the food be approximated.

Even with careful label reading, however, the consumer must be very aware. In a study conducted by Washington State University and the U.S. Department of Agriculture, a cereal recently test-marketed by one food manufacturer was shown to contain granulated table sugar, brown sugar and corn syrup. Also contained as ingredients were four cereal grains — refined white flour, corn flour, degermed corn meal and rice flour. The food manufacturer circumvented the listing of sugar as the main ingredient by grouping the four flours into a single "cereal grain" category and by listing the three sugars separately, thus giving the impression that the cereal was made up chiefly of grain. The label did not change the fact that concentrated sugar was the primary ingredient in the cereal; it only served to confuse the consumer about the real sugar content of the product.

Label reading is further complicated because concentrated sugar can be identified under various names: sugar, sucrose, glucose, maltose, dextrose, lactose, fructose, malt, corn solids, corn syrup, honey, molasses and invert sugar. A good rule is to avoid the food if any of these items are among the first three on the list of ingredients.

Two other areas of concern were alcoholic beverages and soft drinks. Alcohol is a concentrated sugar and one which can quickly saturate the sugar storing capacity of the body while providing little nutritional value. And soft drinks contain non-nutritive carbonated water, colorings, flavorings, and in the case of colas, caffeine. In addition, they are about 9% concentrated sugar. One can contains 5-9 teaspoons.

There is no short cut to achieving a low-sugar diet. Where processed foods and beverages, snack foods, candy and alcohol constitute much of the diet, high sugar intake is assured. It is only through the elimination of these sugar sources and the institution of fresh foods in their place that a permanent reduction in concentrated sugar intake can take place.

SUMMING UP SUGAR

The Positive Diet is not totally free of concentrated sugar. However, it is designed to restrict excessive sugar consumption through the use of a few simple rules:

▶Remove refined sugar from the table; avoid using concentrated sugar as a sweetener.

▶Reduce concentrated sugar called for in homemade recipes by ⅓.

▶Avoid sugary foods, such as candy, soft drinks, ice cream, cake.

▶Use more fresh fruit.

▶Drink alcohol only in moderation.

▶Read food labels carefully. If concentrated sugar is listed as one of the first three ingredients, avoid the food. Know all the names for concentrated sugar.

Sugar Content in Common Breakfast Cereals

Cereal	Percent of Sugar
All-Bran	20.0%
Alpen	3.8%
Alpha Bits	40.3%
Apple Jacks	55.0%
Baron Von Redberry	45.8%
Boo Berry	45.7%
Bran Buds	30.2%
40% Bran Flakes (Kellogg)	16.2%
40% Bran Flakes (Post)	15.8%
Brown Sugar-Cinnamon Frosted Mini Wheats	16.0%
Buck Wheat	13.6%
Cap'n Crunch	43.3%
Cheerios	2.2%
Cinnamon Crunch	50.3%
Cocoa Krispies	45.9%
Cocoa Pebbles	53.5%
Cocoa Puffs	43.0%
Concentrate	9.9%
Corn Chex	7.5%
Corn Flakes (Food Club)	7.0%
Corn Flakes (Kellogg)	7.8%
Corn Flakes (Kroger)	5.1%
Corn Total	4.4%
Count Chocula	44.2%
Crisp Rice	8.8%
Crispy Rice	7.3%
Crunch Berries	43.4%
Fortified Oat Flakes	22.2%
Frankenberry	44.0%
Fruit Loops	47.4%
Frosted Flakes	44.0%
Frosted Mini Wheats	33.6%

Cereal	Percent of Sugar
Fruity Pebbles	55.1%
Granola	16.2%
Granola (w/almonds & filberts)	21.4%
Granola (w/dates)	14.5%
Granola (w/raisins)	14.5%
Grape Nut Flakes	3.3%
Grape Nuts	6.6%
Heartland	23.1%
Heartland (w/raisins)	13.5%
Honeycomb	48.8%
King Vitamin	58.5%
Life	14.5%
Lucky Charms	50.4%
Orange Quangaroos	44.7%
Peanut Butter	5.2%
Pink Panther	49.2%
Post Toasties	4.1%
Product 19	4.1%
Puffed Rice	2.4%
Puffed Wheat	3.5%
Quisp	44.9%
Raisin Bran (Kellogg)	10.6%
Raisin Bran (Skinner)	9.6%
Rice Chex	8.5%
Rice Krispies (Kellogg)	10.0%
Shredded Wheat (large biscuit)	1.0%
Shredded Wheat (spoon size biscuit)	1.3%
Sir Grapefellow	40.7%
Special K	4.4%
Sugar Frosted Corn Flakes	15.6%
Sugar Frosted Flakes	29.0%

Cereal	Percent of Sugar
Sugar Pops	37.8%
Sugar Smacks	61.3%
Sugar Sparkled Corn Flakes	32.2%
Super Sugar Chex	24.5%
Super Orange Crisp	68.0%
Team	15.9%
Total	8.1%
Trix	46.6%
Uncle Sam Cereal	2.4%
Vanilla Crunch	45.8%
Wheat Chex	2.6%
Wheaties	4.7%

Source: American Society of Dentistry for Children

Sugar Content in Common Foods

Beverages   Sugar Content in Teaspoons

Cola Drinks — 6 oz.	3½
Orange-ade — 8 oz.	5
Root Beer — 10 oz.	4½
Kool-Aid — 8 oz.	6
Seven-Up — 6 oz.	3¾
Soda Pop — 8 oz.	5
Ginger Ale — 6 oz.	5
Chocolate Milk — 8 oz.	6
Eggnog — 8 oz.	8

Cakes and Cookies

Angel Food — 4 oz. piece	7
Applesauce Cake — 4 oz. piece	5½
Cheesecake — 4 oz. piece	2
Chocolate Cake — 4 oz. piece (plain)	6
Chocolate Cake — 4 oz. piece (iced)	10
Coffeecake — 4 oz. piece	4½
Cupcake (iced) — 1	6
Fruitcake — 2 oz. piece	2½
Pound Cake — 4 oz. piece	5
Brownies (plain) — 1	3
Chocolate Cookies — 1	1½
Fig Newtons — 1	5
Ginger Snaps — 1	3
Macaroons — 1	6
Oatmeal Cookies — 1	2
Chocolate Eclair — 1	7
Cream Puff — 1	2
Doughnut (plain) —1	3
Doughnut (glazed) — 1	6

Candy   Sugar Content in Teaspoons

Milk Chocolate Bar — 1½ oz.	7
Chewing Gum — 1 stick	½
Chocolate Cream — 1 piece	2
Butterscotch Chew — 1 piece	1
Chocolate Mint — 1 piece	2
Fudge — 1 oz. square	4½
Gum Drop — 1	2
Hard Candy — 4 oz.	20
Lifesaver — 1	½
Peanut Brittle — 1 oz.	3½
Marshmallow — 1	1½

Canned Fruit and Juices

Canned Fruit Juices — ½ cup sweetened	2
Canned Peaches 2 halves with syrup	3½
Canned Apricots 4 halves with syrup	3½
Stewed Fruits — ½ cup	2
Fruit Cocktail — ½ cup	5

Dairy Products

Ice Cream — 3½ oz.	3½
Ice Cream Bar — 1	1-7
Ice Cream Cone — 1	3½
Ice Cream Soda — 1	5
Ice Cream Sundae — 1	7
Malted Milkshake — 10 oz.	5

Desserts   Sugar Content in Teaspoons

Apple Cobbler — ½ cup	3
Custard — ½ cup	2
French Pastry — 4 oz. piece	5
Jello — ½ cup	4½
Apple Pie — 4 oz. piece	10

Jams, Jellies and Sauces

Apple Butter — 1 tbsp.	1
Jelly — 1 tbsp.	1½
Orange Marmalade — 1 tbsp.	1½
Strawberry Jam — 1 tbsp.	1½
Maple Syrup — 1 tbsp.	2½
Honey — 1 tbsp.	3
Chocolate Sauce — 1 tbsp.	4½

Source: Reprinted with permission from Dr. Kurt W. Donsbach, copyright 1975.

CHAPTER SIX

THE SECRET TO SUCCESS: TIMING

Figuring out what to do about eating healthfully was not the whole solution, I then had to make it work — I had to relearn how to eat.

I found it very discouraging to face so many negative areas — fat, cholesterol, sugar, salt, and total calories. I was concerned that in my enthusiasm and new found knowledge, I might attempt too much. The result could then resemble that of a fad diet: immediate success, long-term failure.

It seemed reasonable to start the Positive Diet slowly, establish a firm foundation, and then build gradually. Steady progress should be the name of the game. If it took me a year or two to make the changes permanent, that was all right. After all, whom was I racing against?

My decision was to initiate each of the basic principles individually. This approach allowed me to select one principle, practice it over a period of time, and make it a permanent part of my diet pattern. During that time I would not worry about the other basic principles. I had to feel comfortable with one before I was ready to go on to another. As the Chinese say, "A journey of a thousand miles starts with a single step."

A second decision was to adopt each of the basic principles in three distinct stages: the Planning State, the Practice Stage and the Refinement

Stage. Each of these stages represented a different level of achievement. During the Planning Stage, I familiarized myself with the basic principle involved and outlined a plan as to how to proceed. The Practice Stage, which signaled the start of the diet, was when the plan was implemented. It was the period during which the principle was put to work, the time in which the basic tools were implemented. The Practice Stage was extremely important because it led to permanent dietary change. Finally, the Refinement Stage was an opportunity to "fine tune" the use of the basic principle.

I began with the first basic principle, focusing on red meat as the starting point. In the Planning Stage, I decided to eat red meat at no more than three dinners and one lunch per week. As the Practice Stage began, I found that this plan was a dramatic change for me. But because I was concerned exclusively with red meat at this point, all of my efforts could be concentrated.

After a few weeks I began to feel comfortable with this adjustment. I continued to work with meal planning and creative substitution, and I became increasingly confident in my ability to accept the red meat reductions. Soon a month had passed, and I knew that eating less red meat could be accomplished without a problem. My diet pattern had fundamentally changed.

Since that time, I have been in the Refinement Stage, constantly attempting to reduce the frequency and the size of my red meat meals. It was only after reaching the Refinement Stage that some other aspect of the Positive Diet was attempted. This way I never felt rushed, harried or under stress, and the progress made, while slower than that of fad diets, was permanent. Once the change was accomplished, it was for good.

The time that an individual must spend in each of these stages will differ from person to person. No two people will find success on exactly the same schedule. The important thing to keep in mind is not the speed of the progress, but the continuance of it — not quick results, but permanent change.

THE FIRST BASIC PRINCIPLE: REDUCE ANIMAL FAT AND CHOLESTEROL

Planning and Practice Stages

▶Institute meal planning and creative substitution.
▶Learn to read labels.
▶Eliminate meats rich in saturated fat, such as sausage, bacon, hot dogs and luncheon meats.
▶Eliminate fatty processed foods, convenience foods and commercially baked goods.
▶Eliminate deep-fried foods.
▶Eliminate frying or sautéing in lard, bacon fat or margarine; use a non-stick pan or use broth, wine, vermouth, water, flavored vinegar or lemon juice.
▶Eliminate the use of animal fat and oil; instead, use olive oil or unsaturated liquid vegetable oil such as safflower, corn or soybean.
▶Eliminate stick margarine; use soft tub-style margarine made from safflower oil or corn oil.
▶Eliminate foods rich in cholesterol, such as organ meats.
▶Reduce red meat meals to 3 dinners and 1 lunch per week.
▶Use only extra-lean meat, trimmed of all visible fat; use more poultry, fish and vegetables.
▶Reduce whole eggs to 3 per week; use egg substitute.
▶Beware of fatty restaurant food, especially fast food and food with sauces.
▶Increase complex carbohydrates.

Refinement Stage

▶Reduce the portion size of red meat.
▶Reduce red meat meals to 2 dinners and 1 lunch per week.
▶Increase portion size of complex carbohydrates.

THE SECOND BASIC PRINCIPLE: REDUCE BUTTERFAT

Planning and Practice Stages

▶Eliminate whole milk and whole milk products; use skim milk and low-fat dairy products.
▶Eliminate butter; use soft tub-style margarine made from safflower oil or corn oil.
▶Eliminate convenience foods made with cream, butter or a butter sauce.
▶Eliminate frying or sautéing in butter; use a non-stick pan or use broth, wine, vermouth, water or flavored vinegar.
▶Beware of fatty restaurant food, especially food with cream sauces.

Refinement Stage

▶Reduce the portion size of all dairy products consumed.

THE THIRD BASIC PRINCIPLE: REDUCE SALT

Planning and Practice Stages

▶Remove the salt shaker from the table.
▶Reduce salt in cooking, first by ¼, later by ½.
▶Eliminate obviously salty foods, such as potato
  chips, salted peanuts, pickles, ham.
▶Eliminate foods with hidden salt, such as
  canned soups and vegetables, hot dogs, com-
  mercial salad dressings, certain cheese.
▶Beware of high-salt restaurant foods.

Refinement Stage

▶Reduce salt in cooking by ¾

THE FOURTH BASIC PRINCIPLE: REDUCE SUGAR

Planning and Practice Stages

▶Eliminate the use of table sugar.
▶Eliminate the use of soft drinks; drink fresh fruit juices, mineral water or tap water with a slice of fresh lemon or lime.
▶Eliminate high sugar foods, such as sugared cereal, hot chocolate mixes, commercial pastry and baked goods.
▶Eliminate candy and sugared snacks; use more fresh fruit.
▶Reduce alcohol consumption.
▶Reduce the amount of sugar used in homemade recipes by ⅓.
▶Beware of high-sugar restaurant food.

Refinement Stage

▶Further reduce the amount of sugar used in homemade recipes.

TIMING SEQUENCE CHART

WEEK	1	2	3	4	5	6	7	8	9	10	11	12	13	14	15	16	17	18	19	20	21	22	23	24	25	26	27	28	29	30
FAT CONTROL	□	□	▨	▨	▨	▨	■	■	■	■	■	■	■	■	■	■	■	■	■	■	■	■	■	■	■	■	■	■	■	■
BUTTERFAT CONTROL								□	▨	▨	▨	▨	■	■	■	■	■	■	■	■	■	■	■	■	■	■	■	■	■	■
SALT CONTROL													□	□	▨	▨	▨	▨	■	■	■	■	■	■	■	■	■	■	■	■
SUGAR CONTROL																			□	□	▨	▨	▨	▨	■	■	■	■	■	■

□ PLANNING STAGE ▨ PRACTICE STAGE ■ REFINEMENT STAGE

As a guide in the construction of a personal timing schedule, this chart outlines how I moved through the various stages of the Positive Diet.

CHAPTER SEVEN

WEIGHT CONTROL

The Duchess of Windsor once remarked that in America a person can be neither too rich nor too thin. Her statement, while perhaps not complimentary, is certainly a perceptive view of one of our most cherished national fantasies — to be thin. Everyone seems to be concerned about weight, but the irrefutable fact is that as a people, Americans are fat. That should be no surprise to anyone familiar with the American diet pattern of fatty meat and dairy products, sugar and alcohol. After all, when you eat too much, when you eat too often, when what you eat is too high in calories . . . you get fat! And that is what has happened to many Americans.

The United States is a victim of the disease of over-consumption. Although the decrease in energy needed in our present lifestyle has played a part in our national condition, most health professionals cite the American diet as the single most significant influence upon our national and individual corpulance.

A number of scientific studies have been concluded which have illustrated the magnititude of the overweight problem in America. In one such study, conducted by Dr. Ancel Keys, it was found that over 60% of American males in the 40-49 year age bracket are obese, meaning that they carry a greater-than-average body content of fat for their age, weight and sex. This compared with 30% in the Netherlands and Yugoslavia, 28% in Italy, 11% in Greece and just 2% in Japan.

But one does not have to rely exclusively on the data from such studies to draw conclusions about our overweight national condition. Just look around. The country has an abundance of double chins, rolls around the waist, and spreading buttocks. And the problem is not confined merely to middle-aged people, either. Pudgy children and porky adolescents can be found everywhere, a Big Mac in one hand and a double-scoop ice cream cone in the other. Rotundity has become a national characteristic. America — the land of the free and the brave . . . and the fat!

OBESITY IS A CARDIAC RISK FACTOR

Obesity is a condition in which a person carries excessive body fat. According to Dr. Covert Bailey, a specialist in this field, an adult male should carry no more than 15% of his total body weight as fat; an adult female, no more than 22%. Yet the averages for Americans are 23% for males and 32% for females.

Most people are concerned with being overweight due to social implications. They wish to be thinner for reasons of appearance, attractiveness and self-esteem. While these reasons are important and should not be minimized, clearly the most important reason for weight control is good health. In a series of tests spanning a number of years, insurance companies have found that the death rate from all causes increases as weight rises, and that this risk becomes substantial for people who weigh more than 30% above their ideal weight.

PERCENT OF MALES (40-49)
WHO ARE OVERWEIGHT

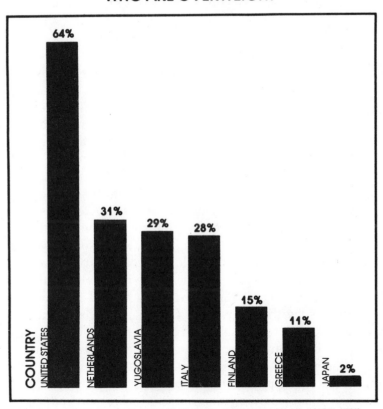

SOURCE: CORONARY HEART DISEASE IN SEVEN COUNTRIES BY DR. ANCEL KEYS

One of the most significant health problems with weight concerns the heart, for excessive body fat constitutes a cardiac risk factor. Every cell in the body must be supplied with nourishment and oxygen via the bloodstream on a continuous basis. It makes no difference if the cells are productive muscle tissue or deadweight fat; all cells must be served.

When excessive fat cells accumulate in the body, the circulatory system is required to develop miles of additional arteries and capillaries to move blood to these cells. As a result, the heart is forced to pump the blood over much greater distances, thereby increasing its own workload. This condition places a tremendous strain upon the heart and causes a notable drain on cardiac energy.

In addition, since the blood in a fat person must be pumped over greater distances, an increase in blood pressure is necessary to insure that the blood will reach the farthest point in the circulatory system. The combination of increased workload and elevated blood pressure can often decrease the blood supply to the heart. So, while the heart is compelled to work harder, it is forced to do so with less oxygen. The result can be a heart attack.

There are other reasons why obesity is a cardiac risk. A fat person is frequently prevented from participating in an exercise program which can burn calories, tone muscle tissue and reduce body fat. Such exercise is needed to condition the heart as a muscle. Recent research, not as yet definitive, has shown that excess ·fat cells may play an important role in the transportation of artery-blocking cholesterol and triglycerides in the blood stream. While there is still controversy in the scientific community over the lack of hard test data to prove that weight reduction can prevent cardiovascular disease, most physicians recommend weight reduction as a prudent measure for those concerned about cardiac health.

QUICK WEIGHT LOSS

The American desire to be thin, which borders on obsession with many people, has in recent years spawned a many-faceted, multi-million dollar industry dedicated to the immediate loss of weight. The "quick weight loss" industry — complete with its own clubs, diet books, diet foods, pills and sometimes gimmicks — is now represented in every American community. The industry is concered with one thing: immediate weight loss. For many people this approach has produced short-term success, but not permanent weight control.

Anyone who is able to drastically alter caloric intake by going on a diet can drop a few pounds in a short time; as long as the caloric intake remains low, weight will be lost. But as soon as the normal eating pattern is re-established by going off a diet, the increase in calories will cause the lost weight to reappear. Most people are susceptible to this cycle due to the high caloric makeup of the contemporary American diet. The "on again, off again" cycle has been the key to the growth of the quick weight loss industry. Their best customers return again and again and again. They do so because no fundamental change in their diet pattern has been made which would allow for permanent weight control.

A number of people with a sincere desire to permanently cut calories have looked to so-called "diet foods" for their salvation. But many diet foods are misleading and ineffective. According to the Food and Drug Administration's Bureau of Foods, if a food is to be classified as a diet product, its label must show how or why the food differs from the conventional product. It does *not* mean the diet food must contain fewer calories.

In a study conducted by *Consumer Digest*, it was reported that some diet products that contain sugar substitutes, such as sorbitol or fructose, contain approximately the same number of calories as their counterpart products made with refined sugar. According to the report, an Estee Dietetic cookie contains 50 calories and costs 4.75¢; an Oreo cookie also contains 50 calories but costs only 2.7¢. Featherweight low-calorie chicken noodle soup contains 60 calories per half cup and costs 8.2¢. Campbell's also contains 60 calories but costs only 3.3¢. In many instances "diet" foods cost more money, yet contain no fewer calories than conventional foods. Indeed, many of the so-called "lite" and "lean" boxed meals are over 50% fat.

The quick weight loss approach can never provide permanent weight control because it does not fundamentally change the diet pattern, and without such a change, short-term success eventually ends in long-term failure.

THE POSITIVE DIET APPROACH TO WEIGHT LOSS

While I understood that being overweight was a cardiac risk, I did not design the Positive Diet for weight control. Frankly, at the time the diet was first being developed, my hands were full with the identification and elimination of cholesterol, saturated fat, salt and sugar from my eating pattern. I did not have time for weight control. The last thing needed was to further complicate life by counting calories. My priority was to institute a way of eating which would decrease my blood fat level and consequently minimize the potential for life-threatening artery blockages to form.

However, after practicing the Positive Diet for a short period of time, an unexpected benefit occurred: I lost weight and kept it off. Without a conscious effort to diet for weight reduction, some fifteen pounds had disappeared. Hydrostatic weighing tests a year after surgery also indicated that my body fat content had concurrently been reduced to just over 15%. How did it happen? After all, there was nothing in the Positive Diet that called for twenty glasses of water a day, or three meals of grapefruit and coffee, or pills to dull the appetite. The Positive Diet was not a fad diet, yet permanent weight loss had been accomplished.

The answer is that the Positive Diet fundamentally and permanently changes eating habits. In the process it provides for weight loss and weight control in three ways:

1. Calorie Control
2. Portion Control
3. Attitude

Calorie Control

Gaining or losing weight is a consequence of the balance between calories consumed and calories used. When more calories are taken in than are burned up, weight gain occurs. It is the opposite for weight loss. This basic fact is rarely considered relevant in food selection on the American diet with the exception, of course, of those on a quick weight loss diet. Food is selected and consumed for reasons of taste, convenience or status.

Caloric value is not a factor. Consequently, the contemporary American diet is made up of foods not only rich in fat, cholesterol, sugar and salt, but which are also extremely high in calories.

The Positive Diet systematically removes or reduces the foods rich in fat, cholesterol, sugar and salt, and replaces them with foods which are more conducive to cardiac health. In the process the Positive Diet dictates a natural decrease in the total amount of calories consumed. Many of the fat-rich foods eliminated are high in calories, since fat contains 9 calories per gram compared to 4 per gram for protein and carbohydrates.

By replacing high-fat foods with low-fat foods, the caloric content of the meals decrease. Four ounces of sirloin steak contain 463 calories; the same amount of light meat chicken, a low-fat alternative, is only 206 calories. And four ounces of trout at 115 calories is lower still. A half cup of french fries has 228 calories; a medium baked potato has 92 calories. The switch from whole milk to skim milk saves 60 calories per cup. No-cholesterol egg substitute is 40 calories for ¼ cup (2.1 oz.); a large egg (1.8 oz.) is 81 calories.

The same relationship holds true when dealing with sugar-rich foods. These foods are calorically dense; they pack a lot of calories into a small amount of food. An average size piece of chocolate cake with icing represents 365 calories; a 4-ounce Mr. Goodbar contains 620 calories; 2 ounces of whiskey has 148 calories. A fresh apple by comparison has just 66 calories. A cup of strawberries has 55 calories. And a glass of mineral water has no calories.

By eliminating or reducing foods rich in refined sugar, salt, fat and cholesterol, the Positive Diet acts to reduce the amount of calories consumed naturally. And because it is a permanent way of eating, the weight lost stays off.

Portion Control

A side effect of the Positive Diet is to keep caloric intake down. By eating bulky, low-calorie complex carbohydrates — especially vegetables and whole grains — one can feel full before the higher-calorie foods are served.

Dinner, for example, is generally a problem because it is the main meal of the day. Most people are hungry, if not ravenous, by dinnertime. The problem is exaggerated by pre-dinner cocktails, which create a false hunger that is very difficult to control. The typical American dinner includes a small helping of salad and vegetable, and a large helping of the entrée — usually beef, pork or other red meat. Second helpings of the entrée are accepted as a matter of course. This pattern maximizes the high-fat portion of the meal (the entrée) and dictates a high caloric intake. And when portion control is exercised — no second helpings — often the hunger craving goes unsatisfied.

The Positive Diet reverses the position of the low-fat and high-fat foods. Salad, starch and vegetable portions become large, and the entrée portion, small. Second helpings are of the low-fat foods only. The result is that much of the hunger craving is satisfied by bulky, low-fat foods even before the entrée is served. Filling up on salad and vegetables can allow an 8-ounce serving of beef to be replaced by a 4-ounce serving. The difference in caloric intake over time with such a change is substantial. And because the foods recommended on the Positive Diet satisfy, smaller entrée portions become a permanent way of eating. When this happens, long-term weight control is the result.

Attitude

Attitude, the key to making the Positive Diet work, is one of the most important ingredients in a permanent weight control program. Too often a weight loss diet is started for less than significant reasons: to look good for the holidays or to fit into a new pair of jeans. Because these reasons are not truly substantial, an individual generally has little problem in rationalizing why he can go off the diet. And when he does, his efforts at weight control cease.

It is not so on the Positive Diet. In order for the diet to be effective, a real commitment to a new way of eating must be made. But unlike the weight loss diet, the commitment is made for a substantial reason: cardiac health. French fries, or a large helping of prime rib or a chocolate sundae are not passed up for the sake of appearance, but to increase the chances for a long and healthy life. Anyone who approaches the Positive Diet with this commitment has a good chance for success. The self discipline and the common sense used to control diet as a risk factor will also provide a means to weight loss and permanent weight control.

Weight Control Tips

There are certain actions which can be taken to enhance the opportunity for weight control on the Positive Diet.

▶Make a commitment to staying on the Positive Diet. Too often a healthy, weight reducing approach to eating is defeated not by the stomach but by the head.

▶Use meal planning for all regular meals. This will enable you to plan to avoid foods which are high in calories.

▶Eat balanced meals. Be sure to include fresh fruits and vegetables at every meal; they are low in calories and high in bulk and will keep you satisfied between meals.

▶Avoid second helpings. If you must have seconds, they should be of vegetables and fruits rather than of the entreé.

▶Watch out for hunger between meals. Often times it is a false hunger brought on by nervousness about the dietary change. Combat it with fresh raw vegetables. Keep a bowl of cut up vegetables on ice in the refrigerator for snacks. When hunger or nervousness moves you to eat between meals, vegetables can keep your jaws occupied.

▶Ban calorically dense foods from the house. Why tempt yourself with cookies, cakes and candy? For desserts, use fresh fruit.

▶Moderate the use of alcohol. Instead of pre-dinner cocktails and hors d'oeuvres, drink mineral water and munch on raw vegetables with pot cheese or tomato salsa. This provides the relaxation and satisfaction of the cocktail hour at only a fraction of the calories.

▶If you are counting calories closely, use a food scale to weigh your food. This will give you exact portions and maximum calorie control.

▶Beware of restaurant food, especially at the beginning of the diet. A single high-calorie meal can undo a week or more of successful weight reducing efforts.

CHAPTER EIGHT

HOW TO HANDLE EATING IN A RESTAURANT

Americans enjoy restaurants. Ethnic, gourmet, family style, fast food, deli . . . more people are eating out than ever before. In fact, according to the American Restaurant Association over 50% of all meals in the United States today are consumed in restaurants. And that figure is predicted to climb to 75% by the 1990's.

Pleasurable as the experience may be, dining out can pose a serious problem for cardiac health. Restaurant foods generally contain oil, butter, cream, lard, meat drippings, fatty meat, cheese, cheese sauce and other saturated fats in liberal amounts. In addition, many items are sautéed, fried, pan fried, or deep fried. As a result, restaurant meals can be extremely high in saturated fat, as well as in salt, sugar, cholesterol and total calories. Such meals are in direct opposition to healthful eating.

The alternatives available in this situation are few. A person can eat what the restaurant serves and suffer the health consequences; or he can avoid restaurants altogether and in doing so eliminate a pleasurable experience. Or he can apply the basic principles of the Positive Diet to menu selections in order to make intelligent and healthy food selections.

The first two alternatives are unrealistic and unacceptable in the long term. The third alternative — the use of a low-fat, low-cholesterol, low-salt, low-sugar criterion against which restaurant food must be measured — is the only way to reconcile dining out with eating right. When this alternative is exercised, dining in a restaurant can be both an enjoyable and a healthful experience.

How is this accomplished? By following three guidelines:

▶Have an understanding of the basic principles and be familiar with their application.

▶Be inquisitive. Ask questions at the restaurant about ingredients and methods of preparation. Know what you are ordering.

▶Be innovative. Use creative substitution to replace the unhealthy elements in restaurant foods with healthy ones.

Knowing the basic principles and how they apply to food selection is fundamental to success in restaurant dining. This comes, of course, with the practice of the Positive Diet at home. Often I will recommend to a person just beginning the Positive Diet that he should stay away from restaurants until he feels comfortable with the diet. This gives him time to concentrate his total effort on understanding and practicing the diet at home and allows him to make the principles for healthful eating a permanent fixture in his life. When that occurs, he is in a better position to handle restaurant menus. But regardless of whether or not this course is taken, a person needs to be totally familiar with the Positive Diet before he can apply its precepts to restaurant food.

The second guideline is to be inquisitive. Find out what the restaurant offers and how the food is prepared. Ask questions of the personnel. It does no good to understand the low-fat principle, for example, if you cannot put it into effect in a restaurant. And you cannot put it into effect if you do not ask questions.

I remember an early visit to a restaurant which was made soon after the start of the Positive Diet. Being conscious of the fat content of marbled red meat, I avoided the prime rib, the sirloin steak, and the spareribs in favor of a broiled salmon filet. But when the fish arrived, it was swimming in a fat-laden buttersauce. And the same sauce covered the vegetables and the rice. I hadn't reduced fat consumption by one whit! This discouraging episode took place because I did not question the preparation of the food before ordering. Had I realized that buttersauce came "automatically," I could have avoided the problem by asking that the sauce be held.

The same key questions which are posed by the Positive Diet at home must be asked in restaurants: is the dish made with butter, oil, cream, or animal fat? Is it fried or deep-fat fried? Is the dressing made with cream? Are large quantities of salt or sugar added to the food in the cooking process? The practice of the Positive Diet at home can provide you with these and other logical questions. Often restaurant personnel are very knowledgable about food content and cooking methods, and can be helpful in the attainment of dietary goals. But they cannot help if you do not ask questions and tell them what you want.

Finally, be innovative. The basic principles will tell you what is not acceptable fare. Even a neophyte practitioner of the Positive Diet knows enough to avoid foods such as fried hamburgers, fried chicken, French fries and milkshakes; salami sandwiches, pickles and potato chips; fried eggs, bacon, fried potatoes and toast with butter; fatty spareribs, sour cream as a condiment for baked potatoes, Thousand Island dressing and cheesecake. Such foods are to be avoided in res-

173

taurants, just as they are to be avoided at home.

Often creative substitution can be used on a restaurant menu to strip away the unhealthy elements, yet preserve much of the taste and the semblance of the dish. Order a club sandwich, for example, without the bacon. Skip cream soups in favor of beef or chicken broth. Then ask the waiter for fresh mushrooms, spinach, pasta or a slice of tomato to add to the soup. Instead of sour cream on a baked potato, ask for salsa. Instead of butter on steamed clams or lobster tails, ask for fresh lemon wedges. If you're out for breakfast and must eat eggs, order them poached, boiled or shirred, but never fried. Or have Eggs Benedict — without the hollandaise sauce.

There are many enjoyable restaurant foods which conform to the Positive Diet. Do not take a "doom and gloom" approach, but rather open your mind to the endless possibilities available. If your attitude is positive, and if you are mentally and emotionally committed to making the Positive Diet work, then neither the menu choices offered nor the food selection of others will negatively affect your decision to eat healthfully.

Tips for Ordering in a Restaurant

Appetizers: Avoid those made with saturated oil, butter and cheese, or those which are pickled or salted. Acceptable choices are oysters (raw, baked or steamed); steamed mussels; clam, crab, oyster and lobster cocktails; seviche; steamed or raw vegetables, such as fresh artichokes with lemon juice or salsa or a vegetable antipasto.

Soups: Skip the cream and meat soups. Order gazpacho, oxtail soup, consomme, beef or chicken broth.

Entrees: Avoid fatty meat, deep-fried fish and foods containing sauces and gravies. Acceptable choices include broiled or poached fish, such as salmon, halibut, cod or trout; shellfish, such as clams, crab, lobster, oysters and scallops; baked, roasted or broiled chicken; roasted turkey; broiled veal. On occasion, broiled lean red meat, such as rack of lamb or New York steak are acceptable.

Vegetables: Avoid pickled vegetables or those prepared with butter, cream or cheese sauces. Order fresh vegetables, such as asparagus, broccoli or mushrooms, either raw or slightly steamed. Baked or mashed potatoes, rice and pasta are acceptable but beware of butter, sour cream and bacon bits.

Breads: Avoid commercial bakery products made with butter, shortening and sugar, as well as salted items, such as crackers, saltines and pretzels. Acceptable choices include plain breadsticks, hard rolls, rye crisp, melba toast, sourdough rolls, bagels and English muffins.

Salads: Many savory salads are available with lettuce, spinach, romaine, green peppers, waterchestnuts, mushrooms, tomatoes, onions and sprouts. Use oil and vinegar (make sure that the oil is not palm or coconut), fresh lemon and pepper, or plain vinegar dressing. Avoid creamy dressing such as sour cream, Thousand Island and Blue Cheese. Avoid salads with strips of meat and cheese. A good innovation is to order a chef's salad without the ham; specify that the cheese be low-fat (mozzarella, for example) and that the dressing be oil and vinegar and served on the side. There are many appetizing salads made with

175

chicken, tuna, turkey, and crab. With a little picking and choosing, these can be heart-healthy fare. For innovation, order a Salad Niçoise and omit the anchovies or pickled vegetables. Fruit salads offer a wide range of possibilities. No matter what the season, fresh fruit is always available.

Sandwiches: Avoid fatty processed meats, hard cheese, fried foods, and foods with sauces and gravies. Order sandwiches made with tuna, sliced chicken or turkey (white meat), crab, lobster or vegetables. Be conscious of the mayonnaise. Any cheese should be low-fat. Innovate by ordering a bacon, lettuce and tomato sandwich without the bacon; or crab on an English muffin with a low-fat cheese, such as mozzarella; or a French Dip without the dip. Use different breads — Armenian, rye, French, sourdough, whole wheat — to provide variety.

Desserts: Avoid commercial pastries, pies, cakes and candy. Fresh fruit, gelatin, sherbert, sorbet, ices and unfrosted angel food cake are good alternatives to high calorie desserts. Occassionally, a piece of carrot cake without the frosting is acceptable.

Breakfasts: Avoid fatty meats, whole eggs, fried foods and sugared cereals. Maximize the use of fresh fruit. If you must eat eggs, do it only occasionally, and order them poached, boiled or shirred, but never fried. If you must eat breakfast meats, Canadian bacon or a small broiled steak are better than regular bacon, sausage or ham. For innovation, try Eggs Benedict without the hollandaise sauce or bagels without the cream cheese. Even an omelet can be acceptable if cooked in a non-stick pan or an unsaturated oil.

Beverages: Avoid drinks rich in sugar, alcohol or salt. Acceptable choices include fruit juice, mineral water, herbed tea, decaffeinated coffee or skim milk. Drink wine in moderation. For innovation, make your second drink a Virgin Mary or a glass of mineral water with a slice of lime.

Remember, you can eat better and with more control at home. But when you do dine out, you can eat as healthfully as possible by using the Positive Diet as your guide.

COOKBOOK

CHAPTER NINE

COMMENTS FROM THE COOK

by Bernie Piscatella

Learning to cope with the Positive Diet has been no small challenge. After open-heart surgery, Joe had a list of foods which he was to avoid: bacon, sausage, hot dogs, shrimp, spareribs, luncheon meats, eggs, avocados, olives, whole milk, cheese made from whole milk and cream, sweet cream, sour cream, ice cream, chocolate, butter, lard, hydrogenated margarine, hydrogenated vegetable shortening, hydrogenated peanut butter, most frozen dinners, commercial baked goods, French fries, crackers, most sauces and gravies, fast foods, such as hamburgers, fish, chicken, tacos, and pizza. In addition red meat was to be limited to 5 meals per week; out of a total of 21 meals that, in itself, was to be quite a switch! The forbidden list seemed to contain most of the best tasting foods on the market and all the foods that we most enjoyed eating. If we couldn't eat these foods, what was left?

The list of forbidden foods did not offer much help in finding replacements. Meal preparation was further complicated because our new way of eating affected not only the adults in our family (who could understand the grave necessity for the change), but also our young children. They were likely to go on a hunger strike if I began substituting carrot sticks for French fries and poached fish for Big Macs. I was also concerned that our friends might dread a dinner invitation to our house for fear of being served a Third World diet.

As a result, those were difficult months for the entire family and many of the meals turned out to be real disasters. But it was also during those months that I made a commitment to somehow master such a diet. I became determined to discover foods and create meals which not only would be heart-healthy, but appetizing and appealing to our entire family and to our guests as well.

Not until Joe's research made clear the risks posed by eating unhealthy foods — the risks to everyone in our family, not just Joe — did I really accept the Positive Diet. Then I could understand why certain foods are acceptable while others must be avoided.

This understanding was instrumental in developing more realistic and appetizing meals. I learned to take a familiar recipe which I had used for years, analyze it, and identify the "good" and the "bad" ingredients. I could then substitute good heart-healthy ingredients for the bad, not-so heart-healthy ingredients. If a recipe called for sour cream, for example, I would substitute nonfat yogurt. If it called for eggs, I would use egg substitute. It took some months of experimentation, failure, and a lot of adjustment, to develop the Positive Diet. But ultimately a low-fat, low-cholesterol, low-salt and low-sugar program developed, including specific meal plans, menus and recipes. Today the Positive Diet is an integral part of our lifestyle.

Undertaking the Positive Diet is a lifestyle change, and no lifestyle change is easily accomplished. But we have done it, and so have others. It is possible for you to master it too.

Remember, it is a long range plan. If you blow it on one day, don't be discouraged. Simply vow to start over again the next day. The important thing is to make steady progress. Work the problems one day at a time.

Take some time to read and to understand the basic principles. Until I understood what a high-fat diet did to the heart, as well as to the whole body, I felt no real motivation to change our diet pattern. I went through the motions, but I feared that our new way of cooking and eating would be short-lived and that we might eventually revert to our old familiar ways. Once I understood the basic principles, however, I knew that there was no turning back. It was only then that I was able to face the challenge of creative and healthful cooking.

Understand the value of meal planning; it is essential to the successful practice of the diet. Without taking time to plan meals in advance, I often became frustrated and the meals were disasters. Either the Positive Diet meal would not turn out or I would get in a hurry and then serve a familiar, but not so healthful meal.

Because I did not take the time to plan what to serve sometimes until the last minute, I would find myself grocery shopping just before the dinner hour. I knew I should not serve food that wasn't good for our cardiac health, but I would be caught short, unable to recall what to serve for a heart-healthy meal.

At the start of the Positive Diet, meal planning was an invaluable tool. It provided the time and forethought necessary to implement a dietary change. Now this way of cooking and eating has become second nature and it is easy and natural to prepare meals and even to grocery shop at the last minute without pre-planning.

183

Understand the role of substitutions. It is unrealistic to totally discard the old ways of cooking and eating; rather, it is better to remove the unhealthy ingredients and replace them with healthful ones. Then, you have the best of both worlds. There is a list of substitutions in this book. Take time to study it.

Learn to read labels. The information contained on the food label is the key to knowing what is contained in the food. The food processor is required by law to list all of the ingredients on the label in descending order by weight. Thus, if a chocolate drink mix lists its ingredients as sugar, cocoa, lecithin, salt, and artificial flavors, you can be sure that sugar is the main ingredient in the food.

The label also lists the serving size in cups or ounces, the number of servings in the container, the number of calories, and the amount of protein, fat and carbohydrates in each serving. When reading labels, it is important to identify the amount of fat, the amount of unsaturated fat versus the amount of saturated fat, and whether or not sugar or salt is a main ingredient. If fat, sugar or salt is a primary ingredient, do not buy the product. If there is saturated fat, avoid the product or at least be sure the amount of unsaturated fat is no less than twice that of saturated fat. Since food processors may change the make-up of their products, it is important to continually check food labels.

Learn to calculate the percentage of fat in the food. The label will identify the total calories and the amount of fat in grams. Each gram of fat equals 9 calories. Multiplying the number of grams of fat by 9 will provide you with the calories provided by fat in the food. Then divide the fat calories by the total calories to arrive at the percentage of calories from fat. This calculation will tell you if the food is high-fat or low-fat. As an example, if a product contains 100 calories and 8 grams of fat, the 8 grams represent 72 calories of fat (8 x 9). Divide this figure (72) by the total calories (100), and the result illustrates that 72% of the calories come from fat. That food could certainly be classified as high-fat. If, however, the food contained only 2 grams of fat, then it would contain only 18 calories of fat (2 x 9) or 18% of the total calories. Any food that is less than 20% fat can be considered low-fat.

Learn the difference between saturated and unsaturated fats and oils. Remember that saturated fats and hydrogenated oils tend to elevate blood cholesterol levels. Many processed foods, commercially baked goods and fast foods contain either saturated fats or hydrogenated oils, sometimes both.

A quick way of distinguishing between saturated (harmful) and unsaturated (not harmful) fats and oils is that the saturated fats, such as butter, lard, suet, bacon, salt pork, chicken fat, meat fat, hydrogenated margarine, hydrogenated shortening, hydrogenated vegetable oil, vegetable shortening, palm oil and coconut oil, will harden at refrigerator temperature. Polyunsaturated oils, such as safflower oil, soybean oil, sunflower oil, corn oil, cottonseed oil and sesame oil will remain in a liquid state. Of these oils, safflower is the most highly recommended for Positive Diet purposes because it is the most unsaturated, followed in order by soybean, sunflower, corn, cottonseed and sesame.

As a word of caution, a label that simply lists "vegetable oil" as an ingredient (and does not specify which vegetable oil) should not be purchased because coconut oil and palm oil, which are saturated and must be avoided, are also vegetable oils. Coconut oil and palm oil are used frequently by food processors in place of the other vegetable oils because they can be imported and processed more cheaply than can our native oils. Beware of them in crackers, bakery products, convenience foods and non-dairy creamers.

Besides the saturated and unsaturated fats, there are monounsaturated fats. Olive oil is the primary monounsaturated fat (peanut oil is also monounsaturated). Recent studies have shown that olive oil helps to reduce LDL cholesterol without reducing HDL cholesterol. This may be why Mediterranean people such as Italians and Greeks have relatively little coronary heart disease. Many health professionals have designated olive oil as the oil of choice on a healthy diet.

Another term to be aware of is "hydrogenated." Hydrogenation is a process used in processing food whereby an unsaturated oil becomes hardened or hydrogenated and, thus, saturated. An example of hydrogenation can be seen in stick margarine: if it were not hydrogenated, it would not be hard. For this reason, even stick margarine made with an unsaturated oil, such as corn oil, should be avoided.

When it is necessary to use stick margarine, look for one that lists the first ingredient on the label as "liquid oil," as in "liquid safflower oil." The second ingredient listed may be a partially hydrogenated oil, such as "partially hydrogenated soybean oil or cottonseed oil." If the partially hydrogenated oil is listed first, however, the product should not be used.

Whenever possible, choose tub-style safflower margarine, because safflower oil is the most unsaturated of the unsaturated oils. Tub-style margarine is not required to hold its shape and therefore does not have to be hardened or hydrogenated.

Another product where hydrogenation takes place is in pre-stirred hydrogenated peanut butter. Always buy the old fashioned, non-hydrogenated variety where the oil is at the top and must be stirred into the peanut butter. For convenience, store the peanut butter upside down for a few hours or overnight before opening. Very little stirring will be necessary.

When buying mayonnaise always choose one made from an unsaturated vegetable oil, such as safflower oil, soybean oil, sunflower oil or corn oil. Safflower oil, once again, is the most highly recommended. For a delightful taste sensation, try making your own safflower mayonnaise.

Canned soups are often high in saturated fat, as well as sodium. Try to avoid them. Homemade soups are more heart-healthy and more flavorful than the commercial variety. Homemade chicken broth and beef broth should be prepared the day before serving. This allows time to chill the soup in order to remove the congealed fat which will rise to the top.

Many Positive Diet meals are prepared with broths. For greatest convenience, try to keep homemade de-fatted chicken and beef broth on hand in the freezer. Freeze some in ice cube trays; when frozen, remove them from trays to plastic freezer bags. The cubes are a perfect size for sautéing vegetables. Freeze the remainder of the broth in half-pint, pint and quart containers. If you run short, buy a good grade of commercial broth, refrigerate it overnight or place in the freezer for 30 minutes. The fat will congeal and rise to the top, and can then be skimmed. Be certain to reduce the salt in the recipe you are following to compensate for the saltiness of the commercial broth.

Avoid making gravy from fat-laden meat

drippings, which are high in saturated fat. To make lean gravy, place the meat drippings in a bowl, add several ice cubes, and place in the freezer for 15-20 minutes. The fat will congeal around the ice cubes; the fat and the ice cubes can be discarded, and the defatted drippings can then be used in the gravy. A good gravy can be made without meat drippings simply by thickening defatted beef or chicken broth with a little flour, arrowroot or grated raw potato.

Never fry in butter, hydrogenated margarine or meat fat. Many dishes, such as pancakes, French toast or omelets may be cooked in a teflon pan without any liquid or oil added. If a recipe does call for cooking in oil or fat, (for example, sautéing vegetables), use wine, vermouth, broth, lemon juice, water or flavored vinegars.

Always buy tuna fish that is packed in water and preferably one that is salt free. Tuna packed in oil is high in fat and sodium. If it is necessary to use oil-packed tuna, it should be drained and rinsed before using.

Avoid pre-mixed, dehydrated, frozen and packaged convenience foods as these often contain saturated fat. Frozen dinners and ready to eat foods, such as pork and beans and chili, are generally undesirable as they often do not identify the kind of fat used in processing. If the fat is not specifically identified, do not use the food.

Milk chocolate, although made from a vegetable oil, contains fatty acids which are highly saturated and, as such, must be avoided. In preparing recipes calling for baking chocolate, substitute 3 tablespoons of unsweetened cocoa powder plus 1 tablespoon of safflower oil for each ounce of baking chocolate. Cocoa powder does not contain saturated fat and is acceptable on the Positive Diet. It should be used only sparingly, however, because of the sugar and the extra calories often found in chocolate desserts. Instant cocoa mixes do not contain saturated fat, but do contain sugar. As such, their use should be limited.

Buy only the leanest red meats. Remember that grass fed beef, usually classified less than prime, is leaner and contains less fat than grain fed beef. Before cooking red meat, trim all visible fat. Red meat contains a great deal of internal fat which is not visible to the eye; this fat is more than sufficient to lubricate the meat.

Broiling, roasting, baking, barbecuing and stewing are the preferred cooking methods for purposes of the Positive Diet. In recipes where meat needs to be browned, use a teflon pan or use wine, vermouth, chicken broth or beef broth as a substitute for oil. When roasting, place the meat on a rack in a roasting pan to allow the fat to drip away during cooking. The use of low temperatures (about 350°) will increase the fat drip off. High temperatures will sear the meat, sealing in the fat. Broiling also allows meat fat to drip away. Baking is ideal for less fatty meats as it helps to retain moisture. Always cook meats to at least medium, or preferably to well-done, to allow the maximum amount of grease to drip away.

Try to gradually reduce total red meat meals to no more than three per week, including breakfast, lunch and dinner. Make more use of chicken, turkey, veal and fish. Avoid high fat meat items, such as spareribs, hot dogs, sausages, bacon, luncheon meats, variety meats and organ meats. Avoid canned, cured, pickled or smoked meats which are high in fat, as well as sodium.

Get to know your local butcher. It took some searching, but we found a local butcher who not only helps us in our low-fat selection, but also makes special orders of low-fat sausage, bratwurst and knockwurst, using extra lean meats, no salt and no preservatives.

Poultry, except for duck and goose, is lower in fat than is red meat and so is more desirable. Since much of the fat in poultry is concentrated just below the skin, the removal of the skin before cooking takes away most of the fat. The fat that does remain can drip away during cooking. Steamed or poached chicken may be substituted for ground round in dishes such as chili, tacos, taco salad and lasagne. Turkey breasts are available in most food stores; quick and easy to cook, they provide great dinners as well as terrific sandwiches. Often you can buy a whole turkey on sale, have a turkey dinner, freeze some of the leftover meat in sandwich-size portions and then make turkey soup from the carcass.

Increase fish in the diet to at least 7½ ounces a week. Research indicates that this level provides cardiac benefits. Fatty fish such as salmon, tuna and lake trout are excellent as they are rich in Omega-3's. Be sure to bake, steam, barbecue and broil fish; never fry or deep-fat fry. Add fresh lemon instead of butter and tartar sauce. Once regarded as too high in cholesterol, shellfish are now included in a heart-healthy diet because of their beneficial oil.

Whole eggs should be limited to 3 per week, including the whole eggs used in cooking foods, such as cakes, pancakes, mayonnaise and sauces. Egg whites can be used without restriction, as can egg substitute. Egg substitute allows egg dishes such as omelets, huevos rancheros, pancakes, waffles and French toast to be prepared without the disadvantage of high cholesterol. Commercial egg substitutes are available in the frozen-food section of the supermarket. Try to keep some on hand; they do contain preservatives, however, so when time allows, it is preferable to make home-made, which is simple and can also be frozen.

Use skim milk fortified with vitamins A and D. Whole milk and buttermilk made from whole milk as well as the so called "low-fat" 1% and 2% milk all contain too much butterfat and should be avoided. If a recipe calls for 1 cup of whole milk, ¼ cup of nonfat milk powder and 2 tablespoons of safflower oil added to 1 cup of skim milk will produce the same result. If a recipe calls for butter-milk, a low-fat version may be made by heating 1 cup of skim milk to room temperature, adding 1 tablespoon of lemon juice, waiting 5 minutes and beating well. In recipes calling for evaporated milk, use low-fat evaporated milk or fortify 1 cup of skim milk with ⅓ cup of nonfat milk powder. An acceptable whipped cream substitute may be made by beating together ⅓ cup ice water, 1¼ teaspoons lemon juice, ⅓ cup nonfat milk pow-der, 2 tablespoons sugar and ½ teaspoon of va-nilla.

Avoid cheese made from whole milk or cream. In place of creamed cottage cheese, use uncreamed cottage cheese or rinse creamed cot-tage cheese until the water runs clear. A nonfat Ricotta cheese may be made by scalding 4 cups of skim milk, removing it from the heat, stirring in 2 tablespoons of fresh lemon juice, letting it stand 15 minutes, and straining the excess liquid. Many types of cheese are now available in the supermar-ket in low-fat form. Some to look for are low-fat Cheddar, Monterey Jack, Swiss, Danboe, Somer-set and Mozzarella. The specific fat content of low-fat cheese will vary according to brand. If the content is not listed on the label, ask the dairy-man. Unless the cheese is fat-free or less than 20% fat, use it judiciously. Check with the dairyman at regular intervals, as new types of low-fat cheese are becoming more readily available.

Avoid commercially prepared bakery products, such as biscuits, muffins, sweet rolls, cakes, crackers, egg bread, cheese bread and butter rolls. Try to find breads made with a minimum of saturated fat. Label reading is important, as many breads contain lard or hydrogenated shortening as well as sugar and large amounts of salt. It takes some searching, but you can find French breads, rolls, bagels, English muffins, Armenian pocket breads, rye breads, pumpernickels, enriched whites, and whole wheat breads on the market that do not contain lard or hydrogenated shortening. In addition, crackers such as Rye Crisp, Finn Crisp, Matze-Thins, WASA, Scandinavian Flat Bread, and Cracker Bread conform to the Positive Diet.

Many health food stores carry unsalted potato chips and unsalted taco chips that are baked, not fried, using safflower oil. Tortillas are also a good alternative to bread. Always use corn tortillas, as flour tortillas are made with lard. Don't miss the experience of baking your own bread. With the recipes in this book, this is a simple operation and the results are well worth the effort. Moreover, homemade breads can be frozen for future use.

Avoid sugared and coconut cereals. There are some excellent whole grain cooked or dry cereals on the market. Just be certain to read labels so as to select only those containing acceptable Positive Diet ingredients.

Avoid pasta made from whole eggs. When purchasing pasta look for the words *durum* or *granoduro* in the list of ingredients. Durum is the kernel or core of the durum wheat whose outer shell produces semolina flour. It is 100% protein. Pasta is called the "energy food" because it contains important vitamins and minerals, such as thiamine, riboflavin, niacin and iron, plus 8 amino acids, and it is also low in sodium. Always buy a good brand of pasta; a pasta dish, no matter how good the sauce, is only as good as the pasta itself. Sample the many varieties and shapes available, and for a change of pace try the buckwheat (soba) noodles available in Oriental markets and in Oriental sections of the supermarket.

Avoid prepared rice mixes and rice made with heavy sauces. Japanese New Variety Rice, available in Oriental markets and in Oriental sections of the supermarket, and brown long grain rice as well as wild rice are healthy alternatives. And be sure to try barley and the wide variety of dried beans and lentils available.

All fresh vegetables, except olives and avocados, are acceptable on the Positive Diet; for best dollar value, choose from those that are in season. Read the labels of canned or frozen vegetables to insure that they do not have added salt. Avoid those that are packaged in creamy sauces. A vegetable steamer or microwave oven should be used in cooking so that vegetables do not lose as many nutrients and minerals as they do when cooked in water. Another healthful cooking method is stir-frying in a small amount of broth, wine, flavored vinegar or lemon juice. It is important not to over-cook vegetables; they are at their best when on the crisp side.

All fresh fruits are acceptable on the Positive Diet. Whenever possible, use fresh fruit. When buying canned fruit, read the label to make certain it is packed in its own juice and does not contain added sugar. For maximum freshness and sugar control, can your own fruit in a waterpack or very light syrup. And freeze some fruits and berries for out-of-season eating and for garnishes.

Learn to reduce salt in cooking. A relatively

painless way to accomplish this is to reduce in 4-month intervals. When you begin the Positive Diet, reduce the salt in every recipe by ¼; if a recipe calls for 1 teaspoon of salt, use only ¾ teaspoon. After 4 months reduce the salt again by ¼; if a recipe calls for 1 teaspoon of salt, use only ½ teaspoon. Then, after 4 more months reduce the salt by ¾; if a recipe calls for 1 teaspoon of salt, use only ¼ teaspoon. When preparing a recipe, whenever possible, add the salt last and always taste the preparation first to see if the salt is necessary. When purchasing processed foods, such as tomato sauce and tomato paste, look for brands with no salt added. When this is not possible, further reduce the salt used in cooking in order to compensate. Learn to use herbs and spices to flavor a recipe, rather than salt. In addition, be sure always to leave the salt shaker off the table.

Learn to reduce sugar intake. In most recipes, the sugar may be reduced by ⅓ with no noticeable difference. Desserts made with sugar or honey should be prepared only for very special occasions. Remember, the premier natural snack or dessert is fresh fruit.

And, finally, learn to persevere. If you have coronary heart disease (or have a high risk to develop it) and you must change your diet pattern, do not bemoan your fate or adapt a "woe is me" attitude. Learn to live with the disease. Learn to make a new way of eating a permanent part of your lifestyle. Thomas Edison once remarked that genius is 10% inspiration and 90% perspiration. It is the same when making permanent dietary change. The work is hard, especially at the beginning, but it does become progressively easier. And the effort is worthwhile, for the stakes are the longevity and quality of life.

GUIDE TO BASIC FOODS

Recommended	Not Recommended
chicken	duck
turkey	goose
veal	spareribs
fish	mutton
most shellfish	sausage
rabbit	bacon
venison	frankfurters
beef*	luncheon meats
lamb*	heavily marbled meats
pork*	fatty meats
ham*	shrimp
	lox
lima beans	kidney
lentils	liver
chick peas	heart
split peas	sweetbreads
egg whites	egg yolks
egg substitute	(limit to 3 per week)
fortified skim milk	whole milk
fortified skim milk powder	1% milk
non-fat buttermilk	2% milk
evaporated skim milk	evaporated milk
non-fat yogurt	egg nog
non-fat ice cream	chocolate whole milk
	whole milk yogurt
	2% low-fat yogurt
	whole milk buttermilk
	ice cream
	cream
	half & half
	sour cream
	whipped cream
	non-dairy cream substitute

*occasional use only

Recommended	Not Recommended
cheese made from skim or partially skim milk, if lower than 20% fat	cream cheese
	cheese spreads
	creamed cottage cheese
some to look for	whole milk cheese or cheese made with cream
include:	*some to look for*
	include:
Framer's	
Baker's	
Hoop	Swiss
Sapsago	Brie
Dry Cottage Cheese	Camembert
Pot	most Jack
low-fat Danboe	most Cheddar
low-fat Somerset	Roquefort
low-fat Mozzarella	Blue Cheese
low-fat Cheddar	
most vegetables	olives
	avocados
	pickles
	sauerkraut
	all brined vegetables
	all pickled vegetables
most fresh fruits	fruits canned in heavy syrup
safflower oil	coconut oil
soybean oil	palm oil
sunflower oil	hydrogenated vegetable shortening
corn oil	
cottonseed oil	lard
sesame oil	suet
olive oil	chicken fat
peanut oil	pork fat
tub-style safflower oil margarine	meat fat
	cube margarine
safflower oil mayonnaise	butter

Recommended	Not Recommended
non-hydrogenated peanut butter	hydrogenated peanut butter
cocoa powder	coconut
	milk chocolate
	baker's chocolate
bagels	sweet rolls
English muffins	biscuits
Italian bread	doughnuts
French bread	cheese bread
pumpernickel	egg bread
rye bread	flour tortillas
whole wheat bread	(made with lard)
Armenian pocket bread	
Finn Crisp	most crackers
Matze Thins	
WASA	
Scandinavian Flat Breads	
Rye Crisp	
Cracker Bread	
whole grain cereals	sugared cereals
brown rice	coconut cereals
New Variety Rice	prepared rice mixes
barley	
bulgur	
durum or granoduro pasta	egg noodles
angel food cake	packaged cake mixes
most unsalted nuts	commercially baked goods
unsalted, potato or corn chips, baked in safflower oil	most potato and corn chips
	Macadamia nuts
	cashews

TABLE OF SUBSTITUTIONS

Rather Than	Substitute
Whole Egg	Beat together 1 egg white, 2 teaspoons nonfat milk powder, and 2 teaspoons safflower oil *or use* 2 egg whites *or use* commercially prepared egg substitute.
Whole Milk (1 cup)	Fortify 1 cup skim milk with 1 cup nonfat dry milk powder *or combine* 1 cup skim milk plus 2 tablespoons safflower oil.
Evaporated Milk	Lowfat or skim evaporated milk
Buttermilk (1 cup)	Heat 1 cup skim milk to room temperature; add 1 tablespoon lemon juice. Let stand 5 minutes; beat *or make* homemade using a cultured food processor.
Whipped Cream	Combine ⅓ cup ice water, 1 tablespoon lemon juice, ¾ teaspoon vanilla, and ⅓ cup nonfat dry milk powder. Beat 10 minutes or until stiff; add 2 tablespoons sugar.

Whole Milk Yogurt	Prepare homemade nonfat yogurt using an inexpensive yogurt maker or cultured food processor.
Sour Cream	Plain nonfat yogurt *or prepare* lowfat sour cream using a cultured food processor.
Ice Cream	Prepare lowfat using an ice cream freezer.
Whole Milk Cheese	Lowfat cheese — ask your dairyman to verify percentage of fat.
Parmesan Cheese Romano Cheese	Sapsago Cheese, grated *or for a milder flavor* Somerset, Mozzarella or Danboe.
Butter Margarine Shortening	Use tub style safflower margarine *or use* safflower oil.

Proportion	*Proportion safflower oil*
1 tablespoon	1 tablespoon
2 tablespoons	1½ tablespoons
⅓ cup	4 tablespoons
½ cup	6 tablespoons
¾ cup	9 tablespoons

Hydrogenated Peanut Butter	Nonhydrogenated, old-fashioned style peanut butter
Mayonnaise	Homemade safflower mayonnaise *or* Commercially made safflower mayonnaise
Cream Soup	Homemade cream soup *or* thicken homemade chicken or beef broth with flour, arrowroot or grated raw potato.
Chicken Broth Beef Broth	Homemade de-fatted, low sodium broth
Bouillon Cube (1 cube)	1 cup homemade chicken or beef broth — reduce liquid in recipe requiring bouillon cube to compensate.
Bacon Bacon Bits	Canadian Style Bacon (for occasional use only)
Baking Chocolate Baking Chocolate (1 oz. square)	3 tablespoons cocoa powder plus 1 tablespoon safflower oil

SKIM MILK

1½   cups nonfat milk powder
3¾   cups water

Combine milk powder and water in a covered container; shake vigorously.

Note: Always buy milk powder that is fortified with vitamins A and D.
For a creamier flavor increase milk powder by ⅓ cup.

EGG SUBSTITUTE

1   egg white
2¼   teaspoons nonfat milk powder
2   teaspoons safflower oil

Combine ingredients in a blender; whirl.
Yield is the equivalent of 1 egg.

Note: Egg substitute keeps 1 week in the refrigerator and may be frozen. Recipe may be multiplied.

WHIPPED CREAM SUBSTITUTE

⅓ cup ice water
1¼ teaspoons lemon juice
½ teaspoon vanilla
⅓ cup nonfat dry milk powder
2 tablespoons sugar

Combine water, lemon juice and vanilla; stir in nonfat dry milk powder. Beat 5-10 minutes or until stiff; add sugar. Beat 1-2 minutes.

Note: If topping should separate, beat again just before serving.

PLAIN NONFAT YOGURT

1 quart skim milk
⅓ cup nonfat milk powder
1 heaping tablespoon plain lowfat or
    nonfat yogurt

Combine skim milk and dry milk powder in a 2-quart saucepan; heat just to boiling. Remove from heat; cool. Measure milk temperature with the thermometer that accompanies the yogurt maker; when mercury reaches the "add starter" level on the thermometer, stir in 1 tablespoon lowfat or nonfat yogurt. Process according to manufacturer's instructions. Refrigerate several hours before serving.

Note: Yogurt will keep several weeks in the refrigerator. Be sure to save some to use as starter for the next batch.

FRUIT YOGURT

1   recipe plain nonfat yogurt* (page 202)
    fresh or frozen fruits or
      berries, puréed in the blender

Method 1: Fill the bottom of each yogurt cup with ⅓ cup of puréed fruit, such as strawberries, raspberries, blackberries or blueberries. Prepare nonfat yogurt as directed in preceeding recipe; pour over puréed fruits. Process as directed.

Method 2: Prepare nonfat yogurt; process as directed. Chill. Just before serving add ⅓ cup of chilled puréed fruit to each cup of yogurt. Stir.

TIPS ON HERBS

Fresh Herbs greatly enhance the flavor of meats and vegetables and diminish the need to season with salt. Many herbs can be grown in small gardens outdoors or in window pots indoors year round. When seasoning with fresh herbs use twice the amount of fresh as you would of dried. Fresh herbs may be dried for late use.

To Dry Herbs wash and pat dry. Tie in small bundles; hang in a cool, airy attic or shady breezeway. When leaves are brittle, strip leaves from stems and place in an air tight container. After 24 hours check for moisture. If moisture is present, air dry again for a few more days. Store dried herbs in an air tight container in a cool, dark place. To make dried herbs into powder, whirl in blender.

To Dry Herbs in the Microwave wash and pat semi-dry with paper towels; pull off leaves. Place on several layers of paper towel or on a paper plate. Cover with an additional paper towel. Microwave on full power 30 seconds; let stand 10 minutes. Herbs should be brittle. If not, microwave a few seconds longer. Store in an air tight container. Check for moisture the following day. If moisture is present, microwave again for a few more seconds. Store in an air tight container in a cool, dark place.

To Develop the Maximum Flavor of Dried Herbs soak them for 20-40 minutes in some liquid you will be using in the recipe, such as broth, water, wine, safflower oil, olive oil, tomato sauce, vinegar, or lemon juice.

FRESH HERBS AND SEASONINGS

ARTICHOKES:	Lemon, Garlic, Onion, Black Pepper, Safflower Oil, Olive Oil
ASPARAGUS:	Lemon, Vinegar, Garlic, Onion
GREEN BEANS:	Lemon, Dill, Garlic, Tarragon, Black Pepper, Marjoram, Onion, Mushrooms, Waterchestnuts, Tomato
BROCCOLI:	Lemon, Vinegar, Black Pepper, Onion, Tomato, Sesame Seeds, Sesame Oil
CORN ON THE COB:	Garlic Powder, Onion Powder
CUCUMBER:	Chives, Dill, Garlic, Onion, Vinegar

EGGPLANT:	Oregano, Garlic, Black Pepper, Onion, Parsley, Tomato, Green Pepper, Mushrooms
PEAS:	Almonds, Mint, Mushrooms, Onion
POTATOES:	Paprika, Parsley, Dill, Chives, Mace, Rosemary, Black Pepper, Garlic Powder
RICE:	Chives, Saffron, Green Pepper, Onion, Mushrooms
SQUASH:	Cinnamon, Ginger, Black Pepper, Mace, Onion
ZUCCHINI:	Lemon, Parsley, Black Pepper, Tomato, Garlic

BEEF:	Bay Leaf, Dry Mustard, Garlic, Marjoram, Thyme, Mushrooms, Onion, Green Pepper, Parsley, Artichoke Hearts
VEAL:	Thyme, Black Pepper, Bay Leaf, Oregano, Garlic, Curry, Ginger, Marjoram, Tomato, Parsley, Apricot
LAMB:	Garlic, Lemon, Curry, Rosemary, Mint, Tomato, Onion, Mushrooms, Green Pepper
POULTRY:	Lemon, Paprika, Curry, Black Pepper, Oregano, Tarragon, Thyme, Rosemary, Cayenne, Celery, Onion, Garlic, Tomato, Mushrooms, Green Chilies, Parsley
SEAFOOD:	Lemon, Ginger, Celery, Onion, Tomato, Garlic, Safflower Oil, Olive Oil, Fennel, Watercress, Basil, Mushrooms, Tomato

The following combination of herbs, taken from the book *Cooking Without Your Salt Shaker,* published by the American Heart Association, is a tasty and satisfying alternative to the salt taste. Try it in your salt shaker.

HERB SEASONING

1	tablespoon garlic powder
½	teaspoon cayenne pepper
1	teaspoon ground basil
1	teaspoon ground marjoram
1	teaspoon ground thyme
1	teaspoon ground parsley
1	teaspoon ground savory
1	teaspoon ground mace
1	teaspoon onion powder
1	teaspoon black pepper
1	teaspoon ground sage

Combine seasonings; pour into a salt shaker. Use in place of salt.

Reproduced with permission by the American Heart Association.

POSITIVE DIET BREAKFAST SUGGESTIONS

FRESH FRUITS

Cantaloupe	*Fresh Orange Slices*
Honeydew Melon	*Tangerines*
Sliced Peaches	*Tanglos*
Apricots	*Satsumas*
Strawberries	*Sliced Bananas*
Raspberries	*Rhubarb Sauce*
Blackberries	*Applesauce*
Blueberries	*Baked Apple*
Fresh Pineapple Spears	*Fresh Grapefruit*
Papaya	*Kiwi*

HEARTY BREAKFASTS

French Omelet filled with crab, sprouts, mushrooms, tomatoes, onion and low-fat cheese; cottage fries; fresh strawberries.

Marinated Salmon — with sliced onion and fresh tomato on pumpernickel bread; fresh fruit.

Scrambled Eggs with tomato salsa; English muffin; ½ cantaloupe.

Huevos Rancheros; hash brown potatoes; fresh grapefruit.

Breakfast Quiche; warm tortillas; fresh orange juice.

Cheese and Egg Muffins; and ½ fresh papaya.

Waffles with fresh strawberries.

Corn Bread with maple syrup; fresh blackberries.

French Toast with fresh raspberry syrup; apple juice.

Pancakes with fresh blueberries.

Crepes with fresh strawberries and whipped cream substitute.

NOTE: Recipes for the above suggestions are in this book, and are prepared with egg substitute and other heart-healthy ingredients.

LIGHT BREAKFASTS

*Melted low-fat cheese on an English muffin;
fresh orange juice.*

Toasted bagel with peanut butter; apple cider.

*French bread; assortment of low-fat cheese;
fresh fruit.*

*Homemade non-fat yogurt with fresh raspberries;
crumpet.*

*Homemade frozen yogurt with fresh strawberries;
muffin.*

Energy bars; apple juice.

Apple or Berry Cobbler; slice low-fat cheese.

Whole grain dry cereal; sliced bananas.

Homemade granola; fruit shake.

Hot oatmeal with fresh strawberries.

Warm Applesauce; crumpet with peanut butter.

Whole grain toast; sliced low-fat cheese; fresh fruit.

BEVERAGES

Apple Juice

Apple Cider

Grape Juice

Fresh Squeezed Orange Juice

Apricot Nectar

Pineapple Juice

Fruit Shake

Orange Cooler

Strawberry Frost

Herbed Tea

Decaffeinated Coffee

Cappucino

Hot Chocolate

POSITIVE DIET LUNCH SUGGESTIONS

SALADS

Hot Tuna

Crab Louis

Fresh Fruit

Seviche

Chicken

Caesar

Stuffed Lettuce

Taco

Layered

Stuffed Artichoke

Chef's

Salad Niçoise

Tossed Green

Fresh Spinach

Fresh Tomato

NOTE: Accompany salads with fresh bread or rolls, tortillas, cracker bread, bread sticks, Finn Crisp, or Rye Crisp. Garnish with fresh fruits of the season.

SOUPS

Fresh Mushroom

Minestrone

Beef Broth

Beef-Barley-Mushroom

Chicken Broth

Chicken Noodle

Gazpacho

Fresh Tomato

Cream of Cucumber

Cream of Artichoke

Clam Chowder

Seafood Chowder

Oyster Stew

Won Ton

Mexican Chili

NOTE: Accompany soups with Fresh bread or rolls, tortillas, bread sticks, cracker bread, Finn Crisp, or Rye Crisp. Garnish with fresh fruits or the season.

SANDWICHES

Poultry	Seafood
Breast of Chicken	Tuna Salad
Breast of Turkey	Crab Salad
Chicken Salad	Lobster Salad
Turkey Salad	Hot Tuna and Cheese
Club House	Hot Crab and Cheese
	Monte Cristo

Meat	Low-Fat Basics
Hamburger	Toasted Cheese
Cheeseburger	Lettuce and Tomato
Roast Beef	Cheese, Lettuce and
French Dip	Tomato
Cube Steak	Tomato with Melted
Barbecued Beef	Cheese
	Peanut Butter
	Vegie

NOTE: *All the recipes for sandwich suggestions are prepared with heart-healthy ingredients and are in this book.*

SANDWICHES

NOTE: When preparing sandwiches, think variety. Try different breads, such as:

Rye	*Bagels*
French	*Tortillas*
Sour Dough	*Crumpets*
Italian	*Cracker Bread*
Bran Wheat	*Pita*
Raisin Wheat	
Whole Wheat	

Try these breads toasted, untoasted and open-faced.

A variety of garnishes can provide new and different tastes and textures to sandwiches. Water-chestnuts, for example, can give crunch to tuna salad. Sprouts are excellent on sliced breast of turkey. Other garnishes include:

Lettuce	*Green Pepper*
Tomato	*Mushrooms*
Onion	*Almonds*
Green Chilies	*Cucumbers*

All of the recipes for the soup, salad and sandwich suggestions are prepared with heart-healthy ingredients and can be found in this book.

Make interesting combinations by combining soup, from an earlier dinner, and a sandwich; a cup of soup and a hearty salad; or for the lunchbox, simply a sandwich and fresh fruit.

PICNIC LUNCH

French Rolls

Cold Chicken

Hot Chinese Mustard

Sliced Tomatoes and Onions

Marinated Mushrooms

Artichoke Hearts

Baby Corn

Grapes

Cherries

Fruit Juice, Wine or Lemonade

Unsalted Potato or Yogurt Chips

Raisin-Oatmeal Cookies

Wrap all ingredients and place them in a large picnic basket. Include a special table cloth, napkins, cups and paper plates.

POSITIVE DIET DINNER SUGGESTIONS

Gazpacho
Cracked Crab
Caesar Salad
Homemade Chocolate Ice Cream

Barbecued Salmon
Curried Potato Salad
Tomatoes Vinaigrette
Blackberry Pie

Crab Stuffed Zucchini Salad
Tomatoes with Mozzarella
French Rolls
Fruit Sorbet

Barbecued Hamburgers with Lettuce,
Tomato and Onion
Salad Greens Tossed With Mushrooms
Corn on-the Cob
Watermelon

Baked Chicken
Japanese New Variety Rice
Fresh Asparagus
Tomatoes With Fresh Basil

Cube Steak Sandwiches on Sour Dough Rolls
Corn on the Cob
Fresh Green Beans
Artichoke Hearts
Fresh Mushrooms and Cherry
Tomatoes in Vinaigrette
Apple Pie

Steamed Clams with Fresh Lemon
Garden Greens with Dijon Vinaigrette
French Bread
Fresh Fruit and Assorted Low-fat Cheese
Lemon Ice

Chicken Tacos or Enchiladas
Rice
Salad of Assorted Fresh Fruits of the Season

Hamburgers with Lettuce, Tomato and Onion Slices
French Fries
Fresh Fruit

Chicken Soup
Green Salad
French Bread
Fresh Papaya

Hungry Joe Special
Fresh Fruit

Broiled Lamb Chops
Potatoes Arosto
Skewered Mushrooms, Artichokes,
Green Peppers & Onions
Lemon Sorbet

Stir-Fried Chicken With Fresh Vegetables
Buckwheat (Soba) Noodles
Fresh Pineapple, Papaya and
Mandarin Oranges

French Dip Sandwiches
Green Salad
Blackberry Cobbler

Oysters Rockefeller
Hearts of Romaine With Fresh Lemon
Assorted Fresh Fruits of the Season

Chili
Vegetable Antipasto
Fresh Fruit

Roast Chicken
Roast Potatoes and Vegetables
Fresh Strawberries

Meat Loaf
Tossed Salad with Dijon Vinaigrette
Tabbouli Pilaf
Sliced Oranges

Fresh Mushroom Soup
Broiled Scallops
Fresh Spinach Salad with Lemon and
Ground Pepper
Assorted Fresh Fruits of the Season

Pizza
Build Your Own Salad
Watermelon

Chicken Salad
Fresh Pumpernickel or Zucchini Bread
Sliced Low-fat Cheese
Apples, Pears and Bananas

Cioppino
Tossed Green Salad
Crusty French Bread
Fresh Fruits

Roast Beef
Baked Potato with Non-fat Yogurt and Chives
Tossed Green Salad
Chilled Asparagus
Strawberry Shortcake

Cream of Artichoke Soup
Steamed Mussels
Homemade French Bread
Fresh Fruits of the Season

Stuffed Sole
Pea Pods, Waterchestnuts, and
Forest Mushrooms
Rice Pilaf
Lemon Ice

Seafood Chowder
Tossed Green Salad with Oil and Vinegar Dressing
Fresh Fruit

Macaroni and Low-fat Cheese
Fresh Tomatoes
Salad of Fresh Spinach and
Hearts of Romaine

Barbecued Steak
Baked Potatoes with Pot Cheese
Fresh Mushroom Salad
Broiled Tomatoes
Fresh Fruit

Spring Rolls
Won Ton Soup
Salad of Fresh Cucumber and Onion
Watermelon Ice

Pasta Primavera
Crusty French Bread
Assorted Low-fat Cheese
Fresh Fruits of the Season

Barbecued Chicken
French Fries
Fresh Artichokes with
Homemade Safflower Mayonnaise
Watermelon, Grapes, Cherries
and Raspberries

Salad Niçoise
Sour Dough Bread
Fresh Berry Pie

Spinach Salad
Grilled Veal Steaks with
Fresh Lemon and Mushrooms
Parsleyed Potatoes
Sliced Tomatoes
Fresh Pineapple

Taco Salad
Corn on the Cob
Fresh Fruit

THANKSGIVING DINNER

Roast Turkey
Bread Stuffing with Fresh Mushrooms
Mashed Potatoes
Low-fat Gravy
Antipasto
Yams with Pecans
Fresh Cranberry Relish
Homemade Bread
Pumpkin Pie

THE DAY AFTER THANKSGIVING

Turkey Sandwiches
Antipasto Salad
Assorted Fresh Fruits of the Season

TWO DAYS AFTER THANKSGIVING

Turkey Soup
Bread Sticks with Pot Cheese
Fresh Fruits

The preceding dinner menus are meant to show that meals on the Positive Diet need not be dull. All of the recipes for the suggested meals are in this book and are prepared with heart-healthy ingredients. If you desire simpler meals or more elaborate fare, simply follow the Positive Diet guidelines to adapt your own recipes to your own balanced meal plans.

Some of the menus include dessert. This is only to illustrate that desserts need not be denied totally. There are Positive Diet desserts but you must decide for yourself whether or not you want the sugar or the calories.

POSITIVE DIET SNACK SUGGESTIONS

VEGETABLES

Celery   Variations:
Carrots   *Dip Vegetables*
Radishes   *in Tomato Salsa*
Green Onions   *Pot Cheese*
Mushrooms   *or*
Cucumbers   *Peanut Butter*

FRUITS

Apples   *Pears*
Apricots   *Strawberries*
Cantaloupe   *Blackberries*
Watermelon   *Blueberries*
Honeydew   *Raspberries*
Grapes
Cherries   *Frozen Grapes*
Peaches   *Frozen Watermelon*
Plums   *Frozen Berries*
Tangerines
Bananas   *Apples with Low-Fat*
Satsumas   *Cheese*
                              Apples with Peanut
                                  Butter

MUNCHIES

Low-Fat Cheese and Crackers
Pop Corn
Homemade Pretzels
Baked, Unsalted Potato Chips
Homemade Tortilla Chips
Homemade Cheese Tortilla Chips
Homemade Nachos
Homemade Tostados
Homemade Potato Skins
Unsalted Peanuts, Filberts, Soynuts
Almonds, Pecans, Sunflower Seeds
Homemade Toasted Pumpkin Seeds

TO TIDE YOU OVER

English Muffin with Melted Low-Fat Cheese
Toasted Bagel with Peanut Butter
English Muffin with Peanut Butter
Swedish Flat Bread with Cheese or Peanut Butter
Cracker Bread with Pot Cheese

FOR THE SWEET TOOTH

Homemade Popsicles

Homemade Non-Fat Yogurt with Fresh Fruit

Homemade Frozen Yogurt

Homemade Push-Ups

Homemade Low-Fat Ice Cream

Homemade Sorbets and Ices

Tapioca Pudding

Homemade Peanut Butter Cookies

Homemade Molasses Gingersnaps

Homemade Raisin-Oatmeal Cookies

Rice Krispie Cookies

NOTE: When selecting a snack, you must decide for yourself how many calories you can afford. Remember, the most nutritous snack is simply fresh fruit or fresh vegetables.

BEVERAGES

Homemade Lemonade

Fresh Orange Juice

Apple Juice

Hot Apple Cider

Grape Juice

Pineapple Juice

Fresh Grapefruit Juice

Apricot Nectar

Decaffeinated Iced Tea

Herb Tea

Mineral Water

Orange Cooler

Strawberry Frost

Fruit Shake

NOTE: All of the recipes for the suggested snacks and beverages are in this book and are prepared with heart-healthy ingredients.

When planning menus strive for balanced meals. Include a protein portion, such as fish, poultry, red meat, peanut butter, cheese, legumes, egg, or egg substitute; a grain portion, such as potatoes, rice, pasta, bread or cereal; a vegetable portion; and a fruit portion.

Whenever possible choose fresh vegetables and fresh fruits. For best value, select from those which are in season.

According to the American Heart Association, average daily nutritional needs include:

PROTEIN: 2 cups of skim milk or skim milk products; 4-6 ounces of lean poultry, fish or red meat (or the equivalent in vegetable protein)

FRUITS AND VEGETABLES: 2 cups or more of vegetables and fruits, including one good vitamin C source, such as oranges or orange juice and one deep yellow or dark green vegetable

GRAIN: 4 or more servings of whole grain or enriched breads or cereals (one serving is 1 slice of bread, or 1 cup of dry cereal or ½ cup of cooked cereal, pasta or rice).

FATS AND OILS: 2-4 tablespoons of polyunsaturated fats or oils.

COOKING EQUIPMENT AND STAPLES

You need not buy a lot of sophisticated cooking equipment to implement the Positive Diet. A teflon skillet, teflon griddle, teflon baking sheets and teflon cake pans are essential. And an inexpensive yogurt maker is very useful, as is a vegetable steamer, wire whisk, blender and an electric mixer.

The following is a list of staples which are frequently used on the Positive Diet:

Non-fat Milk Powder
Evaporated Low-fat
  Milk
Egg Substitute
Low-fat Cheese
Non-fat Yogurt*
Non-hydrogenated
  Peanut Butter
Water-Pack Tuna Fish
Lemon Juice
Fruit Juices
Fresh Fruits
Chicken Broth*
Beef Broth*
Canned Tomatoes*

Safflower Mayonnaise
Safflower Oil
Olive Oil
Tub Safflower Margarine
Dijon Mustard
Whole Grain Breads
Whole Grain Natural
  Cereals
Flour
Yeast
Fresh Vegetables
Tomato Puree**
Tomato Paste**
Tomato Sauce**

*Preferably Homemade
**Perferably Unsalted or Homemade

COOKING TERMS AND PROCEDURES

SAFFLOWER MAYONNAISE means mayonnaise made from safflower oil. Safflower mayonnaise may be homemade or commercially made.

TO STORE FRESH GARLIC peel the cloves and place them in a jar; cover with safflower oil. Store covered in refrigerator.

GARLIC-SAFFLOWER OIL is the oil that covers the garlic — see preceding tip on storing fresh garlic.

TO STORE FRESH GINGER ROOT peel and cut ginger root and place in a jar; cover with sake. Store in a covered jar in refrigerator.

GINGER JUICE is made by grating a piece of fresh ginger and then squeezing the pulp for the juice.

FOREST OR SHITAKE MUSHROOMS are available in oriental markets or in the oriental section of the supermarket. Use fresh mushrooms or re-constitute the dried by covering them with water and soaking them 20-30 minutes to soften. Always save the soaking liquid as it makes wonderful mushroom soup and may be added to homemade chicken broth or beef broth.

TO CUT INTO STRINGS means to cut the meat or the vegetables into the shape of a long, thin string.

AL DENTE is an Italian term meaning "firm to the tooth." Pasta or vegetables cooked al dente should be just barely tender.

OR LESS SALT means to use less salt if your taste buds permit. The salt content in these recipes is for those people just beginning the Positive Diet. The aim of all should be to continue gradually reducing the salt content of the recipes first by ¼, then by ½ and again by ¾. (Refer to Comments From the Cook for more specifics on gradual salt reduction.)

RECIPE PROPORTIONS: Most recipes in this book serve 4. The proportions are such that they may easily be cut in half and in most cases in half again, or they may easily be doubled.

IMPORTANT: Some recipe ingredients in the Positive Diet Book are followed by an asterisk (*). This indicates that for the recipe to be prepared in the most heart-healthy form, the particular ingredient involved should first be prepared according to instructions in this book. For example, if Chicken Broth* is listed as an ingredient, the asterisk means to use only homemade chicken broth (prepared from the recipe for Chicken Broth in this book).

The most common recipe ingredients followed by an asterisk are Chicken Broth and Non-Fat Yogurt. For this reason, it is convenient to keep some made up and on hand.

CHAPTER ELEVEN

APPETIZERS AND BEVERAGES

STEAMED MUSSELS WITH
WINE AND GARLIC

2 quarts fresh mussels
¾ cup dry white wine
3 cloves garlic

Scrub mussel shell with wire brush or rock full of barnacles to remove beard. Wash and soak mussels in shells to remove sand — follow procedure for steamed clams with fresh lemon* (page 416). Place mussels in a large pot; add wine and garlic. Cover tightly; steam 6-8 minutes, just until shells open. Drain. Serve hot or cold.

Variation: Accompany with Dijon Vinaigrette* (page 361).

STEAMED CLAMS BORDELAISE

2   dozen clams
⅓   cup garlic-safflower oil* (page 232)
3   tablespoons olive oil
¼   cup dry white wine
1   small onion, chopped
2   cloves garlic, minced
1   stalk celery, chopped
    fresh parsley for garnish
    fresh lemon wedges for garnish

Wash and soak clams to remove sand — follow procedure for steamed clams with fresh lemon* (page 416). Place clams in steamer. Add oils, wine, onion, garlic, and celery. Cover; bring to a boil. Reduce heat; simmer 10 minutes — just until shells open. Drain. Arrange on a bed of fresh parsley. Garnish with lemon wedges.

OYSTERS ON THE HALF SHELL

10   small or extra small oysters
¼   cup ketchup
1½   teaspoons fresh horseradish
     fresh parsley for garnish
     fresh lemon wedges for garnish

Shuck oysters. Drain; dry between paper towels. Combine ketchup with horseradish. Chill oysters and sauce. When ready to serve, place oysters in individual shells or ramekins; garnish with fresh lemon and parsley. Accompany with sauce.

OYSTERS ROCKEFELLER

3   bunches fresh spinach
16-20 small or extra small oysters
2   tablespoons dry bread crumbs
2   tablespoons safflower oil or olive oil
1   tablespoon grated onion
½   teaspoon chervil
½   teaspoon or less salt
¼   teaspoon tarragon
      dash pepper
2-3   drops Tabasco sauce
¼   cup low-fat Mozzarella cheese, grated

Steam spinach 2-3 minutes; squeeze dry. Combine bread crumbs, oil, onion and seasonings; toss with spinach. Place 4-5 well-drained oysters in each shell or ramekin and broil 5-7 minutes or until very hot; drain any excess liquid. Top oysters with spinach; broil 3-4 minutes. Sprinkle with cheese; broil 2-3 minutes longer or until cheese is melted and mixture is piping hot.

MARINATED SALMON

¾ cups fresh lime juice
¾ cup onion, finely chopped
1 stalk celery, finely chopped
2 tomatoes, peeled and chopped
¾ teaspoon or less salt
¾ teaspoon pepper
¾ teaspoon sugar
3-4 drops Tabasco sauce
1 pound fresh salmon, boned, skinned, and cut into 1-inch cubes
fresh parsley for garnish
fresh lemon wedges for garnish
cherry tomatoes, halved, for garnish
1 white onion, sliced into rings for garnish

Combine lime juice, onion, celery, tomatoes, salt, pepper, sugar and Tabasco; pour over salmon. Toss; cover. Chill at least 6 hours; drain. To serve, cover a bed of fresh parsley with onion rings. Arrange salmon over top; ring with cherry tomatoes and lemon wedges.

Note: Serve as an hors d'oeuvre with French bread or for a light supper or for breakfast with bagels and fresh fruit.

SEVICHE

1½   pounds fresh scallops
     fresh lime juice—to cover fish
¼   cup chopped white onion
¼   cup chopped fresh parsley
¼   cup chopped green chilies
1   large ripe tomato, chopped
3   teaspoons olive oil
    dash cayenne
    salt to taste
    pepper to taste
    fresh parsley for garnish
    lemon wedges for garnish
    Finn Crisp, Rye Crisp or Melba
      Toast

Cut each scallop into thirds; cover with lime juice. Marinate in refrigerator 4 hours; pour off lime juice. Toss scallops with remaining ingredients. Serve on a bed of parsley in individual shells or ramekins. Garnish with lemon wedges. Accompany with Finn Crisp, Rye Crisp or Melba toast.

Note: To adjust this recipe, plan on 3 scallops per person. Seviche makes a great appetizer or first course and may also be served as a salad by substituting bibb lettuce for parsley.

Variation: In place of scallops, use lobster meat, pompano or red snapper.

CRACKED CRAB

1 large crab, cracked and cleaned
¼ cup ketchup
1½ teaspoons fresh horseradish
fresh parsley for garnish
lemon wedges for garnish
1 loaf crusty French bread

Chill crab. Combine ketchup with horseradish; chill. To serve, arrange crab on a bed of fresh parsley. Garnish with lemon wedges. Accompany with sauce and crusty French bread.

Note: When selecting a brand of ketchup or horseradish, consult a good sodium dictionary. Some brands are relatively low in sodium while others are very high.

CRAB COCKTAIL

½ cup ketchup
3 teaspoons fresh horseradish
1½ cups crab meat
fresh lemon wedges
fresh parsley

Combine ketchup with horseradish; chill. Chill 4 stemmed glasses; place a small amount of sauce in the bottom of each. Add crab meat; top with additional sauce. Garnish with lemon wedge, fresh parsley and an additional piece of crab or a crab leg.

SPINACH AND CRAB COQUETTE

    1   bunch fresh spinach greens
    ¾   pound crab meat
    ¼   teaspoon Dijon mustard
         safflower mayonnaise to moisten
  1-2   drops Tabasco sauce
    ¾   cup grated low-fat Cheddar or
         Mozzarella cheese
         cherry tomatoes for garnish

Tear spinach into bite-size pieces. Toss crab meat
with Dijon and just enough mayonnaise to moisten; dot with Tabasco sauce. Line individual shells
or ramekins with spinach; top with crab. Sprinkle
with cheese. Bake at 375° 5-10 minutes — just until
cheese melts. Cut cherry tomatoes in half; use as
garnish.

CRAB AND ARTICHOKES WITH DIJON

    ½   pound crab meat
    1   15-oz. can artichoke hearts, drained
    2   green onions, minced
         Dijon vinaigrette to moisten*·
            (page 361).
         fresh parsley for garnish
         cherry tomatoes for garnish
    1   loaf crusty French bread, sliced

Combine crab, artichoke hearts and green onion;
toss with Dijon vinaigrette to moisten. Chill. Garnish with fresh parsley and cherry tomatoes.
Serve with crusty French bread.

ARTICHOKES WITH FRESH LEMON

fresh artichokes
fresh lemon juice
safflower mayonnaise* (page 360)

Wash artichokes. Cut 1-inch off top. Cut off stem and tips of leaves. Place upside down in a deep dish.

To Pan-Steam: Place artichokes upright on steamer rack over boiling water. Pour ½ cup fresh lemon juice over artichokes. Cover pan tightly with lid. Steam 30-40 minutes or until tender.

To Microwave: Pour 4 tablespoons of lemon juice and 2 tablespoons of water over each artichoke. Cover dish with plastic wrap; prick a hole in the top of plastic wrap to allow steam to escape. For 1 medium artichoke allow 5-7 minutes cooking time; for 2 medium artichokes allow 7-9 minutes.

To Oven-Steam: Pour ½ cup of lemon juice over each artichoke. Cover dish with aluminum foil. Bake at 350° 30-40 minutes.

Artichokes are done when bottom leaves pull off easily; do not overcook.

Serve with homemade safflower mayonnaise.

Variation: Serve with Dijon vinaigrette* (page 361).

DIJON CUCUMBER STICKS

fresh cucumbers
Dijon vinaigrette* (page 361)

Peel cucumbers; cut lengthwise into eighths.
Serve with Dijon vinaigrette.

MARINATED MUSHROOMS

1   pound fresh mushrooms
    juice of 1 lemon
1   lemon, cut into thin rounds
¾   cup safflower oil
¼   cup cider vinegar
2   cloves garlic
¼   teaspoon pepper
1   teaspoon or less salt
    fresh parsley for garnish

Clean mushrooms; trim stems. Place in a large
saucepan; toss with lemon juice. Add oil, vinegar,
garlic, pepper and salt. Cook over medium-high
heat 20-30 minutes, stirring frequently. Remove
from heat; cool to room temperature. Chill. Drain.
Cover a serving plate with fresh parsley; top with
lemon rounds. Spoon mushrooms over lemons.

Note: Mushrooms will keep several days in the
refrigerator. Remaining marinade may be used
again for marinated mushrooms, as a marinade
for artichoke hearts or as a salad dressing.

STUFFED MUSHROOMS

1 pound large fresh mushrooms
½ cup oil and vinegar dressing*
(page 362)
1 bunch fresh spinach
½ cup safflower mayonnaise
2 tablespoons grated onion
1 tablespoon lemon juice
6 ounces of crab meat
½ cup grated low-fat Cheddar cheese

Clean and stem mushrooms; marinate in oil and vinegar dressing for 1 hour. Drain. Wash spinach leaves; shake, but do not dry. Cook covered in heavy skillet 2-3 minutes or until wilted. Drain; squeeze out excess moisture. Chop. Combine mayonnaise, onion and lemon juice. Toss with crab and spinach. Stuff mushrooms; sprinkle with cheese. Bake at 375° for 15 minutes.

Variations: Omit spinach; or omit crab and double the spinach.

CHEESE PIE

1 4-oz. can chopped green chilies
1 lb. low-fat Mozzarella cheese, grated
¾ lb. low-fat Cheddar cheese, grated
1 cup egg substitute, slightly beaten

Place green chilies in a 9-inch pie plate or a quiche pan; top with cheeses. Drizzle with egg substitute. Bake at 425° 35-40 minutes. Remove from oven; let set 10-15 minutes. Cut into squares. Serve at once.

SPRING ROLLS

2   dozen spring roll (lumpia) wrappers
2   tablespoons ginger juice* (page 232)
3   chicken breasts, diced
1   teaspoon sake
1   teaspoon salt-reduced soy sauce
¼   pound bamboo shoots, washed and
    cut into 2-inch strings
3-4   green onions, cut into thin strings
    2-inches in length
5-6   Shitake mushrooms, thinly sliced
½   cup fresh bean sprouts
½   teaspoon potato starch
½   cup water

Thaw spring roll wrappers. Grate ginger; squeeze juice from pulp over chicken. Sprinkle chicken with sake and soy sauce; let stand 20 minutes. Brown chicken in a teflon skillet over medium heat; set aside. Sauté bamboo shoots and onions in a small amount of water or chicken broth using a wok or heavy skillet; when barely tender, add mushrooms and bean sprouts; cook 2-3 minutes. Cool to room temperature.

In small saucepan, bring potato starch and water to a boil. Remove from heat; cool to room temperature.

Separate spring roll wrappers; lay them flat. Toss vegetables with chicken; place 3-4 table-spoons of mixture in the center of each wrapper. Brush outside edges of wrappers with mixture of potato starch and water; fold edges over envelope style. Seal outside seam with potato starch and water paste.

Brown spring rolls in a teflon skillet over medium heat 10 minutes or until very hot, or
Continued

brown in a heavy skillet using a very small amount of safflower oil — just enough to coat bottom of pan.

To reheat, warm in hot oven or in a microwave oven.

Note: Spring roll (lumpia) wrappers and Shitake mushrooms are available in oriental markets and in oriental section of many supermarkets. If fresh mushrooms are not available, use dried, but first soak them in water to cover for 30 minutes or until soft.

In place of salt-reduced soy sauce an additional teaspoon of sake may be used.

Serve spring rolls on a bed of fresh parsley. Accompany with hot mustard and sesame seeds and ketchup and horseradish sauce.

HOT MUSTARD AND SESAME SEEDS

extra hot Chinese mustard
toasted sesame seeds

Mound hot mustard in center of a salad size plate. Ring with sesame seeds.

Note: Hot Chinese mustard and toasted sesame seeds are available in oriental markets and in oriental sections of many supermarkets.

KETCHUP AND HORSERADISH SAUCE

¾ cup ketchup
¼ cup horseradish

Combine ketchup and horseradish.

247

TUNA ANTIPASTO

1   6½-oz. can water-pack tuna, drained
1   15-oz. can artichoke hearts, drained
    and quartered
3   green onions, sliced
¼   pound fresh mushrooms, sliced and
    steamed 3 minutes
1   8-oz. can tomato sauce
1   tablespoon olive oil
¼   cup red wine vinegar
1   clove garlic

Combine ingredients; chill.
Serve with crusty French bread for dipping.

EGGPLANT ANTIPASTO

1   large eggplant
1   8-oz. can tomato sauce
3   cloves garlic, minced
1   green pepper, seeded and chopped
1-2 teaspoons cumin
¼   teaspoon cayenne
1   teaspoon or less salt
1   teaspoon sugar
¼   cup red wine vinegar

Dice unpeeled eggplant; place in a 4-quart sauce pan. Add remaining ingredients. Cover; cook over medium heat 20 minutes, stirring frequently. Uncover; cook 30 minutes or until thick.

Note: Serve hot or cold with tortilla chips* (page 256), crusty French bread or as a vegetable dip. Especially nice on a picnic with roast chicken.

VEGETABLE ANTIPASTO

cherry tomatoes
fresh artichokes
fresh mushroom caps
carrot sticks
celery sticks
cauliflower flowerets
broccoli flowerets
fresh pea pods
green onions
radishes, flowered
zucchini spears
cucumber spears

Chill vegetables. Pile cherry tomatoes in center of a large basket or tray. Surround with remaining vegetables.

Note: Broccoli and asparagus may be served raw or steamed 3-5 minutes, just until tender.

Serve with tomato salsa*, spinach dip*, Spanish dip*, artichoke dip*, hot mustard and sesame seed dip*, tuna antipasto* or eggplant antipasto* (recipes in appetizer section).

A colorful way to serve dip is to hollow the inside of a purple cabbage, leaving the bottom and the outer leaves intact for a bowl; place in center of a large basket or tray. Fill with dip. Garnish with a mushroom cap. Surround with fresh vegetables.

SKEWERED FRUIT

Summer
watermelon balls
cantaloupe balls
honeydew melon balls
fresh strawberries
fresh mint for garnish

Winter
fresh pineapple chunks
papaya squares
orange segments, skin and membrane
  removed
purple or black grapes
fresh mint for garnish

Alternate fruits on small skewers. Garnish with mint.

FRUIT ANTIPASTO

Summer
cantaloupe wedges
grapes
low-fat Mozzarella or Somerset cheese

Remove rind from cantaloupe wedges. Snip grapes into small clumps. Cut cheese into 1-inch cubes. Arrange cantaloupe wedges on plate or tray. Tuck cheese between wedges. Ring with grapes.

Winter
assortment of low-fat cheese
apples

Cut cheese into 1-inch cubes. Pile in center of basket or tray. Just before serving, slice apples; position around cheese.

EGGPLANT ROUNDS

1   medium eggplant
¾   cup bread crumbs
½   cup skim evaporated milk
1   onion, thinly sliced
2   tomatoes, thinly sliced
¼   pound low-fat Cheddar Cheese,
        thinly sliced
     salt to taste
     pepper to taste

Peel eggplant. Slice lengthwise into quarters; slice quarters crosswise into rounds. Dredge each round in bread crumbs, then dip in milk and back into bread crumbs. Brown on a teflon griddle over medium-high heat, about 5 minutes on each side — just until tender.

Place slices on a teflon baking sheet; top each piece with a slice of onion and a slice of tomato. Bake at 350° for 20 minutes. Remove from oven; top each piece with a slice of cheese. Return to oven for 10 minutes or until cheese melts. Season.

APPETIZER PIZZA

1   1-lb. can tomatoes
2   tablespoons tomato paste
1   tablespoon olive oil
1   loaf French bread
¾   pound low-fat Mozzarella or
      Cheddar cheese, grated

Drain tomatoes; dice. Reserve ½ cup of the juice and mix with diced tomatoes, tomato paste and olive oil. Slice French bread in half lengthwise; spread with sauce and sprinkle with cheese. Bake at 450° 10-15 minutes or until bread is hot and cheese has melted. To serve, slice crosswise into rounds.

MUNCHIES

dry roasted peanuts
Spanish peanuts
toasted soy nuts
dry roasted soy nuts
filberts
almonds
pecans
shelled sunflower seeds
unshelled sunflower seeds
raisins
chopped dates

Poor ingredients into an air tight container. Toss. Cover tightly. Store in refrigerator.

Note: Use only unsalted nuts.

POTATO SKINS

potatoes
low-fat Cheddar cheese, grated

Scrub potatoes; bake at 400° until soft when squeezed. Slice potatoes in half lengthwise; scoop pulp from skins (reserve for mashed potatoes). Cut skins lengthwise into quarters; place skin side down on a teflon baking sheet. Bake at 500° 10 minutes or until crisp; sprinkle with cheese. Return to oven for 2-3 minutes or until cheese melts.

Variation: Sprinkle with chili powder, onion powder, garlic powder or black pepper. Serve with tomato salsa* (page 361).

CHEESE BURRITOS

4   corn tortillas
½   cup low-fat Cheddar cheese, grated
2   tablespoons chopped green chilies
1   tablespoon finely chopped tomato
1   tablespoon finely chopped onion
    tomato salsa* (page 361)
    plain non-fat yogurt* (page 202)

Lay tortillas flat; sprinkle with cheese, green chilies, tomato and onion. Roll into a tight roll. Heat at 350° 5-6 minutes. Serve with salsa and non-fat yogurt.

NACHOS

unsalted taco chips, baked—not
    fried—in safflower oil (available
    in health food stores)
low-fat Cheddar cheese, grated
chopped green chilies
tomato salsa* (page 361)

Note: Homemade tortilla chips* or taco chips* (page 256) may be used in place of store bought.

Variation: In place of taco chips use vegetables such as carrot rounds, celery pieces, green pepper strips, thick onion slices, quartered tomato slices, broccoli flowerets, broccoli stems, cauliflower flowerets, asparagus, and waterchestnuts.

TORTILLA CHIPS

corn tortillas

Cut corn tortillas into 8 wedges; place on teflon baking sheet. Bake at 350° about 10 minutes; turn. Bake 10 minutes longer or until crisp.

Variation: Sprinkle with garlic, onion, or chili powder. Serve with tomato salsa* (page 361).

CHEESE TORTILLA CHIPS

4   corn tortillas
½   cup low-fat Cheddar cheese, grated

Cut tortillas into 8 wedges; place on a teflon baking sheet. Bake at 350° about 10 minutes; turn. Bake 10 minutes longer or until crisp. Sprinkle with cheese; bake at 350° 5 minutes or until cheese melts.

Variation: Sprinkle crisp tortilla chips* (page 256) with chopped green chilies and dot with tomato salsa* (page 361) before adding cheese. Serve with additional salsa for dipping.

CHEESE TOSTADOS

4   corn tortillas
½   cup low-fat Cheddar cheese, grated

Place tortillas on a teflon baking sheet; sprinkle with cheese. Bake at 350° until cheese is melted and tortilla is crisp.

TOMATO SALSA

2   cups canned whole tomatoes with liquid
4   Jalapeno peppers
1-2 fresh tomatoes, chopped

Cut tomatoes and peppers into 1-inch pieces. Combine all ingredients. Serve chilled or at room temperature.

Variation: Add ½-¾ cup raw or sautéed onion.

SPANISH DIP

1½ cups pot cheese
⅔   cup diced green chilies
1   tomato, diced
2   green onions, diced

Warm cheese over vary low heat 2-3 minutes — just until slightly warm. Do not overheat or cheese will separate. Stir in remaining ingredients. Serve at once with French bread, unsalted tortilla chips* (page 256), sliced cucumbers, zucchini strips, celery or carrot sticks, radishes or as a stuffing in mushroom caps.

ARTICHOKE DIP

---

1   8-oz. can artichoke hearts, drained
    and quartered
1   4-oz. can diced green chilies
2   tablespoons safflower mayonnaise
1½ cups low-fat Cheddar cheese,
    grated

Purée artichoke hearts and green chilies in blender
or food processor; stir in mayonnaise. Pour into a
shallow baking dish; sprinkle with cheese. Cover;
bake in a 350° oven 15 minutes. Uncover; bake 5
minutes or until cheese melts.

Serve with French bread, unsalted tortilla chips*
(page 256), sliced cucumbers, zucchini strips, celery sticks, carrot sticks, radishes, or as a stuffing
in mushroom caps.

SPINACH DIP

---

1   cup safflower mayonnaise
1   bunch fresh spinach, chopped
1   cup chopped green onion
1   cup plain non-fat yogurt* (page 202)
1   teaspoon lemon juice
2-3 drops Tabasco sauce
    ground pepper
1   cup chopped fresh parsley

Put mayonnaise in blender; add spinach and
green onion. Whirl 2-3 minutes. Spoon into
medium-size bowl; fold in yogurt and remaining
ingredients, except parsley. Chill. Just before serving, add parsley.

TOASTED PUMPKIN SEEDS

2   cups pumpkin seeds
1½   teaspoons safflower oil
     garlic powder
     onion powder
     chili powder

Remove fiber from unwashed pumpkin seeds. Toss seeds with safflower oil. Spread on foil-lined baking sheet; sprinkle with garlic, onion or chili powder. Toast at 250° for 20 minutes or until seeds are lightly browned. Cool. Store in an air tight container.

Note: Chili powder gives a taco-type flavor.

POPCORN

Pop corn in a hot air popper which requires no oil; or pop in a paper bag in the microwave oven according to manufacturer's instructions; or use traditional stove top or electric corn popper method using safflower oil for the oil portion.

Serve plain, or if buttery flavor is desired, season lightly with melted tub-style safflower margarine.

Variation: Season with garlic, onion or chili powder.

FRUIT SHAKE

2 cups chilled strawberries,
     raspberries, or blackberries
1½ cups skim milk

Frost tall glasses in the freezer for 30-60 minutes. Purée fruits in blender. Add milk; whirl until frothy.

Note: Plums, oranges, peaches, melon, papaya or pineapple may be used in place of berries.

Variation: For additional sweetness, add a piece of banana. For variety, add a jigger of rum. For a creamier taste, omit milk; and fold plain non-fat yogurt* (page 202) into puréed fruits.

FRESH LEMONADE

1 cup fresh lemon juice
4 cups cold water
2 tablespoons sugar or lightly to taste
1 lemon, sliced into rings
     orange slices for garnish
     strawberries for garnish
     fresh mint for garnish

Combine lemon juice, water and sugar in a large pitcher; stir to dissolve sugar. Add lemon slices. Chill. Serve over ice. Garnish with orange slices, strawberries and a sprig of fresh mint.

STRAWBERRY FROST

2   cups strawberries
juice of 2 oranges
juice of ½ lemon
¼   cup apple juice
5-8   ice cubes
whole berries for garnish

Purée berries in blender; add juices. Add ice cubes one at a time; crush. Pour into tall glasses. Garnish with whole berries.

Variation: For a creamier taste, fold in ½-1 cup plain non-fat yogurt*(page 202).

ORANGE COOLER

⅔   cup concentrated orange juice
1   cup skim milk
1   cup water
⅛-¼   cup honey
1   teaspoon vanilla
6-8   ice cubes
orange slices for garnish
fresh mint for garnish

Combine orange juice, milk, water, honey and vanilla in blender; whirl until frothy, gradually adding ice. Serve at once. Garnish with orange slices and fresh mint.

SANGRIA

1   litre red wine
2   ounces brandy
3   ounces fresh orange juice
3   ounces fresh lemon juice
1   cinnamon stick
    sugar to taste
3   oranges with rinds, sliced
3   lemons with rinds, sliced
3   ounces club soda or to taste

Combine all ingredients, except club soda. Chill. Just before serving, add club soda.

Variation: Add any other fruits in season.

HOT CIDER

1 quart apple juice
2 cloves
1 cinnamon stick

Heat apple juice, cloves and cinnamon over medium heat until juice is piping hot; do not boil. Serve at once.

ICED TEA

1 quart cold water
¼ cup decaffeinated tea
  fresh lemon slices for garnish
  fresh mint for garnish

Combine water and tea in a covered jar. Chill overnight. Strain. Serve over ice. Garnish with lemon slices and fresh mint.

CHOCOLATE WHIP WITH CINNAMON

1 tablespoon cocoa powder
1 cup skim milk
ground cinnamon
whipped cream substitute* (page 202)
(optional)

Mix cocoa powder with 1 tablespoon skim milk to make a paste. Heat remaining milk just to scalding; do not boil. Add cocoa paste; stir. Pour into blender; whirl until frothy. Sprinkle with ground cinnamon. Top with whipped cream substitute.

Variation: For iced chocolate whip, chill and serve over ice.

CAPPUCCINO

decaffeinated espresso coffee
skim milk
cinnamon stick (optional)
whipped cream substitute* (page 202)

Brew espresso. Heat milk just to scalding; do not boil. Pour milk into blender; whirl until frothy. Fill mugs with ⅓ coffee to ⅔ milk; garnish with cinnamon stick. Top with whipped cream substitute.

Variation: For iced cappucino, chill and serve over ice.

CHAPTER TWELVE

BREADS
AND BREAKFASTS

ENRICHED WHITE BREAD

2 packages active dry yeast
⅔ cup warm water
6 cups enriched all-purpose flour
3 teaspoons salt
2 cups skim milk
¼ cup safflower oil

Dissolve yeast in ⅔ cup warm water. Combine flour, salt, milk and oil in a large mixing bowl; add dissolved yeast. Mix with a wooden spoon to form a soft dough. Remove to floured surface. Knead 5-10 minutes or until dough is smooth and elastic.

Grease a glass mixing bowl with tub safflower margarine; place dough in bowl and turn to coat top. Cover; let rise in warm place 3-4 hours. Punch down.

Divide dough in half. Put into 2 loaf pans greased with tub safflower margarine. Cover. Let rise in warm place 1-2 hours. Bake at 350° 35-40 minutes. Remove from pans. Cool on wire racks. Yield: 2 loaves.

Variation: To make rolls, divide dough into 4 dozen equal-size balls. Grease muffin pans with tub safflower margarine. Place 2-3 balls in each cup. Cover. Let rise 1-2 hours. Bake at 350° 25-35 minutes.

Helpful Hint: When bread is done it will be well-browned, will shrink slightly away from edges of pan, and will sound hollow when tapped with knuckles. When done, immediately remove bread from pan to prevent a soggy crust. Cool on wire racks. Bread may be frozen

HONEY WHEAT BREAD

2 packages active dry yeast
⅔ cup water
5½ cups whole wheat flour
2⅓ cups skim milk
3 teaspoons salt
½ cup honey
2 tablespoons safflower oil
3 cups enriched white flour
tub safflower margarine

In a large mixing bowl, dissolve yeast in ⅔ cup warm water; add 3 cups whole wheat flour, milk and salt. Stir. Warm honey and oil; pour over flour mixture. Beat until smooth, using low speed of electric mixer. Gradually add remaining whole wheat flour and enriched white flour; stir with a wooden spoon to soft dough stage. Form into a ball.

Knead 5 minutes on a lightly floured surface. Divide dough in half; knead 10 minutes. Cover bread with wax paper brushed with tub safflower margarine. Place dish towel over top. Let rest 20 minutes; uncover. Punch down.

Divide into two loaf pans greased with tub safflower margarine. Cover with oiled wax paper. Place pans in plastic bag; twist closed. Let rest in refrigerator for 24 hours. Remove from refrigerator and let rest 10 minutes. Bake at 375° 40-50 minutes. Remove from pans. Cool on wire racks. Yield 2 loaves.

Variation: To make rolls, divide dough into 4 dozen equal-size balls. Grease muffin pans. Place 3 balls in each cup; brush tops with safflower margarine. Bake at 375° 30-40 minutes.

FRENCH BREAD

1   package active dry yeast
⅓   cup warm water
4   cups unbleached all-purpose flour
2⅛   teaspoons salt
1½   cups lukewarm water
      tub safflower margarine

Dissolve yeast in ⅓ cup warm water. Mix flour with salt; add dissolved yeast and remaining water. Mix with a wooden spoon to form a soft dough. Remove to a heavily floured surface; knead until smooth and elastic.

Place dough in a mixing bowl greased with tub safflower margarine. Cover. Let rise 3 hours or until double in size. Punch down. Knead slightly. Let rise 2 more hours or until double in size. Punch down. Knead slightly. Let rise 1½ hours. Knead slightly. Divide dough in half.

Form into loaves as follows: lay each piece of dough flat. Using a karate-type chop, make a deep seam in the bread dough; roll bread to one side to seal edges; then roll seam to top. Flatten dough. Again using a karate chop, make a deep seam; roll bread to one side to seal edges. Roll seam to bottom. Roll dough out into a long rope. Place in two French bread pans greased with tub safflower margarine. Cover. Let rise 1½-2 hours or until double in size.

Preheat oven to 425°. Spray oven (be sure oven light is off) and bread dough with water. Bake 15-20 minutes or until set. Push loaves out of pans and onto oven racks. Bake 5-10 minutes longer or until brown. Cool on wire racks.

To freeze: Wrap cooled bread tightly in aluminum foil. To reheat, place frozen, foil-wrapped bread in preheated 300° oven for 20 minutes.

GARLIC BREAD

---

1   loaf French bread
    tub safflower margarine
    garlic powder

Slice bread lengthwise; spread with tub safflower margarine. Sprinkle with garlic powder. Put loaf back together; slice crosswise into rounds. Wrap bread in foil. Warm in a 400° oven 10-12 minutes or until hot. Serve in a napkin-lined basket.

CROUTONS

---

1   small loaf of bread, diced

Brown diced bread in a 250° oven 2 hours or to desired crispness, or dry in the microwave 1½ minutes on each side per slice of bread. Store croutons in jar in refrigerator with lid slightly ajar.

Variation: To make seasoned croutons, sprinkle with herbs, garlic powder, onion powder or chili powder.

BREAD CRUMBS

---

1   crouton recipe* (page 270)

Prepare bread as for croutons, making sure that the diced bread is dry enough to float on water. Place dried bread in a plastic bag; roll with a rolling pin to form fine crumbs or grind in a food processor or blender. Store in covered jar in refrigerator with lid slightly ajar.

HEALTH BREAD

3	tablespoons active dry yeast
½	cup warm water
1½	cups oatmeal
¾	cups coarse ground cracked wheat
2	cups wheat germ
¾	teaspoon or less salt
3	tablespoons safflower oil
3½	cups hot water
¾	cup honey
¼	cup molasses
3	cups whole wheat flour
3	cups unbleached white flour

Dissolve yeast in ½ cup warm water. In large mixing bowl, mix oatmeal, cracked wheat, wheat germ, salt, safflower oil, and hot water. Cool to room temperature. Add honey, molasses, dissolved yeast, whole wheat flour and white flour. Stir with a wooden spoon to form a soft dough. Remove to floured surface. Knead for several minutes, adding more flour as needed to reduce stickiness.

Place dough in a bowl greased with safflower tub margarine. Cover with waxed paper and a kitchen towel. Put in a warm place and let rise until double. Divide dough into 3 loaves and place in loaf pans greased with tub safflower margarine. Cover with waxed paper and a dish towel. Put in a warm place and let rise until double. Bake at 350° for 50 minutes or until bread pulls away from edges of pan. Yield: 3 loaves.

Note: Good toasted or spread with peanut butter.

CHALLAH

2	packages active dry yeast
2½	cups warm water
2½	tablespoons sugar
1½	teaspoons salt
½	cup safflower oil
1	cup egg substitute
8-10	cups all-purpose flour
	tub safflower margarine
	sesame seeds or poppy seeds
	egg wash — 1 tablespoon egg substitute plus 1 tablespoon water

Place yeast in large mixing bowl; add warm water. To dissolved yeast add sugar, salt, oil, egg substitute and ½ of the flour. Mix with a wooden spoon until dough is smooth; gradually add remaining flour to form a soft dough.

Knead on a heavily floured surface 10 minutes or until dough is smooth and elastic. Place in bowl greased with tub safflower margarine and turn dough to coat top. Cover with plastic wrap.

Set aside to triple in size, approximately 1½ hours. Punch down. Turn out onto floured board. Knead lightly. Cover. Let rest 10 minutes.

Shape dough into 4 loaves; place in loaf pans greased with tub safflower margarine. Cover. Let rise until double in size.

Brush with egg wash; sprinkle with seeds. Bake at 350° 25 minutes or until golden brown. Cool on wire racks. Makes 4 loaves.

Continued

Variations: To make braided loaves divide dough into 9 parts. Cover parts not being worked on. Roll 3 parts into ropes about 15-inches long; braid ropes together and tuck each end under. Place on teflon baking sheet. Repeat with remaining parts. Cover. Let rise until double. Brush with egg wash; sprinkle with seeds. Bake at 375° 25-30 minutes. Makes 3 braided loaves.

To form braided wreath, divide dough in half. Cut each half into thirds; roll each third into a rope about 24-inches long. Braid 3 ropes together. Place on a teflon baking sheet; form into a wreath about 5-inches in diameter; fold ends of dough under. Braid remaining thirds; form into a wreath. Cover. Let rise until double. Brush with egg wash; sprinkle with seeds. Bake at 375° 45 minutes or until golden brown. Cover with foil if bread gets too brown. Cool on wire racks. Makes 2 braided wreaths.

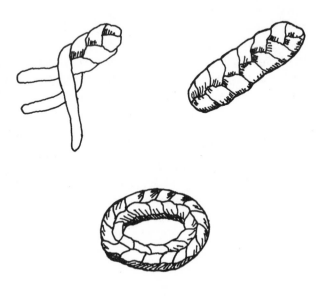

BAGELS

2   packages active dry yeast
⅔   cup warm water
2   cups whole wheat flour
¾   cup water
3   tablespoons sugar
3   teaspoons salt
2   cups enriched all-purpose flour
     tub safflower margarine
1   gallon of water
1   teaspoon sugar
     poppy seeds

Dissolve yeast in ⅔ cup warm water. Add whole wheat flour, ¾ cup water, 3 tablespoons sugar and salt. Blend on low speed of electric mixer. Then beat on high speed for 2 minutes. Lower speed; gradually add white flour. When dough becomes too stiff for mixer, remove from bowl onto well-floured surface and knead by hand until smooth. Place in teflon pan. Cover. Let rest 15 minutes. Divide dough into 12 portions. Shape into balls.

With a nut pick punch a hole in the center of each; pull to enlarge, keeping the shape uniform. Place on a teflon baking sheet. Cover. Let rise for 30 minutes.

Bring 1 gallon of water and 1 teaspoon of sugar to a boil; reduce heat to simmer. Add 6 bagels; simmer 3 minutes. Turn with tongs; simmer 4 minutes. Remove from water; pat dry with paper towels. Place on teflon baking sheet; sprinkle with poppy seeds. Repeat with remaining bagels. Bake at 375° 30 minutes. Serve warm.

Note: Bagels can be frozen.

BREAD STICKS

2	packages active dry yeast
⅔	cup warm water
2¾	cups water
2	tablespoons safflower oil
3	teaspoons salt
3⅓	cups whole wheat flour
4½	cups all-purpose flour
	tub safflower margarine
2	egg whites beaten with 1 tablespoon water until frothy
	sesame seeds or poppy seeds

Dissolve yeast in ⅔ cup warm water. Heat remaining water, safflower oil and salt to lukewarm; pour into large mixing bowl. Add whole wheat flour and dissolved yeast. Mix with a wooden spoon until smooth. Gradually add all-purpose flour. Remove to lightly floured surface. Knead 10 minutes or until smooth and elastic. Form into ball.

Place in medium bowl greased with tub safflower margarine. Cover. Let rise in a warm place about 2 hours or until double in size. Punch down.

Cut dough into 5 dozen equal size pieces. Roll each between palms into a 6-8-inch rope. Place 2-3 inches apart on a teflon baking sheet. Cover. Let rise in a warm place 30-60 minutes or until double in size. Brush with beaten egg whites; sprinkle with seeds. Bake at 375° 10 minutes. Reduce heat to 300°; bake 20-35 minutes. Cool on wire racks.

Variation: Instead of bread sticks, form the dough into the shape of cars, trucks, airplanes, animals, angels, flowers, trees or gingerbread boys. Bake at 375° 25-30 minutes. Slice the bread characters lengthwise between front and back; fill with chicken, peanut butter or other sandwich filling.

SOFT PRETZELS

1	package active dry yeast
1½	cups lukewarm water
1	teaspoon salt
3	teaspoons sugar
4	cups flour
1	egg, beaten

Dissolve yeast in water; add salt, sugar and flour. Knead 5-10 minutes, add more flour as necessary to reduce stickiness. Twist dough into shape of cars, trucks, airplanes, animals, flowers, trees, gingerbread boys, numerals or circles. Place on teflon baking sheet. Brush with beaten egg. Bake at 425° 15 minutes or until lightly browned.

CHEESE BREAD

2	cups warm water
2	packages active dry yeast
2	tablespoons sugar
1	tablespoon salt
¼	cup safflower oil
6	cups flour
3¼	cups grated low-fat Cheddar cheese

Dissolve yeast in water; add sugar, salt, oil and ½ of the flour. Mix. Add remaining flour; knead into a soft dough — about 5 minutes. Divide dough into 2 loaves; knead 1½ cups of cheese into each loaf. Shape into round loaves; flatten slightly. Bake on a teflon baking sheet or in individual loaf pans at 375° for 30-35 minutes. Makes 2 loaves.

MUFFINS

1 cup enriched white flour
½ cup whole wheat flour
½ cup oatmeal
2 teaspoons baking soda
    dash salt
½ cup wheat germ
1 cup raisins
1 egg or ¼ cup egg substitute
½ cup safflower oil
1 cup skim milk
¼ cup honey

In a large bowl combine flour, oatmeal, baking soda, salt, wheat germ, raisins and egg. In a separate bowl combine oil, milk and honey; add to flour mixture. Blend with a wooden spoon. Pour into paper-lined muffin cups. Bake at 400° for 25 minutes.

CORN BREAD

¾ cup corn meal
1 cup flour
3 teaspoons baking powder
¾ teaspoon or less salt
¼ cup molasses
¾ cup skim milk
1 egg or ¼ cup egg substitute, beaten
2 tablespoons safflower oil

Sift together corn meal, flour, baking powder and salt; add remaining ingredients. Mix with a spoon. Bake in a 9"-round teflon pan at 375° for 30 minutes.

COFFEE CAKE

1½ cups all-purpose flour, sifted
2¼ teaspoons baking powder
¼   teaspoon or less salt
⅓   cup sugar
½   cup safflower oil
½   cup skim milk
1   egg

Topping
½   cup brown sugar
2   tablespoons flour
2   tablespoons safflower oil
2   teaspoons cinnamon
¾   cup raisins

Sift together flour, baking powder, salt and sugar. Blend oil, milk and egg with a fork; add to dry ingredients. Stir with a wooden spoon until flour mixture is moistened. Set aside. Combine ingredients for topping.

Spread half of the batter in an 8-inch round teflon cake pan; sprinkle with half of the topping. Add the remaining batter; sprinkle with remaining topping. Bake at 375° for 30 minutes.

Variation: To glaze combine ⅓ cup confectioners sugar, 1 tablespoon skim milk and ⅛ teaspoon vanilla. Spread over cooled coffee cake.

NOTE: Because sugar reduction is essential to good cardiac health, coffee cake, cinnamon rolls and other sweet breads should be used sparingly and only for very special occasions.

CINNAMON BREAD

1   recipe enriched white bread* (page 267)
¾   cup brown sugar
¼   teaspoon safflower oil
3   teaspoons cinnamon
1   cup raisins
    tub safflower margarine

Follow procedure for enriched white bread until after the first rising. Divide dough in half; flatten and pull each half into as large a square as possible. Combine sugar, oil and cinnamon; sprinkle over dough. Top with raisins.

Roll dough lengthwise as for jelly roll. Arrange dough in 3 loaf pans greased with tub safflower margarine. Cover. Let rise in warm place 1-2 hours. Bake at 350° 35-40 minutes.

Variation: To make cinnamon rolls, slice the rolled and filled dough crosswise into rounds 1½-inches wide. Place rolls in round or square teflon baking pans. Bake at 350° 35-40 minutes.

Note: There will be enough dough for 1 loaf of cinnamon bread, 1 pan of cinnamon rolls and 1 loaf of white bread.

BANANA-RAISIN BREAD

1½	cups all-purpose flour
1	teaspoon baking soda
1	cup sugar
½	teaspoon or less salt
3-4	bananas, mashed (about 1½ cups)
½	cup egg substitute or 2 eggs
1	teaspoon vanilla
½	cup safflower oil
¾	cup plain non-fat yogurt* (page 202)
⅔	cup raisins
	tub safflower margarine

Sift together flour, soda, sugar and salt. Set aside. Whirl bananas, egg substitute, vanilla and oil in blender; fold in yogurt. Add raisins. Pour over dry ingredients. Blend with wire whisk until smooth. Pour into a loaf pan greased with tub safflower margarine. Bake 1 hour at 350°.

ZUCCHINI BREAD

¾ cup egg substitute, beaten
1 cup safflower oil
2 cups sugar
2 cups grated zucchini
3 teaspoons vanilla
3 cups all-purpose flour
¾ teaspoon or less salt
1 teaspoon soda
3 teaspoons cinnamon
½ teaspoon baking powder
1 cup raisins
  tub safflower margarine

Using low speed of electric mixer, combine egg substitute, oil, sugar, zucchini and vanilla. In separate bowl, combine remining ingredients, except raisins. Gradually add to zucchini mixture. Blend. Stir in raisins. Pour into 2 loaf pans that have been greased with tub safflower margarine. Bake at 350° for 1 hour. Yield: 2 loaves.

Note: Bread may be frozen.

ENERGY BARS

⅔   cup whole wheat flour
⅔   cup safflower oil
1   egg or ¼ cup egg substitute
⅓   cup packed brown sugar
1   teaspoon vanilla
½   teaspoon cinnamon
½   teaspoon baking powder
½   teaspoon or less salt
1½   cups uncooked rolled oats
1   cup unsalted, low-fat Cheddar
      cheese, grated
¾   cup raisins
1   cup apples, peeled and chopped

Mix flour, oil, egg, sugar, vanilla, cinnamon, baking powder and salt with a wooden spoon; stir in oats, cheese and raisins. Add apples; stir. Drop by heaping tablespoons onto teflon baking sheets. Bake at 375° for 20 minutes or until golden brown. Store in tightly covered jar in refrigerator.

Note: Perfect for breakfast with fresh orange or apple juice.

GRANOLA

3½   cups rolled oats
½   cup sunflower seeds
½   cup unsalted peanuts
½   cup soybeans
¼   cup almonds
¼   cup pecans
¼   cup sesame seeds
¼   cup honey
¼   cup safflower oil
⅛-¼   cup water or more as needed to
      moisten
½   cup raisins
½   cup dates, dried apples, or dried
      apricots, chopped

Combine all ingredients, except raisins and dates in a large bowl; toss. Add just enough water to moisten. Pour granola onto a teflon baking sheet. Bake at 300° for 30 minutes or until golden brown, stirring occasionally. Cool. Stir in dates and raisins. Store in covered jar in refrigerator.

PANCAKES

---

    1   cup egg substitute
    1   cup skim milk
    1   cup cold water
  2½   cups flour, sifted
   ¼   cup safflower oil
   ¾   teaspoon sugar
   ¼   teaspoon salt

Lightly beat egg substitute, milk and water; add remaining ingredients. Blend with a wire whisk. Bake on a pre-heated teflon griddle. Turn pancakes when top side is bubbly and a few bubbles have broken.

Variation: To make blueberry pancakes, just after bubbles have broken, sprinkle pancakes with blueberries. Turn, brown on other side.

YOGURT PANCAKES

---

    1   cup egg substitute
    2   cups plain non-fat yogurt* (page 202)
   ½   cup flour, sifted
   ¼   teaspoon salt
    1   teaspoon baking soda

Lightly beat egg substitute; fold in yogurt. Combine dry ingredients; blend with eggs and yogurt using a wire whisk. Bake on a pre-heated teflon griddle, turning when top side is bubbly and a few bubbles have broken.

CRÊPES

½   cup egg substitute
½   cup skim milk
½   cup cold water
1   cup flour, sifted
2   tablespoons safflower oil
½   teaspoon sugar
⅛   teaspoon salt

Lightly beat egg substitute, milk and water. Add remaining ingredients; blend with a wire whisk. Pour enough batter into a pre-heated, 5-inch teflon crêpe pan to coat bottom of pan; tilt pan to spread batter. Cook 1 minute or just until set. Turn. Cook 1 minute longer or until browned.

Note: Especially good with fresh strawberries and whipped cream substitute* (page 202).

Crêpes may be prepared in advance, layered between wax paper, and wrapped in aluminum foil for freezing. Bring to room temperature for easy separation before using. To reheat, remove wax paper layers; wrap in aluminum foil. Heat in a 200° oven for about 10 minutes or until warm.

Some crêpe fillings may be prepared in advance and refrigerated or frozen for later use.

FRENCH TOAST

- ½ cup egg substitute
- ⅓ cup skim milk
- ⅛ teaspoon sugar
- ½ teaspoon cinnamon
- 6 slices day-old crusty French bread

Beat eggs; add milk, sugar and cinnamon. Blend. Heat teflon griddle over medium-high heat. Dip bread one slice at a time into egg mixture, coating both sides evenly. Brown 2-3 minutes; turn and brown 2-3 minutes more.

WAFFLES

- ¾ cup egg substitute
- 1½ cups skim milk
- ⅓ cup safflower oil
- 2 cups all-purpose flour
- 2 teaspoons baking powder
- 2 teaspoons sugar
- ½ teaspoon or less salt

Whirl eggs in blender; add milk and oil. Blend 2 minutes; add dry ingredients and whirl. Bake in pre-heated teflon waffle iron. Makes 4 large waffles.

Note: For a thinner batter, add more milk.

FRUIT SYRUP

2   cups raspberries, strawberries, blackberries or blueberries

Purée fruit in blender. Serve warm or cold over pancakes, waffles, French toast, corn bread, ice cream or sherbet.

Variation: For a sweeter syrup, warm ¼ cup honey with fruit.

For a more tart syrup, add 1 teaspoon lemon juice.

For a thicker syrup, warm fruit and gradually stir in 2 tablespoons corn starch; heat and stir until mixture thickens.

MAPLE SYRUP

1½   cups corn syrup
¼   cup sugar
2   tablespoons water
1   teaspoon maple flavoring

Combine ingredients in medium saucepan. Bring to a boil; boil 2 minutes. Cool to room temperature. Store in refrigerator. Warm slightly before reusing. Yield: 1 pint.

Variation: Substitute brown sugar for granulated sugar.

Helpful Hint: For a truly heart-healthy syrup, simply purée fresh or frozen berries and use in place of syrup.

FRENCH OMELET

Select desired fillings per person

2 teaspoons chopped onion
¼ cup sliced mushrooms
1 teaspoon minced green pepper
   wine, broth or water
1 teaspoon minced chives
2 teaspoons chopped parsley
2 teaspoons diced green chilies
2 tablespoons crab meat
2 tablespoons low-fat Cheddar cheese, grated
2 tablespoons chopped tomato

¼-½ cup egg substitute per person
1 tablespoon water per person
   dash salt
1-2 slices tomato per person for garnish
   fresh parsley for garnish

Sauté onion, mushrooms and green pepper until tender in small amount of wine, broth or water.

Beat eggs, water, salt and pepper with a fork until mixture is well-blended, but not frothy. Heat an 8-inch teflon skillet over medium heat until a drop of water sizzles when sprinkled on the pan. Pour in eggs. Tilt pan to spread evenly throughout and at an even depth.

Using a fork, stir rapidly through top of uncooked eggs. Shake pan frequently to keep eggs moving. When egg is set, but still shiny, remove pan from heat. Spoon desired fillings across center. Flip sides of omelet over, envelope style, to hold in filling. Tilt pan and roll omelet over onto plate. Garnish with sliced tomatoes and fresh parsley.

HUEVOS RANCHEROS

    1   4-oz. can whole green chilies, drained
    ½   cup low-fat Monterey Jack cheese,
           grated
    1½   cups egg substitute, beaten
    ¼   cup grated low-fat Cheddar cheese
         corn tortillas
         tomato salsa* (page 361)
         sliced tomatoes for garnish

Gently slit each chilie lengthwise and remove
seeds. Stuff with shredded Jack cheese. Press slit
edges together to keep in cheese. Cut stuffed
chilies into bite-size pieces.

Heat teflon skillet over medium heat. Arrange
chilies in pan. When cheese begins to melt, pour
in beaten eggs. When eggs start to firm, lift chilies
slightly to allow uncooked eggs to run underneath. When almost fully cooked, sprinkle grated
Cheddar cheese on top. When cheese melts, remove skillet from heat and serve.

Serve with corn tortillas and tomato salsa. Garnish with sliced tomatoes.

SCRAMBLED EGGS

¼-½   cup egg substitute per person

Beat egg substitute lightly with a fork. Heat teflon skillet over medium heat. Pour in egg substitute. Stir rapidly until egg is cooked throughout but still glossy and moist.

Variation: Just as egg substitute begins to set add any of the following: chopped fresh parsley, chopped green chilies, chopped green onion, or grated low-fat Cheddar cheese. Top with tomato salsa* (page 361).

BREAKFAST QUICHE

1   4-oz. can chopped green chilies
1¾   pound low-fat Mozzarella cheese
1½   cups egg substitute

Sprinkle green chilies in bottom of a quiche pan or pie plate. Grate cheese; sprinkle over chilies. Lightly beat egg substitute; drizzle over cheese. Bake at 350° for 45 minutes. Let set 10 minutes before serving.

Serve with tomato salsa* (page 361) and plain non-fat yogurt*(page 202). Accompany with warm corn tortillas.

Note: Serves 6–8.

CHEESE AND EGG MUFFINS

1   whole English muffin per person
2   slices low-fat Cheddar cheese per
        muffin
1   slice tomato per muffin (optional)
1   slice white onion per muffin (optional)
1   egg or ¼ cup egg substitute per muffin

Split and toast muffins. Slice cheese. Cover bottom half of muffin with tomato, onion and one slice of cheese. Soft boil an egg, or fry an egg over easy in a teflon pan, or scramble egg substitute in a teflon pan. When nearly done, place muffins under the broiler or in a microwave oven until cheese melts. Place egg on bottom half of muffin. Top with remaining half of muffin.

CHAPTER THIRTEEN

SOUPS
AND SANDWICHES

CHICKEN BROTH

1	large chicken
3	quarts cold water
2	stalks celery with leaves
2	carrots, peeled
1	large onion, quartered
2	cloves garlic
¼	teaspoon basil
4	peppercorns
1	tablespoon or less salt
⅛	teaspoon pepper

Put chicken and water in a stock pot. Cover; simmer 2½ hours or until chicken is tender and pulls away from bone. Strain. Remove meat from bones; (freeze for later use). Refrigerate broth overnight; fat will float to the top. Skim and discard fat.

Heat broth to boiling; add vegetables and seasonings. Simmer 2 hours; strain. Reserve vegetables for soup or later use; use broth within 2 weeks or freeze.

Variation: For a richer broth, add another chicken or additional chicken parts.

Note: For maximum economy, when a recipe calls for cooked chicken breasts, buy a whole chicken. Skin and debone breasts. Discard skin. Freeze the bones along with the giblets, necks, wings and backs in a plastic freezer bag. When 5-6 pounds accumulate or when you have a chicken carcass — after a meal of roast chicken — remove bones from freezer bag to a stock pot, add water to cover by 2 inches. Add vegetables and seasonings as in above recipe. Bring to a boil. Cover. Reduce heat. Simmer 5-6 hours. Strain. Discard bones and vegetables as they will be greasy. Refrigerate broth overnight. Skim and discard fat

CHICKEN SOUP WITH
CHINESE VEGETABLES

      1   recipe chicken broth* (page 295)
     ½   pound fresh mushrooms, sliced
    1-2 bunches fresh spinach, torn into
           bite-size pieces
      1   cup fresh bean sprouts
    2-3 drops hot sauce

Heat chicken broth to boiling. Add mushrooms, then spinach; cook 2 minutes. Add bean sprouts and hot sauce. Serve at once with homemade bread or rolls.

CHICKEN SOUP WITH TOMATO
AND GREEN ONION

      4   cups chicken broth* (page 295)
      4   green onions with tops, thinly
           sliced
      1   tomato, thinly sliced

Heat broth to boiling. Ladle into soup bowls. To each bowl, add one green onion, sliced, and one slice of tomato.

CHICKEN SOUP WITH LEMON

3   cups chicken broth* (page 295)
2   tablespoons fresh lemon juice

Heat broth to boiling; add lemon juice. Serve.

Note: Especially nice as a first course with a sea-food entrée.

CHICKEN SOUP WITH SPINACH AND SAIFUN

1   package Saifun noodles
1   recipe chicken broth* (page 295)
2   bunches fresh spinach, washed and
      torn into bite-size pieces

Cook saifun in boiling water 3-5 minutes (texture will be gummy). Rinse. Drain. Heat broth to boiling. Spoon saifun into bowls. Sprinkle with spinach. Ladle broth over. Serve at once.

Note: Saifun noodles are available in oriental markets.

WON TON SOUP

¾ lb. extra lean boneless pork chops
black pepper to taste
sage to taste
6 Shitake forest mushrooms, chopped
10 green onions, chopped
2 dozen won ton wrappers, thawed
1 recipe chicken broth* (page 295)

Grind pork in meat grinder, blender or food processor; sprinkle with black pepper and sage. Toss with mushrooms and green onions. Place mixture by teaspoonful into center of won ton wrappers; squeeze top of wrapper together to seal.

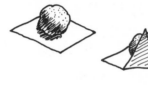

Drop won tons into 3½ quarts of boiling water; bring to a second boil. Boil 2 minutes; add 2 cups cold water. Bring to a third boil; boil 2-3 minutes. Drain. Bring chicken broth to a boil. Add won tons. Serve

Note: Won tons may be cooked ahead and refrigerated. To reheat drop into boiling broth. If fresh Shitake mushrooms are not available, the dried can be purchased in oriental markets or in the oriental section of the supermarket. To reconstitute dried mushrooms soak them in enough water to cover for 30 minutes or until soft; remove and squeeze out the excess water. Remove and discard stems. Reserve soaking liquid; add to chicken broth.

EGG DROP SOUP

---

4   cups chicken broth* (page 295)
¼   cup egg substitute, beaten
6-8 cherry tomatoes, thinly sliced
4   green onions with tops, thinly
        sliced

Heat chicken broth to boiling. Pour egg through a wire strainer into hot broth. Ladle broth into soup bowls; add 1-2 sliced cherry tomatoes and 1 sliced green onion to each bowl. Serve at once.

CHICKEN VEGETABLE SOUP

---

2   cups fresh green beans
2   tablespoons fresh lemon juice
1   2-pound can tomatoes
1   onion, chopped
6   carrots, peeled and diced
2   stalks celery, diced
¼   teaspoon pepper
¼   head chopped cabbage
1½ cups cooked chicken, cubed
1   cup cooked rice, barley, or pasta
2   tablespoons chopped fresh parsley

Cut beans diagonally into thirds; toss with lemon juice and steam until tender. Combine tomatoes, onions, carrots, celery and pepper in stock pot; bring to a boil, reduce heat, and simmer 1-2 hours or until vegetables are tender. Add beans and cabbage; simmer 15 minutes. Add chicken and rice, barley, or pasta; heat. Sprinkle with parsley.

CHICKEN NOODLE SOUP

1 recipe chicken broth* (page 295)
1½ cups cooked chicken, diced
4 cups cooked pasta

Heat broth to boiling; add chicken and pasta. Heat.

Variation: Add cooked carrots, celery or other vegetables.

For Chicken With Rice Soup, substitute rice for pasta.

CHICKEN SOUP WITH
BUCKWHEAT NOODLES

1 recipe chicken broth* (page 295)
1 package Chinese Buckwheat (Soba) noodles

Heat broth to boiling; add uncooked noodles, and bring to a second boil. Cook 2-3 minutes or until noodles are tender. Do not overcook.

Note: Chinese Buckwheat (Soba) Noodles are found in oriental markets or in the oriental section of the supermarket.

TURKEY BROTH

1 turkey carcass with meaty bones
  water to cover (about 3 quarts)
2 cloves garlic
¼ teaspoon basil
4 peppercorns
1 tablespoon or less salt
⅛ teaspoon pepper
4 stalks celery with leaves
4 carrots, peeled
1 large onion, quartered

Place turkey carcass in stock pot; add water to cover. Add seasonings; bring to a boil. Add vegetables. Cover, reduce heat, and simmer 6-8 hours. Strain, discard bones and vegetables as they will be very greasy. Remove meat from bones and reserve for later use. Refrigerate broth overnight. Skim and discard fat which floats to the top. Reheat broth or freeze for later use. Broth will keep up to two weeks in the refrigerator.

HEARTY TURKEY SOUP

1 recipe turkey broth* (page 301)
3 carrots, peeled and diced
2 stalks celery, peeled and diced
4 cups cooked pasta or barley
½ pound fresh mushrooms, sliced

Heat broth to boiling; add carrots and celery. Cover; reduce heat and simmer until carrots and celery are tender. Add pasta and mushrooms. Heat.

BEEF BROTH

6	pounds beef bones or 2-3 pounds beef shank or short ribs
9	cups water
3	stalks celery with leaves, diced
2	carrots, diced
1	onion, chopped
1	tomato, quartered
2	bay leaves
2	cloves garlic
¼	teaspoon thyme
¼	teaspoon marjoram
8	peppercorns
2	teaspoons salt

Put meat, bones and water in stock pot. Simmer uncovered for 3 hours (do not boil). Strain. Remove any meat or marrow from bones. Add marrow to stock; reserve meat for soup. Chill stock overnight; skim and discard fat which floats to the top. Bring stock to boiling; add remaining ingredients, and simmer uncovered 2 hours. Strain. Reserve vegetables for soup or later use. Use broth within 2 weeks or freeze for later use.

Note: For a hearty soup, do not strain broth. Add 2-3 cups cooked pasta.

BEEF BROTH PARISIAN

1   leek, finely chopped
3   cups beef broth* (page 302)
½   cup fresh mushrooms, thinly sliced
¼   teaspoon tarragon or thyme
¼   cup finely chopped fresh parsley

Sauté leek in small amount of broth; add mushrooms and stir over high heat for 1 minute. Add beef broth, tarragon or thyme. Bring to a boil; cover; reduce heat, and simmer 20 minutes. Just before serving, sprinkle with parsley.

MUSHROOM-BARLEY SOUP

1½   cups barley
1   recipe beef broth* (page 302)
½-¾   pound fresh mushrooms, sliced

Soak barley for several hours or overnight in enough water to cover. Heat broth to boiling, add barley with its soaking liquid. Cover and simmer 2-2½ hours or until barley is tender, add mushrooms. Simmer 10-20 minutes.

Variation: Add ¾-lb. extra-lean ground round, cooked and drained, to broth. Serve at once.

FRESH MUSHROOM SOUP WITH MOZZARELLA CHEESE

1 onion, chopped
1 carrot, quartered
1 cup celery, chopped
6 cups beef broth* (page 302)
¾ lb. fresh mushrooms, thinly sliced
  juice of 1 lemon
½ teaspoon or less salt
¼ teaspoon pepper
¼ cup sherry (optional)
1 cup grated low-fat Mozzarella cheese
3 tablespoons chopped fresh parsley

Boil onion, carrot and celery in beef broth until vegetables are tender; purée in blender or food processor. Return to stock pot and simmer. Sauté mushrooms in lemon juice until tender. Add mushrooms, salt, pepper and sherry to simmering broth. Heat. Ladle into soup bowls. Sprinkle with cheese and parsley.

Variation: Place a slice of toasted French bread in each bowl; ladle broth over bread.

MINESTRONE SOUP

1 cup dried white beans
4 cloves garlic, minced
1 medium onion, chopped
2 stalks celery, diced
6 cups chicken broth* (page 295)
1 1-lb. can plum tomatoes
1 tablespoon olive oil
½ cup red wine
1 tablespoon basil
1 tablespoon oregano
salt to taste
¼ teaspoon pepper
3 medium-size red potatoes, diced
¾ pound fresh green beans, cut
    diagonally into thirds
2 carrots, diced
1½ cups cooked macaroni

Soak white beans for 6 hours in 1 quart of water; pour beans with soaking liquid into a stock pot. Bring to a boil and add garlic, onions and celery. Cook 1½ hours or until beans are tender; add chicken broth, tomatoes, olive oil, wine, basil, oregano, salt and pepper. Heat to boiling; add potatoes in their jackets, green beans and carrots. Reduce heat to simmer; cook 30-45 minutes or until vegetables are tender. Add macaroni.

FRESH TOMATO SOUP

3½	pounds ripe tomatoes, chopped
1	large onion, chopped
1½	teaspoons dill weed
3	tablespoons tomato paste
3	cups beef broth* (page 302)
1½	teaspoons sugar
	ground pepper
2-3	drops Tabasco sauce
	dash salt
2-3	sprigs fresh basil

Combine tomatoes, onion, dill weed and tomato paste in a stock pot. Bring to a boil, stirring often; reduce heat, cover and simmer 15 minutes. Cool to room temperature. Pour into blender or food processor; whirl until smooth. Return to stock pot; add remaining ingredients. Heat to serving temperature.

Variation: Add 1 cup cooked macaroni.

GAZPACHO

1   fresh ripe tomato
1   green pepper
3   stalks celery
1   cucumber
1   small onion
3   tablespoons parsley flakes
4   green onions
2   cloves garlic
¼   cup red wine vinegar
3   tablespoons safflower oil
1   tablespoon olive oil
½   teaspoon salt
6   cups canned tomatoes, chopped
¼   teaspoon horseradish

Combine all ingredients except horseradish; purée in blender. Chill at least 3 hours. Just before serving, stir in horseradish.

MEXICAN CHILI SOUP

4   cups chicken broth* (page 295)
1   28-oz. can plum tomatoes
1   small onion, diced
1   clove garlic, crushed
1   4-oz. can diced green chilies
1   1-lb. can pinto beans
1   15-oz. can garbanzo beans
1½ cups cooked chicken, diced
2   cups cooked macaroni

Heat chicken broth and tomatoes just to boiling; immediately reduce heat. Add onion, garlic and green chilies; simmer 1 hour. Add beans, chicken and macaroni; simmer 20 minutes.

Note: Serve with corn tortillas.

CHILLED PEA SOUP

2   10-oz. packages frozen peas
¾   cup water
½   teaspoon or less salt
2   cups chicken broth* (page 295)
2-3 drops Tabasco sauce
2   cups plain non-fat yogurt* (page 202)
    paprika
    chopped chives

Combine peas, water and salt in medium sauce-pan; bring to a boil, cover and simmer 15 minutes, stirring occasionally. Purée in blender; add broth and Tabasco and whirl. Chill. Just before serving, stir in 1 cup yogurt. Ladle into soup bowls. Top with generous dollops of non-fat yogurt. Sprinkle with paprika. Garnish with chives.

SEVICHE SOUP

½ pound scallops, chopped
½ cup fresh lime juice
⅓ cup chopped onion
¼ teaspoon salt
½ teaspoon olive oil
1½ cups tomato juice
2 cups chicken broth* (page 295)
1 teaspoon chopped parsley
4 tablespoons chopped green chilies
fresh parsley for garnish
lime wedges for garnish

Combine scallops, lime juice, onion, and salt; marinate overnight in refrigerator. Toss with olive oil, tomato juice, chicken broth and green chilies. Chill several hours. Garnish with fresh parsley and lime wedges.

OYSTER STEW

1	pint small oysters with liquid
1½	tablespoons flour
1	teaspoon or less salt
2	tablespoons cold water
	dash Tabasco sauce
2⅓	cups non-fat milk powder
3¾	cups water

Place oysters with liquid in medium saucepan. Combine flour, salt, Tabasco and 2 tablespoons cold water; blend to a smooth paste and add to oysters. Simmer and stir over very low heat about 5 minutes — just until edges of oysters begin to curl. Combine non-fat milk powder with remaining cold water; heat to scalding, but do not allow to boil. Stir in oysters. Remove from heat; cover. Let stand 15 minutes to blend flavors. Reheat stew briefly to serving temperature.

SEAFOOD CHOWDER

1   pound clams
1   pound mussels
1   cup dry white wine
1   1-lb. can plum tomatoes
3   cloves garlic
2   tablespoons safflower oil
2   tablespoons olive oil
¼   teaspoon or less salt
⅛   teaspoon pepper
1   6½-oz. can chopped clams
¼   pound red snapper, cut into 3-inch
      cubes
¼   pound cod, cut into 3-inch cubes
¼   pound scallops
¼   pound crab legs
2   tablespoons chopped fresh parsley

Wash and soak clams and mussel shells following procedure for steamed clams with fresh lemon* (page 416). Heat wine, tomatoes, garlic, safflower oil and olive oil; simmer 15-20 minutes. Add salt, pepper, and chopped clams; simmer 15-20 minutes. Heat just to boiling, but do not allow to boil. Add clams and mussels; cover and steam just until shells begin to open. Add remaining seafood; cook 5 minutes or until most clams and mussels have opened and red snapper and cod are cooked. Do not overcook seafood. Ladle into soup bowls. Sprinkle with fresh parsley.

Variation: Add 1 cup cooked sea shell shaped pasta or 2-3 red potatoes sliced and steamed in their jackets until just tender.

MANHATTAN CLAM CHOWDER

1   28-oz. can plum tomatoes
1   large white onion, chopped
3   stalks celery, thinly sliced
1   teaspoon thyme
1   tablespoon chopped fresh parsley
½   teaspoon or less salt
2   pounds fresh clams, steamed and
    chopped plus 1½ cups nectar
2   peppercorns
⅛   teaspoon ground pepper
⅛   teaspoon Tabasco sauce
1   bay leaf
3   medium potatoes, pared and diced
2   carrots, thinly sliced

Put all ingredients except potatoes and carrots into stock pot; bring to a boil, reduce heat and simmer 1 hour. Bring to a second boil; add potatoes and carrots, reduce heat and simmer 45-60 minutes or until vegetables are tender.

Note: Three 6½-oz. cans of chopped clams with their liquid may be used in place of fresh clams.

Variation: Put all ingredients in crock pot. Cook on low 8-10 hours.

NEW ENGLAND CLAM CHOWDER

2 pounds fresh clams in shells
4 new potatoes with jackets, diced
½ cup chopped onion
2 cups chicken broth* (page 295)
2 cups clam nectar
2 cups skim milk
½ cup flour
¼ teaspoon pepper or to taste
½ teaspoon salt

Soak and steam clams according to procedure for steamed clams with fresh lemon* (page 416); reserve nectar. Remove cooked clams from shells; chop and set aside. Steam potatoes; set aside. Bring onion, chicken broth and clam nectar to a boil in a stock pot; cover, reduce heat and simmer 30 minutes or until onion is tender. Bring to a second boil. Shake milk and flour in a covered jar to form a smooth paste; gradually add to boiling broth, stirring constantly until thick. Add seasonings, potatoes and clams. Heat thoroughly, but do not allow to boil.

Note: Serve with French bread or cracker bread.

HEARTY CLAM NECTAR

2½	lbs. fresh clams
4	cups clam nectar
½	cup flour
1	cup water
2	stalks celery, cooked and diced
3	carrots, cooked and diced
4	red potatoes or new potatoes, cooked and diced
¾	teaspoon or less salt
⅛-¼	teaspoon black pepper

Steam clams — follow procedure for steamed clams with fresh lemon* (page 416) reserve nectar and bring to a boil. Shake flour and water in covered jar to form a smooth paste; gradually add to boiling broth. Reduce heat and cook 10-15 minutes, stirring constantly. Add remaining ingredients. Heat to serving temperature.

Variation: 1½ cups grated raw potato may be used as a thickener in place of flour and water. Add grated potato directly to boiling broth. Simmer 10-15 minutes — until potato is tender and broth thickened; add remaining ingredients.

Two 6½-oz. cans canned clams with their liquid may be used in place of fresh clams. Add chicken broth* (page 295) if necessary to yield 4 cups nectar.

CREAM OF ASPARAGUS SOUP

2 cups chopped asparagus
3 tablespoons chopped onion
1 recipe cream of chicken soup*
   (page 316)

Steam asparagus and onion; purée in blender. Heat cream of chicken soup gradually over low heat; add asparagus and onion. Heat to serving temperature.

CREAM OF ARTICHOKE SOUP

1 medium onion, chopped
3 celery ribs, chopped
2 leeks with tops, chopped
1 new potato with skin, quartered
6 cups chicken broth* (page 295)
1 15-oz. can artichokes hearts,
   drained and quartered
1½ cups broccoli flowerets, cooked
   until just crisp-tender
   freshly ground pepper

Cook onion, celery, leeks and potato in chicken broth until all vegetables are tender; pour into blender and purée. Return to stock pot; simmer ½ hour. Add artichoke hearts; simmer 10 minutes, add broccoli. Heat to serving temperature. Pass ground pepper.

Variation: Use ¾-pound cooked fresh artichoke hearts in place of the canned.

315

CREAM OF CHICKEN SOUP

2 cups chicken broth* (page 295)
¾ cup grated raw potato

Heat chicken broth to boiling; gradually add grated potato. Simmer 10-25 minutes, stirring frequently until potato is tender and broth has thickened. Pour into blender and purée. Keeps several days in refrigerator.

Variation: As a thickener in place of potato, shake ¼ cup flour and ½ cup water in a covered jar to form a smooth paste; gradually add to boiling broth, stirring constantly until broth has thickened.

HEARTY CREAM OF CHICKEN SOUP

1 recipe cream of chicken soup* (page 316)
½ cup cooked chicken, diced
2 carrots, cooked and diced
2 red potatoes with skins, cooked and diced

Heat cream of chicken soup over low heat; add remaining ingredients and heat to serving temperature.

CREAM OF CELERY SOUP

2 cups chopped celery with leaves
3 tablespoons chopped onion
1 recipe cream of chicken soup*
  (page 316)

Sauté celery and onion in water or small amount of broth until tender. Purée in blender; add to cream of chicken soup; heat to serving temperature.

CREAM OF CUCUMBER SOUP

1½ medium cucumbers, peeled
1 clove garlic
3 tablespoons chopped fresh parsley
1½ tablespoons onion
½ cup chicken broth* (page 295)
1½ tablespoons white wine vinegar
1 cup plain non-fat yogurt* (page 202)

Purée cucumbers, garlic, parsley, and onion in blender; add broth and vinegar. Fold in yogurt. Cover and chill 2 hours. Will keep up to 24 hours in refrigerator.

Variation: Garnish with croutons, sliced green onions, parsley, fresh mint, chopped tomatoes or sunflower seeds.

Note: Refreshing on a hot afternoon.

CREAM OF PEA SOUP

1   10-oz. package frozen peas
½   cup water
¼   teaspoon salt
1   cup chicken broth* (page 295)
2   cups skim milk

Combine peas, water and salt in a medium sauce-pan; bring to a boil, cover and simmer 15 minutes, stirring occasionally. Purée in blender. Heat broth to boiling; combine with peas and pour into soup tureen. Heat milk just to scalding, but do not boil; whirl in blender until frothy. Add to peas and broth.

CREAM OF MUSHROOM SOUP

2   cups beef broth* (page 302)
1   cup grated raw potato
1½ cups diced mushrooms
⅛   teaspoon pepper

Heat broth to boiling; gradually add grated raw potato. Simmer 10-25 minutes, stirring frequently until potato is tender and broth has thickened. Pour into blender and purée. Return to saucepan; add mushrooms. Season. Simmer 15 minutes.

CREAM OF ZUCCHINI SOUP

1½   pounds zucchini, sliced
¼   cup chopped onion
¾   cup water
1   teaspoon or less salt
½   teaspoon sugar
½   teaspoon basil
¼   cup flour
2   cups skim milk
    chopped fresh parsley for garnish

Bring zucchini, onion, water, salt, sugar, and basil to a boil; cover and simmer 15 minutes or until onion is tender. Purée in blender. Return to stock pot. Shake flour and water in a covered jar to form a smooth paste; slowly whisk into zucchini. Heat to serving temperature over low heat. Serve at once or refrigerate until ready to serve.

SANDWICHES

When preparing sandwiches, be creative.

Try a variety of breads, such as Pumpernickel, French, Italian, Sour Dough, Bran Wheat, Whole Grain, Whole Wheat, Bagels, English Muffins, Crumpets, Tortillas, Pita Bread, Cracker Bread and Scandinavian Flat Bread.

Serve breads toasted, untoasted or open-faced.

Top with lettuce, tomato, onion, sprouts, green peppers, mushrooms, safflower mayonnaise and mustard.

Garnish with fresh fruits of the season.

BREAST OF CHICKEN SANDWICH

choice of bread
mayonnaise
cooked chicken breast, thinly sliced
lettuce
sliced tomato

Spread bread with mayonnaise; layer remaining ingredients between slices.

Variation: Substitute turkey for chicken.

CHICKEN SANDWICH FILLING

1   cup cooked chicken, finely chopped
½   cup finely chopped celery
¼   cup finely chopped almonds or waterchestnuts
⅓   cup safflower mayonnaise

Combine ingredients in medium bowl. Toss.

CLUB HOUSE SANDWICH

3   slices toast per sandwich
    lettuce leaves
    cooked chicken breast, sliced
    safflower mayonnaise
    sliced tomato

Top first slice of toast with lettuce, chicken and mayonnaise. Top with second slice of toast; add tomato slices and top with third slice of toast. Slice diagonally into quarters.

FRENCH DIP SANDWICH

    horseradish (optional)
    French rolls
    prime rib, thinly sliced
    beef broth* (page 302)

Spread horseradish lightly over French rolls; top with prime rib. Heat broth to boiling; ladle into shallow bowls for dipping.

BARBECUED BEEF SANDWICH

prime rib, thinly sliced
barbecue sauce
French rolls

Place beef in saucepan; cover with sauce. Warm over low heat. Serve on French rolls or hamburger buns.

Note: Be certain to read the label before selecting a barbecue sauce. There are several acceptable brands on the Positive Diet.

CUBE STEAK SANDWICH

cube steaks
French bread
safflower mayonnaise
white onion slices
tomato slices
lettuce leaves

Place cube steaks on a rack in a broiling pan; broil 3 inches from heat 2-3 minutes on each side. Serve on French bread with mayonnaise, onion, lettuce and tomato.

HOT TUNA SANDWICH

1   6½-oz. can water pack tuna,
      drained
2   tablespoons finely chopped green
      pepper
2   tablespoons finely chopped celery
2   tablespoons finely chopped onion
⅓   cup safflower mayonnaise
      English muffins, halved and toasted
      low-fat Cheddar cheese slices

Combine tuna, green pepper, celery and onion; moisten with mayonnaise. Spread on muffin halves. Place under pre-heated broiler 2-3 minutes. Top with cheese; broil 2-3 minutes or until cheese melts.

TUNA SANDWICH FILLING

½   teaspoon fresh lemon juice
1   6½-oz. can water pack tuna,
      drained
3   tablespoons minced onion
2   tablespoons minced celery
2   tablespoons waterchestnuts, finely
      chopped
⅓   cup safflower mayonnaise
      dash prepared mustard (optional)

Sprinkle lemon juice over tuna; toss with onion, celery and waterchestnuts. Moisten with mayonnaise. Mix with mustard.

HOT CRAB AND CHEESE SANDWICH

- ½ teaspoon fresh lemon juice
- ½ pound crab meat
- 2 tablespoons minced white onion
- 2 tablespoons safflower mayonnaise
  English muffins, halved and toasted
- 1 tomato, sliced
  low-fat Cheddar cheese, sliced

Squeeze lemon juice over crab; toss with onion. Moisten with mayonnaise. Spread over toasted muffin halves. Place under pre-heated broiler 2-3 minutes or until hot; top with tomato and cheese. Broil 3-5 minutes longer or until cheese melts.

CRAB SANDWICH FILLING

- ½ pound crab meat
- 2 tablespoons minced celery
- 2 tablespoons minced white onion
- 3 tablespoons safflower mayonnaise
- ½ teaspoon lemon juice

Combine ingredients in medium bowl. Toss.

LOBSTER SANDWICH FILLING

6   oz. lobster meat
1   teaspoon lemon juice
2   stalks celery, minced
     safflower mayonnaise to moisten

Sprinkle lobster with lemon juice; toss with celery.
Moisten with mayonnaise.
Serve on rye or sourdough bread.

CRUNCHY PEANUT BUTTER SANDWICH

     bran wheat bread
     non-hydrogenated peanut butter
     sunflower seeds

Spread each slice of bread with peanut butter.
Sprinkle with sunflower seeds.

Variation: Add sliced bananas.

TOASTED CHEESE SANDWICH

sliced bread
tub safflower margarine
prepared mustard (optional)
low-fat Cheddar cheese slices

Spread each slice of bread with tub safflower margarine (butter one side only). Spread unbuttered side with mustard; top with cheese. Heat a teflon griddle over medium-high heat; brown sandwiches on both sides until cheese melts.

Variation: Top cheese with sliced tomato and white onion.

MONTE CRISTO

1   6½-oz. can water packed tuna,
        drained
¼   cup safflower mayonnaise
¼   cup egg substitute, beaten
        sliced bread

Moisten tuna with mayonnaise. Dip one slice of bread into beaten egg; place on pre-heated teflon griddle. Spread with tuna. Dip second slice of bread into beaten egg; place over tuna. Brown sandwiches on both sides, turning only once.

Variation: Add sliced tomato or white onion.

LETTUCE AND TOMATO SANDWICH

bread
safflower mayonnaise
tomato slices
black pepper
lettuce

Toast bread; spread with mayonnaise. Sprinkle tomato slices with black pepper. Layer lettuce and tomato between toast slices. Serve at once.

Variation: Top tomatoes with sliced white onion and low-fat Cheddar or Mozzarella cheese slices.

VEGIE SANDWICH

whole grain bread
mayonnaise
sliced cucumber
lettuce
sliced tomato
sliced white onion
sprouts
sunflower seeds
low-fat Cheddar or Mozzarella
    cheese slices

Spread bread with mayonnaise. Layer with remaining ingredients.

CHAPTER FOURTEEN

SALADS AND SALAD DRESSINGS

ANTIPASTO

cherry tomatoes
low-fat Cheddar cheese, cubed
garbanzo beans
baby corn
green onions
asparagus spears, steamed 2-4 minutes
broccoli flowerets, steamed 2-4 minutes
whole string beans, steamed until
    tender
whole baby carrots, steamed until
    tender
cauliflower flowerets
whole baby peppers
artichoke hearts
marinated mushrooms* (page 244)
low-fat Mozzarella cheese, cubed
turkey breast, thinly sliced and rolled
roast beef, thinly sliced and rolled
crab legs
dressing of oil and vinegar* (page 362)
    (optional)
Dijon vinaigrette* (page 361) (optional)

Chill ingredients. Pile cherry tomatoes, Cheddar cheese, or garbanzo beans in the center of a large basket or tray. Surround with remaining vegetables, cheeses and meats.

If desired, drizzle with dressing of oil and vinegar or accompany with Dijon vinaigrette.

Note: For a lighter antipasto, omit meats and cheese.

Variation: In place of artichoke hearts, cook whole artichokes (follow procedure page 243). Cut into quarters or eighths.

331

ANTIPASTO SALAD

bibb lettuce
romaine
red leaf lettuce
dressing of oil and vinegar with
 lemon* (page 362)
cherry tomatoes
baby corn
 marinated mushrooms* (page 244)
peppers
artichoke hearts
crab legs (optional)

Toss equal amounts of bibb lettuce, romaine and red leaf lettuce; moisten with dressing. Serve on chilled salad plates. Arrange tomatoes, baby corn, mushrooms, peppers, artichoke hearts and crab legs on a chilled tray. Pass with salad.

SWEET AND SOUR SALAD

1   bunch fresh spinach
1   cup bean sprouts
1   8-oz. can sliced waterchestnuts,
     drained
    Garlic-French dressing* (page 364)

Chill ingredients. Tear spinach into bite-size pieces; toss with bean sprouts and water-chestnuts. Moisten with dressing.

Variation: Warm dressing. Pour over vegetables.

CAESAR SALAD A LA POSITIVE DIET

1	head romaine, torn into bite-size pieces
1	tablespoon garlic-safflower oil* (page 232)
1	tablespoon olive oil
1¼	tablespoons red wine vinegar
⅓	lemon
2	tablespoons egg substitute
¾	cup croutons
	ground pepper
	dash salt
5-6	tablespoons Sapsago or Somerset or low-fat Mozzarella cheese

Drizzle romaine with garlic-safflower oil, olive oil and vinegar. Squeeze lemon over. Add egg substitute; toss. Add croutons. Season. Sprinkle with cheese. Toss. Serve on chilled salad plates.

Note: Sapsago cheese is closer in flavor to Parmesan; Somerset is milder.

SEVICHE SALAD

Prepare seviche* (page 240) according to recipe, substituting bibb lettuce for parsley.

OVERNIGHT SALAD

1	small head iceberg lettuce, finely chopped
½	cup green onion, thinly sliced
1	cup celery, thinly sliced
1	8-oz. can sliced waterchestnuts, drained
1	10-oz. pkg. frozen baby peas
1½	cups safflower mayonnaise
¼	teaspoon garlic powder
¼	teaspoon pepper
	dash salt
1	cup low-fat Cheddar cheese (optional)
1	tomato, thinly sliced

Using a shallow glass bowl, layer vegetables, except tomatoes, in order given. Spread mayonnaise over top and tightly to edges to seal. Cover; refrigerate overnight. Just before serving, season, sprinkle with cheese and spread tomatoes over top. Do not toss; serve layered.

Variation: Omit garlic powder and pepper. Use ½ teaspoon curry powder.

LAYERED SALAD

½	head cabbage, shredded
½	head lettuce, shredded
½	zucchini, sliced
½	white onion, sliced
10-15	fresh mushrooms, sliced
5	stalks celery, sliced
½	green pepper, chopped
½	red pepper, chopped
2-3	slices crisp-broiled Canadian bacon, finely chopped (optional)
1	bunch broccoli flowerets
1	8-oz. can sliced waterchestnuts drained
½	cup slivered almonds
1	10-oz. pkg. frozen baby peas
1½	cups safflower mayonnaise
1½	cups low-fat Cheddar cheese, grated

Using a large salad bowl layer ingredients, except mayonnaise and cheese, in order given. Spread mayonnaise over top and tightly to edges of bowl to seal. Sprinkle with cheese. Cover with plastic wrap. Chill overnight. Toss before serving. Serves 6 as a main course.

Note: Makes great luncheon fare or light supper. Use the leftovers as the salad course for following dinners. Will keep up to 2 days after being tossed.

STUFFED LETTUCE

1	large head iceberg lettuce
1/2	cup safflower mayonnaise
1/4	teaspoon curry powder
1/2	cup cooked chicken breast
1/4	cup chopped celery
3/4	cup sliced waterchestnuts
1/2	cup chopped onion
1	cup grated, low-fat Cheddar cheese
	tomato salsa* (page 361)

Wash lettuce; remove core and hollow out center, leaving a 1/2"-3/4" shell. Combine mayonnaise and curry powder; toss with waterchestnuts and onion. Spoon into lettuce shell. Chill several hours. Just before serving, slice into wedges. Top with cheese and salsa.

WILTED LETTUCE

2	bunches leaf lettuce
1/3	teaspoon or less salt
1/4	teaspoon pepper
1/3	teaspoon sugar
1/2	white onion, thinly sliced
2	tablespoons olive oil
1/4	cup cider vinegar
2	tablespoons water

Tear lettuce into bite-size pieces; toss with salt, pepper, sugar and onion. Warm olive oil; add vinegar and water, heat to boiling and pour over lettuce. Serve at once.

SPINACH SALAD

1 bunch fresh spinach greens, torn into
    bite-size pieces
¼ pound fresh mushrooms, sliced
3-4 green onions, sliced diagonally
    dressing of fresh lemon and
    olive oil* (page 363)

Combine spinach, mushrooms and onions. Add enough dressing to moisten; toss.

FRESH SPINACH SALAD WITH SESAME SEEDS

1 bunch fresh spinach
½ teaspoon sesame oil
4 teaspoons lemon juice
4 tablespoons toasted sesame seeds

Wash spinach in ice water; dry. Remove and discard thick stems. Tear spinach into bite-sized pieces; toss with sesame oil. Sprinkle with lemon juice and sesame seeds; toss again.

SALAD OF TOMATOES, MOZZARELLA AND BASIL

3 large ripe tomatoes
¾ pound low-fat Mozzarella cheese
3 teaspoons fresh basil
2 tablespoons fresh lemon juice
⅓ cup olive oil
  fresh spinach leaves
  ground black pepper

Cut tomatoes in half; slice each half into 3 wedges. Cut cheese into 1-inch cubes. Mix basil with lemon juice and olive oil; pour just enough over spinach to moisten. Arrange spinach on chilled salad plates. Toss cheese and tomatoes with remaining dressing; arrange over spinach. Sprinkle with black pepper.

Note: To use fresh basil, rather than dried, double the amount and omit the lemon juice.

TOMATO AND CUCUMBER SALAD

½ cup safflower mayonnaise
½ teaspoon finely chopped white onion
1 large ripe tomato
1 medium cucumber, peeled and diced
  lettuce greens
  ground black pepper

Combine mayonnaise and onion; toss with tomato and cucumber. Serve over lettuce. Sprinkle with freshly ground pepper.

TOMATOES VINAIGRETTE

⅓   cup safflower oil
2½ tablespoons olive oil
2½ tablespoons red wine vinegar
¼   teaspoon or less salt
1   clove garlic, minced
¼   teaspoon pepper
¼   teaspoon dry mustard
¾   teaspoon oregano
3   large ripe tomatoes
1   tablespoon finely chopped fresh
       parsley
2   tablespoons finely chopped onion
       salad greens

Combine safflower oil, olive oil, vinegar and seasonings; pour over tomatoes. Refrigerate 3-4 hours or overnight. Just before serving, drain off some of the dressing and toss with the salad greens. Place on chilled salad plates. Toss parsley and onion with tomatoes; arrange over greens.

FRESH TOMATOES WITH ROAST PEPPERS

---

roast peppers* (page 399)
bibb lettuce
sliced tomatoes
roast pepper marinade* (page 399)

Prepare roast peppers according to instructions on page 399. Place lettuce on chilled salad plates; cover with sliced tomatoes. Top with roast peppers; drizzle with roast pepper marinade.

SALAD OF TOMATOES, SPINACH AND CHICKEN

1   medium tomato, diced
½   pound fresh spinach, cut into 2-inch
       pieces
½   pound cooked chicken breast, cut
       into 2-inch cubes
       dressing of fresh lemon and ground
       pepper* (page 363)

Chill tomato, spinach and chicken. Layer spinach on individual salad plates. Cover with diced tomato. Top with chicken. Serve with dressing of fresh lemon and ground pepper.

CUCUMBER AND ONION SALAD

1   cucumber, peeled and thinly sliced
¾   teaspoon salt (to be rinsed off)
½   cup plain non-fat yogurt* (page 202)
2   tablespoons cider vinegar
⅛   teaspoon sugar
1   small white onion, halved and cut into
       rings
2-3 drops Tabasco sauce

Sprinkle cucumber with salt; let stand 30 minutes. Rinse; drain and pat dry. Combine yogurt, vinegar and sugar; pour over cucumbers and onion. Chill 30-60 minutes. Sprinkle with Tabasco sauce.

Variation: Sprinkle with dill seed.

FRESH MUSHROOM SALAD

¼ cup safflower oil
¼ cup olive oil
    juice of ½ lemon plus 3 tablespoons
      lemon juice
½ teaspoon or less salt
¼ teaspoon pepper
1 clove garlic, minced
1 pound fresh mushrooms, thinly
      sliced
4 green onions, thinly sliced

Combine safflower oil, olive oil, 3 tablespoons of lemon juice, salt, pepper and garlic; let stand. Squeeze juice of ½ lemon over mushrooms and green onion; toss with dressing. Serve at once.

SALAD OF FRESH MUSHROOMS AND WATERCHESTNUTS

½ pound fresh mushrooms, sliced
1 8-oz. can sliced waterchestnuts,
      drained
2 tablespoons chopped green onion
3 tablespoons fresh lemon juice
5 tablespoons olive oil
    salt and pepper to taste

Combine all ingredients in a glass salad bowl; let stand 20 minutes. Serve.

SALAD OF GREEN BEANS, TOMATOES, ARTICHOKES AND MUSHROOMS

1   pound fresh green beans, cooked
1   15-oz. can artichoke hearts
1   6-oz. can sliced waterchestnuts
½   pound fresh mushrooms, steamed
      2-3 minutes, sliced
     dressing of oil and vinegar with
      lemon* (page 362)
15   cherry tomatoes, chilled

Drain beans, artichokes, waterchestnuts, and mushrooms. Chill. Just before serving, moisten with dressing; toss with chilled tomatoes.

MEXICAN SALAD

2   ripe tomatoes, chopped
1   3½-oz. can chopped green chilies
4   green onions, chopped
     tortilla chips* (page 256)
1   bunch leaf lettuce, torn into
      bite-size pieces
     dressing of oil and vinegar with
      lemon* (page 362)
¼   pound fresh mushrooms, steamed
      2-3 minutes, sliced

Combine tomatoes, green chilies and onions. Chill for 3 hours. Prepare tortilla chips. Just before serving, moisten lettuce with dressing. Toss with tomatoes, green onions, chilies and mushrooms. Garnish with chips.

ZUCCHINI SALAD

2 small zucchini, peeled and sliced
     lengthwise into julienne strips
     Dijon vinaigrette* (page 361)
     bibb or iceberg lettuce leaves
3 cherry tomatoes, halved, for
     garnish

Toss zucchini with vinaigrette. Line a salad bowl with lettuce; fill with zucchini. Garnish.

ZUCCHINI STUFFED WITH CRAB

4 medium zucchini
2 cups dry white wine
¼ pound fresh mushrooms, sliced
1 teaspoon lemon juice
1 tablespoon grated onion
6 ounces of crab meat
8 artichoke hearts, halved and chilled
½ cup safflower mayonnaise
     cherry tomatoes for garnish

Cut zucchini in half lengthwise; hollow centers by scraping and removing seeds with a spoon. Poach zucchini in wine just until tender, add mushrooms during the final 3 minutes of cooking; drain, sprinkle with lemon juice and chill. Combine mushrooms, onions, crab, artichokes and mayonnaise; chill. Spoon into zucchini boats. Serve on crisp lettuce greens. Garnish with cherry tomatoes.

Variation: Substitute chicken or water-pack tuna for crab.

PAPAYA, CRAB AND CUCUMBER SALAD

```
2    tablespoons safflower oil
1    tablespoon olive oil
1½   teaspoons lemon juice
1½   teaspoons red wine vinegar
1½   teaspoons Dijon mustard
     dash tarragon
1    thinly sliced English cucumber
1¼   cups crab meat
1    fresh papaya halved
1    bunch watercress
```

Shake safflower oil, olive oil, lemon juice, vinegar, mustard and tarragon in covered jar; pour just enough over cucumbers to moisten. Marinate 30 minutes. Just before serving, moisten crab with dressing. Arrange papaya halves on watercress. Fill with crab. Garnish with cucumber.

CRAB STUFFED PEPPERS

1	cup crab meat
1	teaspoon minced onion
1	teaspoon lemon juice
1	cup finely chopped celery
3-4	green peppers
	safflower mayonnaise to moisten
¾	cup hearts of lettuce, diced

Combine crab meat, onion, lemon juice and celery. Chill. Remove tops from green peppers; hollow out insides. Just before serving, toss mayonnaise and lettuce with crab mixture; spoon into green peppers.

Variation: Chicken or salmon may be substituted for crab. Tomatoes may be substituted for peppers.

GREEN GODDESS SALAD

head lettuce, leaf spinach and romaine
yogurt dressing to moisten* (page 365)
croutons
crab legs for garnish

Tear equal amounts head lettuce, leaf spinach and romaine into bite-sized pieces; toss with yogurt dressing. Top with croutons. Garnish with crab legs.

STUFFED ARTICHOKE SALAD

2   fresh artichokes, cooked
1   cup crab meat
3   tablespoons chopped green pepper
2   tablespoons finely chopped onion
1   teaspoon lemon juice
¼   cup safflower mayonnaise
½   cup grated low-fat Cheddar cheese
    tomato slices for garnish

Remove small center leaves of each artichoke, leaving a cup; carefully remove choke. Toss crab meat, green pepper, onion, lemon juice, mayonnaise and cheese; stuff artichokes. Place in baking dish; add water — just to cover bottom of dish. Cover and bake at 375° 35 minutes or until hot. Garnish with tomato slices.

Note: This is also delicious cold. To serve cold, chill ingredients. Fill artichokes just before serving.

Variation: Cooked chicken may be substituted for crab.

Helpful Hint: To make a giant, colossal tossed green salad for a large group or party, tear the lettuce, romaine, spinach or Swiss chard apart as usual. Place loosely in a pillow case, knot, and put in the washing machine on the cold water setting of the rinse cycle. Then, spin dry. If leaves are still too wet, repeat the spin dry cycle a second time. The greens will be cold, crisp, and ready to break into bite-size pieces.

Note: Before doing this, I disinfect the washing machine and run it through the rise and spin dry cycle.

CRAB LOUIS

1 head lettuce
½ pound crab meat
¼ cup sliced waterchestnuts
2 stalks celery, thinly sliced
3 green onions with tops, thinly
   sliced
½ green pepper, chopped
2 tomatoes, cut into wedges
1 bunch asparagus spears, steamed
   2-4 minutes
   lemon wedges

Dressing:
¾ cup safflower mayonnaise
2 tablespoons lemon juice
2 tablespoons grated onion

Combine mayonnaise, lemon juice and onion; chill 30 minutes. Line chilled salad bowls with outside leaves of lettuce; shred remaining lettuce. Toss shredded lettuce, crab, waterchestnuts, celery, green onion and green pepper with dressing to moisten; spoon into lettuce-lined bowls. Garnish with tomatoes, asparagus and lemon wedges.

SALAD NIÇOISE

3	red potatoes, cooked *al dente*, and thinly sliced
½-¾	pound fresh green beans, cooked *al dente*, and sliced diagonally into thirds
8-10	artichoke hearts, quartered
3	carrots, cooked *al dente*, and thinly sliced
½	white onion, thinly sliced and separated into rings
½	green pepper, cut into rings
½	red pepper, cut into rings
1	bunch leaf lettuce, torn into bite-size pieces
1-2	cans water-packed tuna fish, drained and flaked
1½	tablespoons chopped fresh parsley ground pepper
6-8	cherry or plum tomatoes, halved

Dressing:

½	cup olive oil
½	cup safflower oil
¼	cup tarragon-flavored vinegar
2	tablespoons fresh lemon juice
1	clove garlic, chopped
1½	teaspoons dry mustard
¾	teaspoon or less salt
½	teaspoon pepper

Combine ingredients for dressing; pour over vegetables. Chill 3-4 hours, stirring often. Arrange lettuce on a medium tray; mound tuna in center. Drain vegetables, reserving dressing, and arrange in piles around tuna. Sprinkle with parsley and ground pepper. Garnish with tomatoes. Drizzle with reserved dressing.

HOT TUNA SALAD

2 cans water-packed tuna, drained
3 stalks celery, thinly sliced
½ green pepper, chopped
½ cup waterchestnuts, sliced
1 tablespoon fresh lemon juice
1 tablespoon grated onion
⅔ cup safflower mayonnaise
2 cups grated low-fat Cheddar cheese
½ cup crushed corn flakes (optional)

Combine ingredients except cheese and corn flakes. Place in individual baking shells. Broil 10 minutes or until hot. Top with cheese; sprinkle with corn flakes. Bake 3-5 minutes or until cheese melts.

Variation: Chicken may be substituted for tuna fish and Mozzarella cheese for Cheddar.

CHICKEN SALAD

2 teaspoons lemon juice
2 cooked chicken breasts, cubed
2 stalks celery, diced
¼ cup slivered almonds
safflower mayonnaise
salt and pepper to taste
4 small tomatoes or green peppers
fresh spinach greens

Squeeze lemon juice over chicken, add celery and almonds; toss. Moisten with mayonnaise. Season. Cut tops from tomatoes; hollow out centers and fill with chicken. Serve on spinach-lined plates.

CHEF'S SALAD

- ½ lemon
- 1 clove garlic, cut
  ground pepper
- 1 bunch leaf lettuce, torn into bite-size pieces
- 1 cup cooked chicken, turkey or roast beef
- ½ cup low-fat Mozzarella cheese
- ½ cup low-fat Cheddar cheese
- 1 bunch radishes, flowered
- 2 tomatoes, cut into wedges
- 1 bunch cooked asparagus, chilled

Chill salad plates; rub with lemon and garlic and sprinkle with pepper. Cover with lettuce. Cut meat and cheese into thin strips; arrange over lettuce. Garnish with radishes, tomatoes and asparagus. Serve with selected dressing.

TACO SALAD

1   pound extra-lean ground round
1   onion, chopped
2   tomatoes, chopped
1   head lettuce
2   cups grated low-fat Cheddar cheese
    tortilla chips* (page 256)
    plain non-fat yogurt* (page 202)
    tomato salsa* (page 361)

Brown ground round with onion; drain. Toss with tomatoes. Line salad bowls with outside leaves of lettuce; shred remaining lettuce and add to bowls. Cover with ground round and tomatoes. Top with cheese. Line rim of bowl with chips. Pass with yogurt and salsa.

Note: One package unsalted, baked in safflower oil, taco chips may be used in place of homemade chips.

SUPER TACO SALAD

1	1-lb. can tomatoes with liquid
¼	teaspoon or less salt
¾	teaspoon dry mustard
1¼	teaspoons chili powder
1	small clove garlic, minced
¾	pound cooked chicken breast, cubed
1	1-lb. can kidney beans with liquid or 1½ cups homecooked kidney beans plus ½ cup liquid
½	head lettuce, chopped
1	medium onion, chopped
2	cups low-fat Cheddar or Mozzarella cheese, grated
	tortilla chips* (page 256)
	tomato salsa* (page 361) (optional)
	plain non-fat yogurt* (page 202) (optional)

Combine tomatoes, salt, mustard, chili powder and garlic; heat just to boiling. Reduce heat and simmer 5 minutes; add chicken. Simmer 5 more minutes; add kidney beans. Heat. Spoon into bowls. Top with lettuce, onion, cheese, tortilla chips, salsa and yogurt, as desired.

Note: Prepare tortilla chips according to instructions in appetizer section or use 1 package unsalted, baked in safflower oil, taco chips.

Variation: Substitute 1-lb. extra lean ground round for chicken.

POTATO SALAD

4	new potatoes, with skins, cooked and diced
¾	cup chopped white onion
1½	cups finely chopped celery
½	green pepper, chopped
½	cup chopped green onion
1	8-oz. can sliced waterchestnuts, drained
1	tablespoon prepared mustard
¾	cup safflower mayonnaise
½	teaspoon or less salt
¼	teaspoon pepper
¼	teaspoon dill weed
1	tablespoon finely chopped parsley

Toss potatoes, onion, celery, green pepper, green onion, and waterchestnuts; chill. Combine mustard, mayonnaise, salt, pepper, dill weed, and parsley; chill. One hour before serving, toss potatoes and vegetables with dressing (use dressing sparingly, just to moisten).

CURRIED POTATO SALAD

2	pounds new potatoes
1	cup safflower mayonnaise
1	tablespoon lemon juice
¼	teaspoon curry powder

Steam potatoes, drain, peel and slice. Blend mayonnaise, lemon juice and curry. Fold in potatoes. Chill and serve.

HOT POTATO SALAD

4	medium red potatoes, thinly sliced
1	cup chopped onion
3	tablespoons olive oil
2	tablespoons flour
1	teaspoon sugar
½	teaspoon celery seed
½	teaspoon or less salt
	dash pepper
⅔	cup water
⅓	cup cider vinegar

Put potatoes and onion in vegetable steamer basket over boiling water; cover and steam 15-20 minutes or until potatoes are tender. Set aside. Warm oil; blend in flour, sugar, celery seed, salt, pepper, water and vinegar. Bring to a boil, stirring constantly. Boil 1 minute; gently stir in potatoes and onions. Remove from heat; cover, let stand 5 minutes or until ready to serve.

Variation: Crisp-broil 2 slices Canadian bacon; finely chop. Sprinkle over potatoes.

MACARONI SALAD

¾	cup safflower mayonnaise
1	tablespoon prepared mustard
1	tablespoon cider vinegar
1	tablespoon safflower oil
⅓	teaspoon or less salt
¼	teaspoon pepper
¼	teaspoon dill weed
1	tablespoon finely chopped parsley
2½	cups cooked elbow macaroni
¾	cup chopped white onion
½	cup chopped green onion
1½	cups finely chopped celery

Combine mayonnaise, mustard, vinegar, oil, salt, pepper, dill weed and parsley; pour over macaroni, onions and celery. Toss. Chill several hours.

THREE BEAN SALAD

¾	lb. green beans, cooked, drained and sliced on the diagonal into thirds
2	cups cooked kidney beans
1	8-oz. can garbanzo beans, drained
1	white onion, chopped
1	green pepper, chopped
2-3	stalks celery, chopped
¾	teaspoon or less sugar
1	recipe dressing of oil and vinegar* (page 362)

Toss beans with onion, green pepper and celery. Set aside. Add sugar to oil and vinegar dressing; pour over vegetables and toss. Chill 3-4 hours.

Note: A 1-lb. can of cut green beans and a 1-lb. can of kidney beans may be used in place of the fresh.

COLESLAW

½	cup safflower mayonnaise
2	tablespoons rice vinegar
1	teaspoon Dijon mustard
½	head cabbage, shredded
½	green pepper, finely chopped
½	white onion, finely chopped

Combine mayonnaise, vinegar and mustard. Chill. Just before serving, toss cabbage, green pepper and onion; moisten with dressing.

WATERMELON SALAD

1   watermelon
1   honeydew melon
1   cantaloupe
2   pounds grapes
1   quart strawberries
1   quart raspberries
1   quart blueberries
    fresh mint for garnish

Pick a rolly-polly watermelon. Cut lengthwise from each end, toward center, slicing off top third. Leave a center portion 2½" wide for the handle. Using a serrated knife, make big scallops around the top edge of the watermelon.

With a melon baller, form balls from watermelon, honeydew and cantaloupe. Toss with grapes and berries. Scrape inside of watermelon with a spoon to remove excess melon. Fill with fruit. Tie a bow on the basket handle to coordinate with table setting and napkins. Garnish with fresh mint. Serves 8-10.

Note: At the end of the meal, rinse watermelon basket; pat dry and freeze for later use.

SUMMER SALAD

¼	watermelon
½	cantaloupe
½	honeydew melon
1	pound grapes
1	pint strawberries
1	pint raspberries
1	pint cherries
1	pint blueberries

Remove rind from melons. Slice melons into wedges. Stem grapes. Hull strawberries. Pile strawberries in the center of a large basket or tray; surround with watermelon, honeydew, cantaloupe, raspberries and cherries. Garnish with grapes and blueberries. Serves 8-10.

CRANBERRY RELISH

1	pound (4 cups) fresh cranberries
2	oranges, cut into eighths
2	red delicious apples, cut into eighths
⅓	cup sugar or to taste

Wash cranberries (discard any that are soft or blemished). Wash oranges; do not peel. Put cranberries, apples, and oranges through medium blade of a grinder or food processor. Drain off excess juice; reserve. Add sugar; stir. Pour ½-¾ of the reserved juice into the relish (relish should be very moist, but not runny). Chill 24 hours. Keeps 2-3 weeks. Yields 2 quarts.

WINTER SALAD

3 oranges
2 satsumas or tangerines
½ pound purple or black grapes
1 papaya
1 fresh pineapple
2 bananas — dip in lemon juice;
    sprinkle with walnuts
10 figs
10 dates
2 apples — dip in lemon juice
1 cup frozen blueberries for garnish

Peel oranges and tangerines; divide into segments and remove skin and membranes. Stem grapes. Cut papaya in half; scrape seeds. Carefully cut out pulp, leaving shell intact. Slice pulp and return to papaya boat. Lay pineapple on its side. Slice off upper ⅓, leaving stem intact. Using a curved grapefruit knife, remove pineapple from shell; cut into spears. Return to pineapple boat.

To serve: Place pineapple boat in center of a large basket or tray. Position papaya boats on each side. Surround with remaining fruits. Garnish with blueberries. Serves 8-10.

Helpful Hint: To freeze strawberries, raspberries, blueberries, blackberries or huckleberries, wash berries; pat dry. Place in a single layer on a baking sheet. Freeze 2-3 hours. Remove from freezer and quickly place in covered freezer containers. Return to freezer. Berries will not stick together and may be removed individually as needed for garnish. They may also be puréed and used on bread or toast in place of jam.

SAFFLOWER MAYONNAISE

1   egg
1   teaspoon red wine vinegar
2   teaspoons fresh lemon juice
1   teaspoon Dijon mustard
½   teaspoon or less salt
¼   cup olive oil
1¼ cups safflower oil

Combine first six ingredients in blender; whirl. With machine running, add safflower oil, one tablespoon at a time. Refrigerate. Keeps several weeks. Yield: 1½ cups.

Variation: To make herbed mayonnaise, add ½ teaspoon basil, dill, tarragon or parsley just before serving.

PRIMAVERA DRESSING

⅓   cup safflower oil
¼   cup olive oil
¼   cup cider vinegar
½   teaspoon Dijon mustard
    salt to taste
    pepper to taste

Combine oils, vinegar, and mustard in covered jar; shake. Drizzle over salad greens. Season to taste.

DIJON VINAIGRETTE

```
 4   tablespoons Dijon mustard
 3   tablespoons red wine vinegar
 1   tablespoon white wine vinegar
 ¼   teaspoon salt
1-2  cloves garlic
 ½   teaspoon basil
 ⅛   teaspoon black pepper
 2   drops hot sauce
 1   tablespoon grated onion
12   tablespoons safflower oil
```

Combine mustard and vinegar in blender. Add salt, garlic, basil, black pepper, hot sauce and onion; whirl. With machine running, add oil, one tablespoon at a time. Chill. Keeps several weeks. Yield: 1¼ cups.

TOMATO SALSA

```
 4   whole Jalapeno peppers
1-2  fresh tomatoes, chopped
 1   1-lb. can plum tomatoes with liquid
 ¼   teaspoon cumin (optional)
 ¼   teaspoon cayenne (optional)
```

Dice peppers, fresh tomatoes and canned tomatoes into 1-inch pieces. Combine in covered jar. Chill. Season.

Variation: For a hotter sauce, add Tabasco sauce to taste.

Note: Great as a salad dressing or as a dip.

DRESSING OF OIL AND VINEGAR

- ½ cup safflower oil
- ¼ cup olive oil
- ¼ cup cider vinegar
- ¾ teaspoon or less salt
- ¼ teaspoon pepper

Combine ingredients in covered jar; shake. Yield: 1 cup.

Variation: To make creamy Italian dressing, add ⅓ cup safflower mayonnaise.

DRESSING OF OIL AND VINEGAR WITH LEMON

- ½ cup safflower oil
- ¼ cup cider vinegar
- 3 tablespoons fresh lemon juice
- ½ teaspoon or less salt
  dash pepper
- 1 clove garlic

Combine ingredients in a covered jar; shake. Yield: 1 cup.

Variation: Substitute olive oil for safflower oil or add ¼-½ teaspoon dry mustard powder.

DRESSING OF FRESH LEMON

juice of ½ lemon
ground pepper

Squeeze lemon over salad greens or vegetables;
sprinkle with freshly ground pepper.

DRESSING OF FRESH LEMON AND OLIVE OIL

2   tablespoons fresh lemon juice
6   tablespoons olive oil
    ground pepper
    salt to taste

Combine ingredients in covered jar; shake. Drizzle over salad greens and season to taste.

DRESSING OF FRESH LEMON AND DRY MUSTARD

¼   cup fresh lemon juice
¼   teaspoon dry mustard
¼   teaspoon ground pepper
1   teaspoon chopped fresh parsley

Prepare dressing. Use at once.

GARLIC FRENCH DRESSING

⅓ cup safflower oil
⅓ cup olive oil
2½ teaspoons cider vinegar
¼ teaspoon sugar
¼ teaspoon dry mustard
4 cloves garlic
salt and pepper to taste

Combine ingredients in covered jar; shake. Let set 3-4 days before using. Drizzle over salad greens. Season with salt and liberally with pepper. Yield: ¾ cup.

CREAMY FRENCH DRESSING

½ cup safflower mayonnaise
1 tablespoon cider vinegar
1 tablespoon skim milk
½ teaspoon paprika
¼ teaspoon dry mustard
⅛ teaspoon salt

Combine ingredients in medium bowl; beat with wire whisk. Chill

RUSSIAN DRESSING

½ cup safflower mayonnaise
2 tablespoons ketchup
1 teaspoon lemon juice
2 tablespoons grated onion
   dash horseradish

Combine ingredients with wire whisk. Chill.

THOUSAND ISLAND DRESSING

½ cup ketchup
¼ cup safflower mayonnaise
1 tablespoon minced green pepper

Combine ketchup and mayonnaise. Chill. Stir in green pepper.

YOGURT DRESSING

---

1 cup safflower mayonnaise
½ cup plain non-fat yogurt* (page 202)
3 tablespoons chopped green onion
¼ cup dried parsley flakes
2 tablespoons tarragon flavor vinegar
2 tablespoons lemon juice
1 clove garlic, minced
⅛ teaspoon pepper

Combine ingredients with wire whisk. Chill 3 hours.

365

CHAPTER FIFTEEN

VEGETABLES

NOTES ON COOKING VEGETABLES: There is no more heart-healthy fare than vegetables. To preserve the natural sugars and nutrients of vegetables do not wash them until just prior to cooking. The most important rule about cooking vegetables is not to overcook — cook until just crisp-tender and still very colorful.

TO STEAM VEGETABLES: Bring 1-2 inches of water to a boil in a medium saucepan. Place vegetables in a steamer basket and place the basket over the boiling water. Cover saucepan with a tight fitting lid. Steam until vegetables are crisp-tender and still very colorful.

TO BOIL VEGETABLES: Bring a small amount of water or broth to a boil — use the smallest amount possible. Add vegetables; bring to a second boil. Cover; reduce heat. Cook at a gentle boil until crisp-tender and rich in color.

TO COOK FROZEN VEGETABLES: Follow package directions; omit salt.

TO STIR-FRY VEGETABLES: Slice vegetables to a uniform thickness of about ⅛th of an inch. Heat a small amount of chicken broth* (page 295) or beef broth* (page 302) in a wok or heavy skillet over high heat. Add vegetables requiring longest cooking time first; gradually add remaining vegetables. Stir rapidly with long chopsticks or flat wooden spoon until vegetables show signs of wilting slightly. Lower heat. Cover with lid — leave on only briefly, just until vegetables are crisp-tender. Serve at once.

TO OVEN-ROAST VEGETABLES: Pare and quarter such vegetables as potatoes, celery, carrots, onions and green peppers. Place on rack in baking dish; add ½ cup water, wine or broth. Cover. Steam 30-40 minutes or until tender. If using mushrooms, tomatoes or artichoke hearts, they should be added the last 15 minutes.

TO MICROWAVE VEGETABLES: Vegetables cooked in the microwave retain their bright color and freshness as well as their vitamins and minerals since they are usually cooked with little or no additional water. For correct cooking procedure and timing for individual vegetables, consult a microwave manual.

TO BLANCH VEGETABLES: Bring 1-2 inches of water to a boil in a medium saucepan. Place vegetables in a steamer basket and place the basket over the boiling water. Cover saucepan with a tight fitting lid. Reduce regular cooking time by ¾. For example, regular cooking time for fresh peas is 3-5 minutes, so the blanching time would be 45-80 seconds — at this point vegetables will be rich in color and translucent. Immediately plunge vegetables into ice water to stop additional cooking. Consult a vegetable blanching and freezing chart for blanching times for individual vegetables.

FRESH ARTICHOKES

2-3	fresh artichokes
3	tablespoons chopped onion
3	cloves garlic
1½	cups dry white wine
2	tablespoons olive oil
¼	cup safflower oil
	dash salt
⅛	teaspoon pepper
1	lemon, sliced

Wash artichokes. Cut 1-inch off of top; cut off stem and tips of leaves. Brush cut edges with lemon juice. Combine remaining ingredients. Bring to a boil. Place artichokes upright in mixture; cover and simmer until bottom leaves pull off easily. Drain. Serve hot or cold with homemade safflower mayonnaise* (page 360) or Dijon vinaigrette* (page 361).

Note: Artichokes are delicious cooked in the microwave. Follow the recipe Fresh Artichokes With Lemon* (page 243).

ARTICHOKE HEARTS WITH LEMON, GARLIC AND OLIVE OIL

fresh artichoke hearts
fresh lemon juice
2 cloves garlic
olive oil
black pepper

Cook artichokes. Remove hearts; quarter. Squeeze lemon juice over. Set aside. Heat garlic and enough olive oil to cover artichokes; pour over artichokes. Toss gently to coat. Sprinkle with black pepper.

BREADED ARTICHOKE HEARTS

¼ teaspoon sage
¼ teaspoon thyme
dash pepper
¼ cup bread crumbs
1 15-oz. can artichoke hearts
½ cup egg substitute

Mix sage, thyme, pepper and bread crumbs. Set aside. Rinse artichokes; drain. Dip in egg, then into bread crumbs. Cook in a teflon skillet over medium-high heat until lightly browned.

FRESH ASPARAGUS WITH LEMON

1   pound fresh asparagus
     juice of ½ lemon

Wash asparagus; snap stalks. Place on vegetable steamer rack over boiling water; cover and steam 5-6 minutes — just until barely tender.

To microwave, arrange asparagus in a single layer, tender tips toward center, in a microwave-proof baking dish; cover with plastic wrap, prick with a fork to allow steam to escape. Cook 3-4 minutes — just until barely tender. Drizzle with lemon juice.

Variation: Omit lemon juice. Serve with homemade safflower mayonnaise* (page 360) or Dijon vinaigrette* (page 361).

CELERY REMOULADE

1   pound fresh celery root
1   recipe Dijon vinaigrette* (page 361)
     fresh parsley
     ripe tomatoes, sliced into wedges

Steam celery root until tender; drain. Toss with just enough Dijon vinaigrette to moisten. Chill 2-3 hours. Garnish with fresh parsley and ripe tomatoes.

GREEN BEANS WITH FRESH LEMON AND TARRAGON

¾   pound fresh green beans
⅓   cup safflower oil
3   tablespoons olive oil
½   cup fresh lemon juice
2   cloves garlic, minced
1   teaspoon dried tarragon or
    1 tablespoon fresh tarragon
1   teaspoon oregano
⅛   teaspoon salt
⅛   teaspoon black pepper

Wash beans; remove ends and strings. Place in vegetable steamer rack over boiling water; steam 15-25 minutes or until tender. Combine remaining ingredients; pour over cooked beans. Serve hot or cold.

GREEN BEANS, ITALIAN STYLE

1   pound fresh green beans
½   cup chicken broth* (page 295)
2   tablespoons safflower oil
2   cups canned plum tomatoes
    dash oregano
    salt to taste
    pepper to taste

Wash beans. Remove ends and strings; cut on the diagonal into 1-inch pieces. Set aside. Combine remaining ingredients and bring to a boil. Add beans; cook covered 15-25 minutes or until beans are tender.

GREEN BEANS WITH MUSHROOMS AND PECANS

¾ pound fresh green beans
½ pound fresh mushrooms, sliced
3 chopped green onions with tops
¼ cup fresh lemon juice
2 tablespoons safflower oil
2 tablespoons olive oil
½ teaspoon or less salt
¼ teaspoon pepper
½ cup walnut or pecan halves

Wash beans. Remove ends and strings; cut on the diagonal into thirds. Place on a vegetable steamer rack over boiling water; steam until just tender 15-20 minutes (do not overcook). Combine beans with mushrooms and green onions; toss with lemon juice, safflower oil, olive oil, salt and pepper. Stir in walnuts or pecans. Serve hot or cold.

GREEN BEANS WITH LEMON AND BLACK PEPPER

¾ pound fresh green beans
1 sprig dill (optional)
 juice of ½ lemon
 black pepper

Place beans in vegetable steamer rack over boiling water; sprinkle with dill and lemon juice. Steam 4-6 minutes; sprinkle with pepper. Cook 15-25 minutes or until beans are tender.

GREEN BEANS WITH MUSHROOMS AND WATERCHESTNUTS

¾ pound fresh green beans
½ pound fresh mushrooms, sliced
1 8-oz. can sliced waterchestnuts
2 tablespoons lemon juice
¼ teaspoon or less salt
⅛ teaspoon pepper

Place beans in a vegetable steamer over boiling water; cook 15-25 minutes or until beans are nearly tender. Add mushrooms the last 5 minutes, add waterchestnuts the last 3 minutes. Spoon beans into serving bowl; toss with lemon juice, salt and pepper.

STIR-FRIED BROCCOLI

---

1 large bunch broccoli
½ cup chicken broth* (page 295)
1 teaspoon sesame oil
2 teaspoons cornstarch
2 tablespoons water
3 tablespoons sesame seeds

Wash broccoli; cut flowerets from stems and set aside. Peel stems; cut diagonally into ¼-inch pieces. Heat chicken broth and sesame oil in wok or heavy skillet. Stir-fry stems 2 minutes; add flowerets, stir-fry 2 more minutes. Add cornstarch dissolved in 2 tablespoons water and toss quickly to coat and glaze broccoli. Sprinkle with sesame seeds.

FRESH BROCCOLI WITH SAFFLOWER MAYONNAISE

---

1   bunch fresh broccoli
1   recipe safflower mayonnaise*
     (page 360)

Wash broccoli; remove outer leaves and tough part of stalks. Place on a vegetable steamer rack over boiling water; cover and steam 5-10 minutes — just until tender. Do not overcook.

To microwave, arrange broccoli in a single layer, flowerets toward center, in a microwave-proof baking dish. Cover with plastic wrap; prick with a fork to allow steam to escape. Cook 3-4 minutes — just until barely tender. Serve with homemade safflower mayonnaise.

Variation: Serve with Dijon vinaigrette* (page 361) or squeeze the juice of ½ lemon over broccoli.

DIJON VEGETABLES

---

     broccoli flowerets
     cauliflower flowerets
     cherry tomatoes, halved
1   recipe Dijon vinaigrette* (page 361)
     poppy seeds

Steam broccoli and cauliflower until barely tender. Chill. Toss tomatoes and cauliflower in just enough vinaigrette to moisten. Chill 4-6 hours. Just before serving, lightly coat broccoli with vinaigrette. Place tomatoes and cauliflower in serving bowl; ring with broccoli. Sprinkle with poppy seeds.

NIPPY CARROTS

 1   bunch fresh carrots, peeled
 ½   cup chicken broth* (page 295)
      tub safflower margarine
1½ teaspoons horseradish
 ½   cup safflower mayonnaise
      ground pepper
 ¼   cup bread crumbs

Slice carrots diagonally into ¼-inch pieces. Cook in chicken broth until crisp-tender; drain, reserving ¼ cup broth — add more chicken broth if necessary to get ¼ cup. Grease an ovenproof dish with tub safflower margarine; add carrots. Mix broth, horseradish, mayonnaise, and pepper; spread over carrots. Top with bread crumbs. Bake at 375° for 15 minutes

Variation: In place of carrots and black pepper, use 1 large bunch fresh spinach greens and ½ teaspoon nutmeg.

CORN ON THE COB

fresh corn
fresh lemons
ground pepper

Husk corn; remove silks. Place on vegetable steamer rack over boiling water; cover and steam 6-8 minutes.

To microwave, place ears in oblong microwave dish; cover with wax paper. Cook 4-6 minutes for 2 ears; 7-8 minutes for 4 ears. Turn once during cooking time.

Squeeze fresh lemon juice over corn. Sprinkle with ground pepper.

Variation: Sprinkle with garlic powder, onion powder, chili powder or black pepper.

BARBECUED EGGPLANT

1   medium eggplant, unpeeled
⅓   cup olive oil
2   tablespoons tarragon white wine
      vinegar
1   clove garlic, minced
⅛   teaspoon or less salt
¼   teaspoon oregano

Cut eggplant lengthwise into 8 wedges. Combine oil, vinegar, garlic, salt and oregano in a covered jar; shake. Pour over eggplant. Drain excess oil. Grill eggplant slices over hot coals until tender, turning once.

BAKED EGGPLANT

1   medium onion, chopped
1   clove garlic, minced
2   tablespoons red wine
1   1-lb. can plum tomatoes
1   8-oz. can tomato sauce
⅓   cup tomato paste
2   teaspoons oregano
½   pound fresh mushrooms, sliced
1   medium eggplant
⅓   cup flour
1   cup egg substitute, beaten
1   cup bread crumbs
8   oz. Mozzarella cheese, sliced

Sauté onion and garlic in red wine until tender; add tomatoes, tomato sauce, tomato paste, oregano and mushrooms. Bring to a boil; reduce heat and simmer uncovered for 30 minutes.

Cut eggplant crosswise into ¼-inch slices; coat with flour. Dip into egg substitute, then into bread crumbs. Cook in a teflon skillet until lightly browned, turning once.

In the bottom of a 13x9x2-inch baking dish, spread ½ of the tomato mixture, layer half of the eggplant slices, top with cheese and spread with sauce. Repeat layers. Pour remaining sauce over top. Bake uncovered at 350° for 20-30 minutes.

BAKED EGGPLANT PROVENCALE

1	medium eggplant, sliced into ½-inch rounds
3	tablespoons safflower oil
1	tablespoon olive oil
2	cloves garlic, minced
1	medium onion, sliced
2	tomatoes, sliced into ¼-inch pieces
¼	cup safflower mayonnaise
⅛	teaspoon pepper
½	teaspoon oregano
2	tablespoons chopped fresh parsley
¾	cup low-fat Mozzarella cheese, grated

Arrange eggplant slices in a single layer on a teflon baking sheet. Combine safflower oil, olive oil and garlic; brush over eggplant. Bake uncovered at 425° for 15 minutes or until tender. Top with onion; bake 5 minutes longer. Top with tomato, spread with mayonnaise, sprinkle with black pepper, oregano and parsley; bake 10 minutes longer. Top with cheese; bake 3 minutes or until cheese melts.

RATATOUILLE

1   medium eggplant, cut into 1-inch cubes
1   large onion, sliced into rings
3   medium zucchini, cut into ½-inch slices
2   green peppers, seeded and cut into ½-inch pieces
3   large tomatoes, chopped
1   cup minced fresh parsley
½   teaspoon salt
1   tablespoon fresh basil or ½ teaspoon dried basil
4   cloves garlic, pressed
2   tablespoons olive oil
2   tablespoons safflower oil
   ground pepper to taste

Layer vegetables in a deep casserole; sprinkle with parsley, salt, basil and garlic. Drizzle with olive and safflower oil. Chill overnight. Bake covered in a 350° oven for 3 hours. Sprinkle with ground pepper. Serve.

VEGETABLES ORIENTAL

1   10-oz. package green peas
1   6-oz. package pea pods
1   8-oz. can waterchestnuts
¼   lb. fresh mushrooms, steamed 2-3
    minutes and sliced
1   cup bean sprouts

Cook peas and pea pods according to package directions; drain. Add remaining ingredients; heat briefly.

Note: Whenever possible use fresh peas and pea pods in place of frozen.

GRILLED VEGETABLES

    cherry tomatoes
    artichoke hearts
    fresh mushrooms
    onions, cut into 2-inch cubes
    green peppers, cut into 2-inch cubes
⅓   cup safflower oil
2   tablespoons red wine vinegar
¼   teaspoon or less salt
⅛   teaspoon pepper

Marinate vegetables 1-4 hours in oil, vinegar, salt and pepper; drain, reserving marinade. Alternate vegetables on skewers. Broil 4-inches from heat, turning often and basting frequently.

STIR-FRIED VEGETABLES

chicken broth* (page 295)
onions, sliced into 1/16th-inch
    pieces
carrots, cut crosswise into rounds
celery, cut diagonally into 1-inch
    pieces
broccoli flowerets
green peppers, cut into strips
sliced mushrooms
pea pods
sliced waterchestnuts
bean sprouts

Heat small amount of chicken broth in wok or heavy skillet; add vegetables, beginning with those requiring the most cooking time. Stir-fry until all vegetables are just crisp-tender, add more broth as needed.

Note: If using a wok, pull vegetables up onto side of pan as they finish cooking.

Variation: Toss stir-fried vegetables with cooked Buckwheat (soba) noodles, asparagus, scallops or chicken.

SAUTÈED MUSHROOMS

---

3 tablespoons white wine or vermouth
1 clove garlic
1 pound fresh mushrooms, caps or
   pieces

Heat wine or vermouth and garlic in a heavy skillet. Add mushrooms. Cook uncovered over medium heat, stirring frequently 3-4 minutes.

Variations: Use 2 tablespoons wine or vermouth plus 1 tablespoon olive oil or safflower oil.

Use 3 tablespoons lemon juice; omit garlic.

SAUTÈED VEGETABLES

¼ cup white wine or vermouth
1 clove garlic
1 pound fresh mushrooms, caps or
   pieces
1 15-oz. can quartered artichoke
   hearts, drained
10 cherry tomatoes

Heat wine or vermouth and garlic in a heavy skillet; add mushrooms and artichokes. Cook uncovered over medium heat, stirring frequently 3-4 minutes. Add tomatoes; toss.

Variations: Use 2 tablespoons wine or vermouth plus 1 tablespoon olive oil or safflower oil.

Use ¼ cup lemon juice; omit the garlic.

Add chopped onion and chopped green pepper.

ONION RINGS

3 large white onions
1 cup flour
¼ teaspoon or less salt
¼ cup egg substitute
1 cup skim milk
1 tablespoon safflower oil

Cut onions into rings ½-inch thick. Mix flour and salt. Beat egg substitute; add milk and oil. Gradually add to flour; beat with wire whisk until smooth. Dip onion into batter; let drain on wire rack. Heat a small amount of safflower oil in a heavy skillet; cook onions 4-5 minutes. Turn; cook 2-3 minutes.

Variation: In place of onions substitute cauliflowerets, or eggplant cut into strips ½-inch thick and ½-inch long, or carrots cut crosswise into rounds.

ONIONS VINAIGRETTE

1 large white onion
dressing of oil and vinegar* (page 362)
basil
pepper

Slice onions into very thin rings. Drizzle with dressing of oil and vinegar. Sprinkle lightly with basil and freshly ground pepper.

BAKED ONIONS

½ cup safflower oil
3 tablespoons wine vinegar
¼ teaspoon basil
¼ teaspoon thyme
¼ teaspoon oregano
¼ teaspoon pepper
⅛ teaspoon salt
2 large onions, sliced into rings

Combine all ingredients, except onions, in a covered jar; shake. Pour over onions. Chill overnight, turning 2-3 times. Bake covered at 350° for 30 minutes. Uncover; bake 30 minutes longer or until onions are tender.

FRIED ONIONS

⅓ cup chicken broth* (page 295) or
    beef broth* (page 302)
2 medium onions, thinly sliced into
    rings
  ground pepper

Heat broth over high heat in wok or heavy skillet. Add onions; stir-fry until tender. Sprinkle with ground pepper.

ALMOND PEAS

1 lb. fresh green peas, washed, shelled
and steamed
⅓ cup slivered almonds

Drain peas; toss with almonds.

MINTED PEAS

1 pound fresh green peas, washed,
shelled and steamed
fresh mint

Add fresh mint to peas while steaming.

COTTAGE FRIES

1   potato per person
½   teaspoon safflower oil per potato

Boil or steam potatoes in their jackets; peel. Slice thin. Toss with oil. Brown in a teflon skillet over medium heat, turning frequently.

Variation: For Potatoes O'Brien sauté chopped onion and chopped green pepper in a small amount of water or broth until tender. Toss with potatoes and oil. Brown.

FRENCH FRIED POTATOES

1   potato per person

Cut potatoes into strips. Arrange on a teflon baking sheet. Bake at 425° 15-20 minutes or until brown. Turn; bake 15-20 minutes or until tender.

Note: To shorten baking time, parboil potatoes 15 minutes; slice and roast.

Variation: Before cooking brush with safflower oil and sprinkle with garlic powder, onion powder, chili powder or celery seed.

HASH BROWN POTATOES

1   potato per person
¾   teaspoon onion per potato (optional)
½   teaspoon safflower oil per potato
     dash salt
     dash pepper

Boil or steam potatoes in their jackets. Chill. Peel. Shred. Toss with onion, oil, salt, and pepper. Pat into thin patties. Brown in a teflon skillet over medium heat 10-12 minutes. Turn. Brown 8-10 minutes longer or to desired brownness. For extra crispness, using two spatulas, cut horizontally through center of patty; flip one half over the other.

POTATO CHIPS

1   potato per person
     safflower oil

Slice potatoes crosswise into paper-thin rounds; brush with safflower oil. Bake on a teflon baking sheet at 425° 20 minutes. Turn; bake 15-20 minutes or until brown and crisp.

BAKED POTATOES

1   potato per person

Scrub potatoes (do not use new potatoes); prick with fork. Bake at 425° 40-60 minutes or at 350° 60-80 minutes.

Variation: Top with tomato salsa* (page 361) or low-fat Cheddar cheese and green onion.

TWICE-BAKED POTATOES

4   potatoes
¼   cup hot skim milk
½   cup grated low-fat Cheddar cheese
     paprika

Bake potatoes in their jackets (do not use new potatoes). Cut potatoes in half lengthwise; scoop out centers. Mash. Beat with hot milk. Mound back into skins. Sprinkle with cheese. Top with paprika. Bake at 400° for 20 minutes.

POTATOES WITH ONION AND DILL

1   pound small new potatoes, unpeeled
1   small red onion, thinly sliced
1   green pepper, thinly sliced into rings
1   cup plain non-fat yogurt* (page 202)
1   tablespoon chopped fresh dill or
       ¼ teaspoon dried dill
2   tablespoons safflower oil
2   tablespoons olive oil
¼   teaspoon or less salt
⅛   teaspoon pepper

Scrub potatoes; boil or steam until just tender. Place whole or sliced into a serving bowl; tuck onion and green pepper slices among potatoes. Combine yogurt, dill, oils, salt and pepper. Pass with potatoes.

LEMON POTATOES

1   pound small red potatoes
2   tablespoons beef broth* (page 302) or
       chicken broth* (page 295)
¼   cup fresh lemon juice
       zest of ½ lemon
¼   teaspoon pepper
       chopped chives
       chopped fresh parsley
       dash rosemary

Slice potatoes into thin rounds; steam until just tender. Heat broth and lemon juice, but do not boil; pour over potatoes. Season with pepper. Sprinkle with chives, parsley and rosemary.

391

NEW POTATOES AND FRESH VEGETABLES

1	pound new potatoes or small red potatoes
¼-½	lb. fresh green beans, steamed
1	red or green pepper, cut into rings
1	cucumber, sliced
8	cherry tomatoes
½	pound fresh mushrooms
1	cup plain non-fat yogurt* (page 202)
1½	tablespoons Dijon mustard
2	green onions, finely chopped
	dill weed to taste
	fresh parsley for garnish

Boil or steam potatoes with jackets until tender; cut into wedges. Chill potatoes and vegetables. Combine yogurt, mustard, green onion and dill to make dressing. Chill. Just before serving, arrange vegetables on a platter; place yogurt dressing in the center. Garnish with fresh parsley.

PARSLEYED POTATOES

1-2	tiny new potatoes per person
	dash tub safflower margarine
	juice of a fresh lemon wedge
	chopped fresh parsley

Scrub potatoes; steam in their jackets until just tender. Toss with margarine. Sprinkle with parsley. Drizzle with lemon juice.

POTATOES EPICURE

3-4   medium potatoes
       tub safflower mayonnaise
¾   cup cream of chicken soup* (page 316)
1   cup plain non-fat yogurt* (page 202)
¾   cup grated, low-fat Cheddar cheese
3   tablespoons chopped onion
1   tablespoon safflower oil
½   cup crushed corn flakes

Boil potatoes in their skins; cut into cubes. Grease an 8-inch square casserole with tub safflower margarine; add potatoes. Blend soup, yogurt, cheese and onions; pour over potatoes. Mix safflower oil with corn flakes; sprinkle over potatoes. Bake at 350° 30-40 minutes.

MASHED POTATOES

1   potato per person
       hot skim milk

Peel potatoes; cut into quarters. Boil or steam until tender, drain and mash. Beat with electric mixer until light and fluffy, gradually adding hot milk as needed.

FAT-FREE GRAVY

---

2 cups chicken broth* (page 295) or
beef broth* (page 302)
3 tablespoons defatted meat juices and
drippings (optional)
¼ cup flour
½ cup cold water
salt to taste
pepper to taste

Bring broth and defatted meat drippings to a boil. Shake flour and water in a covered jar to form a smooth paste; gradually add to boiling broth. Reduce heat; simmer 5-10 minutes, stirring constantly until thick. Season.

Note: To defat meat juices and drippings, pour the juices and drippings into a bowl; add a few ice cubes. Chill in the freezer 10-15 minutes or until the fat congeals at the top and around ice cubes. Discard ice cubes and congealed fat.

It is not necessary to use meat juices and drippings to make a satisfactory gravy with the above recipe.

Variation: For a gravy that is especially good with poultry, instead of 2 cups broth, use 1 cup milk and 1 cup broth.

CANNED TOMATOES

Thoroughly wash tomatoes. Put 4-5 at a time in boiling water, then dip in cold water. Peel. Cut out stem ends. Tightly pack tomatoes into clean, quart-size canning jars. Add 1½ teaspoons salt (or less) and ½ teaspoon citric acid to each jar. Adjust caps. Slowly lower jars into canner of boiling water. (Be sure there is enough water in the canner to cover tops of jars). When water again comes to a rolling boil, begin timing. Process 45 minutes, keeping water boiling vigorously entire time. Remove jars from canner. Cool upright on a thick cloth. After 24 hours test seal. Label jars. Store.

Note: If you have not canned before, consult a good canning cookbook before proceeding.

Helpful Hint: Many Positive Diet recipes use canned tomatoes. I try to can 2-3 flats of tomatoes each summer in order to have the sodium control that is not possible with commercially canned products.

BROILED TOMATO HALVES

ripe tomatoes
olive oil
ground pepper
fresh or dried basil
bread crumbs

Cut tomatoes into halves; brush lightly with olive oil. Sprinkle with pepper and basil. Top with bread crumbs. Broil 2-3 minutes.

VERA CRUZ TOMATOES

¼ cup chopped onion
  wine, broth or water
1 bunch fresh spinach, chopped
½ cup plain non-fat yogurt* (page 202)
  dash Tabasco sauce
4 medium tomatoes
½ cup grated low-fat Mozzarella
  cheese

Sauté onion in small amount of wine, broth or water until tender; add spinach and cook 3-4 minutes. Cool, drain and squeeze excess water from spinach. Mix spinach and onion with yogurt and Tabasco sauce. Cut tops from tomatoes and remove centers, leaving shells. Fill shells with spinach mixture. Place in a baking dish. Bake at 375° for 20-25 minutes. Top with cheese; bake 2-3 minutes longer or until cheese is melted.

HERBED TOMATOES

1 tomato per person
1 teaspoon red wine vinegar per
   tomato
pinch chopped fresh parsley
pinch thyme
pinch basil
pinch marjoram
dash pepper

Slice tomatoes. Sprinkle with vinegar and herbs.

SESAME SPINACH

1 bunch fresh spinach
½ teaspoon sesame oil
4 teaspoons lemon juice
4 tablespoons toasted sesame seeds

Wash spinach in ice water; remove thick stems. Pat dry; tear into bite-size pieces. Toss with sesame oil; sprinkle with lemon juice and sesame seeds. Toss again.

BAKED SQUASH

acorn squash
safflower oil
ground pepper

Wash squash; remove seeds. Cut into halves or squares; brush with oil. Place cut side down in shallow pan. Bake at 350° for 30 minutes; turn. Brush again with oil; bake 30 minutes longer or until tender. Season lightly with pepper.

HOLIDAY YAMS WITH MARSHMALLOWS

2   red delicious apples, sliced
⅓   cup chopped pecans
⅓   cup brown sugar
½   teaspoon cinnamon
1   28-oz. can yams, drained
    miniature marshmallows to cover

Toss apples and nuts with combined brown sugar and cinnamon. Alternate layers of apples and yams in a 1½ quart casserole. Cover; bake at 350° 35-40 minutes. Sprinkle with marshmallows; broil 6-8 minutes or until lightly browned. Serves 6-8.

ROAST PEPPERS

8   large red and green sweet peppers
3   tablespoons safflower oil
1   tablespoon olive oil
2   cloves garlic
1   tablespoon tarragon wine vinegar
½   teaspoon basil
¼   teaspoon rosemary
¼   teaspoon oregano

Pre-heat oven to broil. Arrange peppers on foil-lined baking sheet. Broil until the skin of the peppers blisters and turns black, turning 2-3 times so that all sides are blistered and blackened. Remove from oven. Place in a glass bowl; cover with a kitchen towel. Cool 1 hour. Slice into strips; remove stem and seeds. Combine remaining ingredients; pour over peppers. Chill 24-48 hours. Serve with tomato slices or add to sandwiches or pizza.

BARBECUED ZUCCHINI

2   small zucchini
juice of ½ lemon
freshly ground pepper

Cut zucchini lengthwise into quarters. Sprinkle with lemon juice and black pepper. Wrap in foil. Grill 15-20 minutes or until hot and crisp-tender.

ZUCCHINI AND CARROTS JULIENNE

    1   medium zucchini
2-3   medium carrots
¼-½   cup chicken broth*(page 295) or
       beef broth*(page 302)
      freshly ground pepper

Cut zucchini and carrots into julienne strips. Heat broth in wok or heavy skillet; add carrots; stir-fry 5-6 minutes. Add zucchini; stir-fry until carrots and zucchini are crisp-tender. Sprinkle with pepper.

CHEESE-STUFFED ZUCCHINI

  3   small zucchini
  ¼   cup egg substitute, beaten
  ½   cup low-fat Ricotta cheese
  ½   cup low-fat Cheddar cheese
  ½   cup chopped fresh parsley
¼-½   cup bread crumbs

Slice zucchini lengthwise into halves. Steam until just barely tender; drain, pat dry and scoop out pulp. Combine egg, Ricotta cheese, Cheddar cheese, and parsley; fill zucchini shells. Sprinkle with bread crumbs. Arrange zucchini in baking dish greased with tub safflower margarine. Bake at 350° for 25 minutes. Place under broiler 2-3 minutes to brown bread crumbs.

ZUCCHINI-MOZZARELLA CASSEROLE

2   pounds zucchini (about 7 cups)
1   cup egg substitute, beaten
½   cup skim milk
¼   teaspoon or less salt
2   teaspoons baking powder
3   tablespoons flour
¼   cup chopped parsley
1   clove garlic, minced
1   small onion, finely chopped
1   7-oz. can diced green chilies
¾   pound low-fat Mozzarella cheese,
      grated
1   teaspoon herb seasoning* (page 208)
1   cup croutons* (page 270)
3   tablespoons safflower oil

Slice zucchini crosswise into ¼-inch thick slices. Whirl egg substitute, milk, salt, baking powder and flour in blender; add parsley, garlic and onion and whirl again. Pour into large mixing bowl; add zucchini, green chilies and cheese. Toss. Spoon into a greased 9x13x2-inch baking dish or 2 square 8-inch pans (the square ones are nice if you want to eat one and freeze the other). Sprinkle with herb seasoning. Toss croutons with safflower oil; sprinkle over top of casserole. Bake uncovered at 350° for 40 minutes or until zucchini is tender and mixture is set in the center. Let stand 10 minutes before serving.

PASTA PRIMAVERA WITH TOMATOES

1	lb. fresh tomatoes or one 1-lb. can plum tomatoes, puréed in blender
2	cloves garlic, minced
3	carrots, sliced into rounds
1	small bunch broccoli (flowerets only)
3	small zucchini, sliced into rounds
3	green onions, chopped
1	fresh tomato, chopped
1½	tablespoons safflower oil
1½	tablespoons olive oil
¼	teaspoon pepper
½	teaspoon dried basil or 2 tablespoons fresh basil
¼	teaspoon or less salt
1	lb. pinwheel or seashell macaroni, cooked

Heat ¼ of the puréed tomatoes in wok or heavy skillet. Add garlic and carrots; stir-fry until carrots are crisp-tender. Add broccoli; stir-fry 2-3 minutes. Add zucchini and green onion; stir-fry 1-2 minutes. Add remaining ingredients; toss and heat. Serve over pasta.

PASTA PRIMAVERA WITH DIJON

1   lb. seashell macaroni, cooked
1   bunch green onions, chopped
2   large fresh tomatoes, diced
1   cup safflower oil
½   cup olive oil
½   cup cider vinegar
1   teaspoon Dijon mustard
    dash garlic powder
    salt and pepper to taste

Toss macaroni with green onions and tomatoes. Combine oils, vinegar and Dijon; pour enough over pasta to moisten. Season. Serve hot or cold.

PASTA WITH FRESH TOMATOES, BASIL, AND CHEESE

7   ripe tomatoes, cut into ½"-chunks
1   cup fresh basil leaves, chopped
2   tablespoons chopped fresh parsley
3   large cloves garlic, minced
¾   teaspoon crushed red pepper
⅛   teaspoon salt (optional)
1   pound low-fat Mozzarella cheese, cubed
⅓   cup safflower oil
2   tablespoons olive oil
1   pound sea shell-shaped pasta

Combine tomatoes, basil, parsley, garlic, red pepper, salt, cheese, safflower oil and olive oil; let stand for 1 hour at room temperature. Cook pasta, drain; toss with tomatoes while still hot.

FETTUCCINI NAPOLI

1	pound fettuccini, cooked
1	cup olive oil
4	cloves garlic, minced
	juice of 1 lemon
¼	cup chopped fresh parsley
1	teaspoon fresh basil or ½ teaspoon dried basil
½	teaspoon oregano
½	teaspoon or less salt
¼	teaspoon pepper

Place fettuccini in large serving bowl. Combine remaining ingredients; pour over fettuccini. Toss.

FETTUCCINI WITH FRESH BASIL AND TOMATOES

2	lbs. ripe tomatoes, peeled and chopped
1	white onion, finely chopped
2	cloves garlic, chopped
¾	cup fresh basil, chopped
½	cup olive oil
	salt and pepper to taste
1	pound fettuccini, cooked
1	cup low-fat Cheddar cheese, grated

Mix tomatoes, onion, garlic, basil, olive oil, salt and pepper; let stand at room temperature for 1 hour. Cook fettuccini; drain. Toss with sauce; sprinkle with cheese. Serve at once.

MACARONI AND CHEESE

2	cups skim milk
3	tablespoons flour
½	teaspoon or less salt
	dash pepper
¼	cup chopped onion
2	cups grated low-fat Cheddar cheese
3½	cups cooked elbow macaroni
1-2	ripe tomatoes, sliced

Combine milk and flour in a covered jar; shake to form a smooth paste. Pour into a large saucepan; cook over medium heat, stirring constantly until thick. Add salt, pepper, onion and cheese. Stir until cheese is melted. Add macaroni. Toss. Pour into a 1½-quart casserole. Arrange tomato slices over top, pushing edge of each slice into macaroni. Bake uncovered at 350° for 45 minutes.

HUNGRY JOE SPECIAL

1 pound extra-lean ground round
1 onion, chopped
½ pound fresh mushrooms, sliced
1 bunch fresh spinach
black pepper
1 cup egg substitute, beaten
½ cup low-fat Mozzarella or Cheddar
cheese, grated

Brown beef; drain off excess fat. Add onions and mushrooms; simmer 10 minutes. Wash spinach; steam 3-4 minutes. Squeeze out excess moisture. Sprinkle with black pepper; toss with ground round. Scramble egg substitute in a teflon skillet; toss with ground round and spinach. Top with cheese. Toss again.

Accompany with sliced tomatoes.

DRIED BEANS, PEAS AND LENTILS

Soak beans using method 1 or method 2.

Soaking Method 1. Stir 1 teaspoon salt into 6 cups of water for each 1 pound of dried beans. Wash beans; add to salted water. Soak overnight. Drain. Rinse. Discard soaking water.

Soaking Method 2. Bring 8 cups of water for each 1 pound of beans to a boil. Wash beans, add to boiling water. Bring to a second boil; boil 2 minutes. Remove from heat; cover and let soak for 1 hour. Drain. Rinse. Discard soaking water.

Cook soaked beans as follows: For 1 pound of soaked beans bring 6 cups of water, chicken broth* (page 295) or beef broth* (page 302), 1 teaspoon salt and 1 onion to a boil. Add beans; boil gently, uncovered, 25 minutes to 2 hours or until tender. Cooking times will vary according to types used. Add more water or broth as necessary during cooking to keep beans covered.

One pound beans yields 6 cups cooked beans.

Note: Dry legumes are important sources of B vitamins, iron, calcium and potassium. They contain no cholesterol, are low in sodium and are good sources of fiber.

BAKED BEANS

3   cups small red beans or pinto beans,
    cooked
1   large onion, chopped
1   8-oz. can tomato sauce
⅓   cup molasses
1   teaspoon dry mustard
1   teaspoon chili powder

Combine beans, onion, tomato sauce, molasses, mustard, and chili powder; pour into a bean pot or casserole dish. Bake uncovered at 350° for 1 hour. Cover and continue baking for 30 minutes.

WILD RICE

1   small onion, chopped
2   cups beef broth* (page 302)
½   pound mushrooms, sliced
½   cup wild rice
1   cup brown long grain rice
2   tablespoons chopped fresh parsley

Sauté onion in small amount of broth until tender; add mushrooms and remaining broth. Bring to a boil; add wild rice and onion. Cover; reduce heat and simmer 20 minutes. Add long grain rice; return to boiling. Cover, reduce heat and simmer 20 minutes longer or until liquid is absorbed and rice is tender. Sprinkle with parsley.

TABBOULI PILAF

---

2   tablespoons safflower oil
1   medium onion, chopped
½   cup chopped celery
½   pound fresh mushrooms, sliced
1   cup uncooked cracked wheat bulgur
¼   teaspoon oregano
¼   teaspoon salt
¼   teaspoon pepper
2   cups beef broth* (page 302)

Warm oil in heavy skillet over medium heat; add onions and celery. Cook 5 minutes. Add mushrooms and bulgar; cook, stirring constantly for 10 minutes or until bulgur is golden brown and vegetables are tender. Add oregano, salt, pepper and broth. Cover and bring to a boil; reduce heat and simmer 15-20 minutes or until broth is absorbed.

Variations: Use chicken broth* (page 295), rather than beef broth.

Sprinkle with chopped fresh parsley just before serving.

Add ¼ teaspoon dill weed to broth.

RICE PILAF

---

uncooked rice
chicken broth*(page 295)
finely chopped fresh parsley

Cook rice as directed on package, substituting chicken broth for the required water. Just before serving, toss rice with parsley. Spoon into ring mold; pat down. Unmold.

JAPANESE NEW VARIETY RICE

1 cup no talc, extra fancy, new variety
   rice (available in oriental section of
   supermarket)
1 cup water

Place rice in a fine wire strainer; wash under cold running water until water runs clear. Put equal amounts rice and water in saucepan; cover and heat to boiling. Reduce heat; simmer 10-20 minutes until water is absorbed and rice is tender. Add additional water, if necessary.

BARLEY AND MUSHROOM PILAF

1¾ cups pearl barley
  1 onion, chopped
  3 tablespoons safflower oil
  ½ pound fresh mushrooms, sliced
  4 cups beef broth* (page 302)

Soak barley several hours or overnight in enough cold water to cover. Drain. Sauté onion and barley in safflower oil until onion is tender and barley is toasted, add mushrooms; cook 2-3 minutes longer. Spoon into large casserole. Heat broth to boiling; pour over barley. Stir. Bake covered at 350° for 1 hour. Uncover; bake 1 to 1½ hours longer or until liquid is absorbed.

BREAD STUFFING

1	large onion, chopped
3	stalks celery, chopped
2½	cups chicken broth* (page 295)
½	pound fresh mushrooms, sliced
10-12	**cups dried bread cubes**
2	tablespoons safflower oil
1¼	teaspoon sage
½	teaspoon or less salt
¼	teaspoon pepper

Sauté onion and celery in small amount of broth until tender. Add mushrooms; cook 2-3 minutes. Add bread cubes. Toss with oil. Gradually moisten with broth, adding a little more or a little less broth as necessary. Season. Toss. Bake covered at 350° 30-40 minutes or until piping hot. Makes enough dressing to accompany a 10-14 pound turkey.

Note: On the Positive Diet, dressing should not be put into the turkey because as the turkey cooks, the fat in the bird drips into the dressing.

CHAPTER SIXTEEN

SEAFOOD

MUSSELS ITALIAN STYLE

5 dozen mussels
1 chopped leek including greens
1 medium onion, thinly sliced
1 large clove garlic, halved
1½ cups dry vermouth
¾ cup water
¾ teaspoon or less salt
1 1-lb. can plum tomatoes
1 tablespoon safflower oil
2 tablespoons olive oil
  chopped fresh parsley

Scrub mussel shells with a wire brush to remove beard. Wash and soak following the procedure for steamed clams with fresh lemon* (page 416). Combine leeks, onion, garlic, vermouth, water and salt in a stock pot; add mussels. Steam over medium-high heat 6-8 minutes — just until shells open. (Discard any mussels that are opened before cooking and any that do not open during cooking).

Remove mussels to serving platter; cover to keep warm. Boil cooking liquid 2-3 minutes to reduce. Remove garlic; add tomatoes, safflower oil and olive oil. Heat to serving temperature; use the edge of a spoon to cut tomatoes into smaller pieces. Pour sauce over mussels. Sprinkle with parsley.

Serve with crusty French bread for dipping.

Note: Serve left-over sauce over pasta on the following night.

STEAMED CLAMS WITH FRESH LEMON

5 dozen clams
water
1 cup salt (for soaking solution)
5 fresh lemons

Wash clams. Cover with salt water or make a solution of ⅓ cup salt to 1 gallon of water; soak 15-20 minutes, drain and rinse. Repeat procedure 2 more times.

Place clams on a steamer rack in a large pot; add 4½-cups water. Cover tightly and steam 5-10 minutes — just until shells open. (Reserve nectar for chowder). Arrange clams on serving platter, garnish with plenty of fresh lemon wedges.

Note: Tossed green salad, garlic bread or a baked potato with plain non-fat yogurt* (page 202), chives and green onion are nice accompaniments.

Helpful Hint: Other excellent seafood recipes to try include Steamed Mussels with Wine and Garlic, Steamed Clams Bordelaise, Seviche, Oysters on the Half Shell, Oysters Rockefeller, Marinated Salmon and Cracked Crab. These recipes can be found in the appetizer section.

CLAMS ITALIAN STYLE

1   onion, chopped
1   clove garlic
2   stalks celery, chopped
1   2-lb. can plum tomatoes
3   tablespoons olive oil
3   dozen clams
    chopped fresh parsley
    fresh ground pepper

Sauté onions, garlic and celery in small amount of tomato liquid until tender; add tomatoes and olive oil. Simmer 30 minutes. Wash and soak clams following the procedure for steamed clams with fresh lemon* (page 416); reserve ⅔ cup of the nectar and add to simmering tomatoes. Fill soup bowls with steamed clams; pour tomato mixture over. Sprinkle with fresh parsley and ground pepper.

BROILED SCALLOPS

¼   cup prepared mustard
¼   cup honey
1¼ teaspoons curry powder
1   teaspoon lemon juice
2   pounds scallops
    fresh lemon wedges

Combine mustard, honey, curry and lemon juice; pour over scallops. Marinate 10 minutes. Broil 4-inches from heat for 10 minutes or until browned; turn. Brush with sauce; broil 10 minutes longer. Serve with fresh lemon.

Variation: Skewer scallops, mushroom caps, cherry tomatoes and green peppers; brush with sauce. Broil.

Instead of mustard sauce, soak scallops in 2 parts olive oil to 1 part lemon juice for 1 hour. Skewer and broil.

LOBSTER TAILS

4   6-8 oz. lobster tails
3   tablespoons safflower oil
1   tablespoon olive oil
1   tablespoon dry white wine
    fresh lemon wedges

With back up, split tail lengthwise half way through the body; spread back open. Remove whole meat from tails. Bend shells backwards until cracked in several places. Replace meat in shells. Insert skewers lengthwise between shell and meat to prevent curling. Baste with safflower oil and olive oil.

Cook over hot coals 5-10 minutes on shell side; turn and cook 5 minutes longer on flesh side. Baste with wine the last 2 minutes. Serve with lemon wedges.

Variation: To broil, place on broiler rack 3-inches from heat; broil 6-8 minutes on shell side. Turn; broil 5-10 minutes on flesh side. Baste with wine the last 2 minutes.

To bake, bake at 475° for 16 minutes; baste.

Note: If using frozen lobster tails, thaw before cooking.

MARINATED FISH

1   pound fillet of halibut, swordfish,
      lingcod, red snapper or other
      white fish
3   tablespoons safflower oil
2   tablespoons olive oil
2   cloves garlic, minced
      dash paprika

Marinate fish in safflower oil, olive oil and garlic for 1 hour; drain. Sprinkle with paprika. Broil 5-10 minutes or until fish flakes, turning only once; do not overcook.

Variation: Serve with herbed mayonnaise* (page 360) or Dijon vinaigrette* (page 361).

Helpful Hint: Correct Timing For Fish: The Canadian Department of Fisheries suggests measuring the fish at the thickest point and allowing 10 minutes cooking time per inch. If a salmon measures 3-inches at its thickest point, the total cooking time would be 30 minutes (10x3); 15 minutes per side. A halibut roast that is 1-inch thick would require 10 minutes total cooking time; 5 minutes per side. Always test fish a few minutes early, just to be on the safe side.

Testing For Doneness: Fish is done the second it loses translucency and flakes easily when probed with a fork at its thickest point. When testing a whole fish, probe an inch or two below the base of the head, and again at the thickest point behind the abdominal cavity. When fish is opaque and milky and detaches easily from the bone, it is done.

STUFFED WHOLE FISH

¾ cup safflower oil
¼ cup olive oil
1 whole salmon, steelhead, trout, cod or
    other whole fish
    sage to taste
    pepper to taste
1 onion, sliced into rings
2-3 stalks celery, cut into 3-inch lengths
¼ pound fresh mushrooms, sliced
2-3 carrots, peeled, quartered and cut into
    2-inch lengths
2 fresh lemons, sliced into rounds

Pour safflower oil and olive oil over fish; add more if necessary to generously cover fish inside and outside. Marinate 1-4 hours.

Remove fish from oil and season with sage and black pepper. Stuff inside cavity to bulging with onions, celery, mushrooms and carrots.

Place fish on aluminum foil; slide a layer of lemon rounds under fish. Place more lemon slices on top of fish; fish should be smothered top and bottom with lemon rounds. Wrap fish in two thicknesses of foil. Bake at 425° or grill over deep coals until fish flakes

CRAB STUFFED TROUT

3	tablespoons safflower oil
1	tablespoon olive oil
2-3	6-8 oz. trout, heads and tails removed
1	small onion, thinly sliced
¼	pound crab meat
¼	pound fresh mushrooms, sliced
	juice of ½ lemon
3	tablespoons dry vermouth
	fresh lemon wedges
	fresh parsley

Place fish in 9x13x2-inch baking dish. Pour safflower oil and olive oil over fish, add more if necessary to generously cover fish inside and outside. Marinate 10 minutes. Pour off oil; stuff inside cavity with onion, crab and mushrooms.

Combine lemon juice and vermouth; pour over fish both inside and outside. Cover baking dish with aluminum foil.

Bake at 400° about 20 minutes or until skin pulls easily away from fish. Baste frequently during cooking. Serve with plenty of fresh lemon; garnish with parsley.

Note: For a refreshing dessert, try Lemon Ice* (page 513).

Variation: Any other type of whole fish may be used in place of trout.

COURT BOUILLON

2 quarts cold water
1 quart dry white wine, clam nectar or
clam juice
¾ cup wine vinegar
2 carrots, cut into 1-inch pieces
2 stalks celery with leaves, cut into
2-inch pieces
2 onions, thinly sliced
4 sprigs parsley
1 lemon, thinly sliced
1 bay leaf
1 teaspoon thyme
2-3 peppercorns

Prepare as for easy court bouillon.

EASY COURT BOUILLON

2 quarts chicken broth* (page 295)
1 quart dry white wine
2 onions, minced
3 sprigs parsley
¼ cup safflower oil
¼ cup olive oil
pinch crushed thyme

Combine all ingredients for court bouillon or for easy court bouillon in a stock pot; bring to a boil. Reduce heat; simmer uncovered 45 minutes.

Note: With the exception of bouillon that has been used to poach salmon, court bouillon and easy court bouillon may be used several times over and they may also be frozen.

POACHED FISH

1   3-6 pound whole fish fillet, head and
       tail removed, if desired
2   tablespoons lemon juice
2   quarts cold water
1   recipe court bouillon* or easy court
       bouillon* (page 423)

Clean and scale fish. Rinse in lemon juice and water. Wrap in cheese cloth; twist ends and tie with string. Place in fish poacher or roasting pan over 2 burners; cover with court bouillon or easy court bouillon and bring to a boil.

Reduce heat to simmer and begin timing; allow 10 minutes of cooking time per inch of thickness, 20 minutes if frozen. Be careful not to overcook; remember the fish will continue to cook some even when removed from heat. Serve hot or cold.

BROILED FILLETS WITH FRESH LEMON

1   pound fillet of halibut, red snapper,
       cod, sole or other white fish
      juice of 1 lemon
      grated rind of 1 lemon
      lemon slices for garnish
      watercress for garnish
      salt and pepper to taste

Marinate fish in lemon juice and lemon rind at least 2 hours and all day, if possible, turning frequently. Broil 10-15 minutes, turning only once. Serve over lemon slices. Garnish with watercress. Season to taste.

BAKED FILLETS WITH LEMON AND FENNEL

> 1 pound fillet of halibut, red snapper, cod, sole or other white fish
> 2 tablespoons safflower oil
> juice of 1 lemon
> 2-3 green onions, finely chopped
> 1 bunch fresh fennel or 2 teaspoons dried fennel

Brush fish with safflower oil; cover with lemon juice. Sprinkle with green onion and fennel (if fresh fennel is available, slice fennel lengthwise and place fish on top). Bake at 375° 10-20 minutes or until fish flakes.

Variation: Serve with homemade safflower mayonnaise* (page 360).

BARBECUED FILLETS

3   tablespoons safflower oil
1   tablespoon olive oil
1   pound fillet of salmon, halibut,
       swordfish, pike or other type fish
    pinch thyme
    pinch fennel
    fresh lemon wedges

Pour safflower oil and olive oil over fish, add more
if necessary to generously cover fish inside and
outside. Season. Marinate 1-4 hours.

Prepare coals — large fish need deep coal beds
that have burned down to gray ash; small fish
require high heat. Generously oil grill. Cook fish
3-4 inches above the coal bed, turning only once.
Baste frequently with oils. Serve with plenty of
fresh lemon.

Variation: Serve with Dijon vinaigrette* (page 361)
or herbed safflower mayonnaise* (page 360).

FILLETS WITH VERMOUTH AND ORANGE SAUCE

1	pound fillet of halibut, red snapper, cod, sole or other white fish
3	tablespoons safflower oil
1	tablespoon olive oil
½	cup fresh orange juice
½	cup dry vermouth
1	orange, thinly sliced for garnish watercress for garnish

Marinate fish for 1 hour in safflower and olive oil. Heat orange juice and vermouth just to boiling; reduce heat and simmer 2-3 minutes. Pour over fish. Bake at 450° 15-20 minutes, basting frequently. When fish is done, pour juices into a saucepan; boil 3-4 minutes to reduce. Spread a serving plate with orange slices; top with fish. Cover with sauce. Garnish with watercress.

FILLETS WITH WINE AND TOMATO SAUCE

    1   onion, chopped
   2-3   stalks celery, chopped
    2   carrots, diced
    1   clove garlic, minced
    1   cup white wine
    2   tablespoons safflower oil
    1   8-oz. can tomato sauce
    3   tablespoons chopped parsley
    1   pound fillet of halibut, red snapper,
            sole, cod or other white fish

Sauté vegetables in small amount of wine until tender; add oil, tomato sauce, parsley and remaining wine. Simmer 15 minutes. Pour ¼ of the sauce into a baking dish; arrange fish on top. Cover with remaining sauce. Bake covered at 350° 15-20 minutes.

FILLETS WITH FRESH VEGETABLES AND CHEESE

¼	pound fresh mushrooms, sliced water, wine or broth
1-2	green onions, finely chopped
1	tomato, diced
¼	teaspoon basil
¼	teaspoon lemon pepper or black pepper
1	egg beaten or ¼ cup egg substitute, beaten
¾	cup grated low-fat Cheddar cheese
1	pound fillet of halibut, red snapper, sole, cod or other white fish
1	teaspoon safflower oil

Steam mushrooms in small amount of water, wine or broth for 2-3 minutes. Toss with green onions, tomato, basil, pepper, egg and cheese; brush fish with safflower oil. Bake at 500° 5-8 minutes or until fish is just barely tender. Cover with vegetables and cheese. Broil 5 minutes or until cheese melts.

FILLET OF SOLE WITH FRESH VEGETABLES AND DIJON

1	pound fillet of sole, cubed
	juice of ½ lemon
¼	pound fresh green beans
1	cup sliced radishes
1	tomato, diced
1	green pepper, diced
¼	teaspoon pepper
1	recipe Dijon vinaigrette* (page 361)
1	bunch leaf lettuce
1	cucumber, sliced
	fresh lemon wedges

Steam fish on vegetable steamer rack over boiling water until tender. Squeeze ¼ of a lemon over fish. Chill.

Steam beans, squeeze remaining ¼ of lemon over beans during cooking. Drain and chill.

One hour before serving combine fish, beans, radishes, tomatoes and green pepper; sprinkle with pepper and toss with enough Dijon vinaigrette to moisten. Chill.

Just before serving, cover a platter with lettuce; spread cucumber over. Top with fish. Garnish with lemon.

Variation: Any type of white fish may be used in place of sole.

CLAM STUFFED SOLE

¼ cup chopped green onion
1 clove garlic, minced
¼ teaspoon olive oil
¾ teaspoon safflower oil
1½ cups fresh mushrooms, sliced
1 6-oz. can chopped clams, drained
2 tablespoons chopped parsley
½ teaspoon oregano
½ teaspoon basil
¼ teaspoon salt
⅛ teaspoon pepper
1 pound sole fillets
1 tablespoon lemon juice
fresh parsley for garnish
fresh lemon wedges for garnish

Sauté onion and garlic in olive oil and safflower oil until tender. Add mushrooms; cook 2-3 minutes. Stir in clams, parsley, oregano, basil, salt and pepper.

Layer half of the sole fillets in a baking dish and drizzle with lemon juice. Cover each with clam and mushroom filling. Stack remaining fillets over top. Bake covered at 350° for 25 minutes. Garnish with fresh parsley and lemon.

Note: Fresh clams may be used in place of canned. Any type of white fish may be used in place of sole.

CRAB STUFFED SOLE

2	green onions with tops, chopped
½	green pepper, chopped
½	cup fresh mushrooms, sliced
2	tablespoons dry white wine
¼	pound crab meat
1	pound fresh sole fillets
1½	tablespoons fresh lemon juice
½	cup chicken broth* (page 295)
¼	cup flour

Sauté green onion, green pepper and mushrooms in wine; drain. Add crab. Lay sole flat; spread crab filling over each fillet. Roll and secure with toothpicks. Pour lemon juice and ¼ of the chicken broth over fish.

Bake at 350° 10-12 minutes or until fish flakes easily when tested with a fork. Transfer to a serving plate to keep warm.

Shake flour and remaining broth in a covered jar to form a smooth paste. Pour liquid that fish was poached in into a saucepan; bring to a boil. Gradually add flour thickening, stirring constantly until sauce has thickened; pour over sole. Serve at once.

Variation: Lobster meat may be used in place of crab. Any type white fish may be used in place of sole.

FRESH SOLE WITH YOGURT AND CHEESE

fresh sole fillets
fresh lemon juice
grated onion
plain non-fat yogurt* (page 202)
Tabasco sauce
low-fat Mozzarella cheese, grated

Arrange sole in a baking dish; drizzle with lemon juice. Top with grated onion; spread with yogurt. Drizzle with Tabasco sauce. Bake at 350° for 10 minutes; top with cheese. Bake 10 minutes longer or until fish flakes and cheese has melted.

TUNA BURGERS

1 6½-oz. can water pack tuna, drained
2 tablespoons chopped onion
2 tablespoons sliced waterchestnuts
1 teaspoon prepared mustard
   safflower mayonnaise to moisten
   hamburger buns
   sliced low-fat cheese
   lettuce
   sliced tomato
   sliced white onion

Mix tuna, onion, waterchestnuts and mustard; moisten with mayonnaise. Toast or warm buns; spread bottom half with tuna. Broil 5-inches from heat about 3 minutes; add cheese. Broil 2 minutes longer or until cheese melts; add lettuce, tomato, and sliced onion. Top with bun.

SZECHWAN FISH ROLLS

1	tablespoon ginger juice
1	pound boneless sole fillets, cubed
2	green onions with tops, finely chopped
⅛	teaspoon white pepper
⅛	teaspoon salt
2	tablespoons safflower oil
1	tablespoon sesame oil
1	tablespoon sake
1	tablespoon potato starch
1	egg white, beaten
½	teaspoon potato starch plus ½ cup water
18	spring roll (lumpia) wrappers

Squeeze ginger juice over fish, let stand 10 minutes; add green onions, pepper, salt, safflower oil, sesame oil, sake and 1 tablespoon potato starch. Toss. Fold in beaten egg white.

Heat ½ teaspoon potato starch and ½ cup water to boiling to form a glue; cool to room temperature.

Lay thawed wrappers flat; place 2 tablespoons of fish filling in center of each. Brush outside edges of each wrapper with glue; fold edges over envelope style and seal outside seam with glue.

Heat a small amount of safflower oil in a heavy skillet; brown fish rolls on one side over medium-high heat for 10-15 minutes. Turn; brown on other side. Prepare sauce.
Continued

Sauce

2	cups chicken broth* (page 295)
1½	tablespoons sesame oil
1½	tablespoons sake
3	tablespoons flour plus ½ cup cold water
3-4	sliced green onions
2-3	drops hot chili oil (La Yu)

Bring broth, sesame oil and sake to a boil. Combine flour and water; gradually add to broth, stirring until thickened. Stir in green onions and chili oil; pour over fish. Serve at once.

FISH ORIENTAL STYLE

1	pound fillet of sole, cod, turbot, halibut or other white fish
6	tablespoons sake
3	tablespoons ginger juice
3	tablespoons lemon juice
	dash salt
6	Shitake mushrooms
1-2	fresh lemons, cut into wedges

Place each fillet on a piece of aluminum foil; fold edges of foil upwards to make a bowl. Cover each fillet with generous amount of sake, ginger juice and lemon juice; top with 1-2 mushrooms. Pinch top edges of foil together to seal, leaving a small amount of space between top of fish and top of foil. Steam in a 350° oven for 20 minutes or until done. Garnish with plenty of fresh lemon.

Note: Shitake mushrooms can usually be found in oriental markets. If fresh are unavailable, reconstitute dried Shitake mushrooms by soaking them in water for 30 minutes or until soft.

SEAFOOD FETTUCCINI

1	pound steamer clams
1	pound mussels
1	medium onion, chopped
1	clove garlic, minced
2	tablespoons safflower oil
3	tablespoons olive oil
1	1-lb. can plum tomatoes
1	1-lb. can tomato puree
1	6-oz. can tomato paste
1	12-oz. can water (2 tomato paste cans)
¼	teaspoon oregano
1	teaspoon basil
1	teaspoon or less salt
½	green pepper, sliced
½	pound red snapper, bass or cod
¼	pound crab legs
1	pound fettuccini

Wash and soak clam and mussel shells following the procedure for steamed clams with fresh lemon* (page 416).

Sauté onion and garlic in safflower oil; add all remaining ingredients except seafood and pasta. Bring to a boil; reduce heat. Simmer 20-30 minutes; add clams and mussels. Cover tightly and steam about 10 minutes — just until shells begin to open. Add white fish and crab legs and continue cooking about 5-10 minutes until fish flakes and clams and mussels have opened. Serve over pasta. Serves 8.

Serve with green salad and plenty of crusty French bread.

LINGUINE WITH CLAM SAUCE

 4-5 cloves garlic
  2 tablespoons olive oil
  2 tablespoons safflower oil
  1 cup dry white wine
  ¼ teaspoon or less salt
  ⅛ teaspoon pepper
  2 6½-oz. cans chopped clams
  ¾ pound linguine, cooked
  1 pound steamer clams with shells
  ¼ cup chopped fresh parsley

Combine garlic, olive oil and safflower oil in a covered jar; let mellow at least 24 hours — several days is even better.

Heat wine with oils and garlic; simmer 15-20 minutes. Add salt, pepper and chopped clams; simmer 15-20 minutes. Wash, soak and steam clams following the procedure for steamed clams with fresh lemon* (page 416).

Ladle linguine into soup bowls; cover with sauce. Top with steamed clams in their shells. Sprinkle with parsley.

Variation: Add a 1-pound can of plum tomatoes to the sauce.

Note: Tossed salad with an oil and vinegar dressing, crusty French bread, fresh fruits and a selection of low-fat cheeses are nice accompaniments.

PAELLA

1	pound steamer clams in shells
1	pound mussels in shells
1	medium red onion
2	green peppers
1	red pepper (for garnish)
4	cloves garlic
2½	cups uncooked long grain rice
1	teaspoon crushed red pepper
¼	teaspoon black pepper
¼	teaspoon saffron
½	teaspoon basil
¾	cup dry white wine
¾	cup water
1	15-oz. can quartered artichoke hearts
1-2	slices broiled Canadian bacon, diced
2	cooked chicken breasts, cubed
1½	pound firm fillets of white fish
1	pound cracked crab legs

Wash and soak clams and mussels following the procedure for steamed clams with fresh lemon* (page 416). Steam clams; reserve 3 cups of the nectar.

Chop onion and one green pepper. Cut remaining green pepper and the red pepper into long strips.

Sauté onion, garlic and diced green pepper in small amount of nectar until tender; add rice, crushed red pepper, black pepper, saffron, basil, reserved nectar, wine and water. Bring to a boil, stirring constantly.

Transfer to a 4-quart casserole; stir in artichokes and bacon. Cover. Bake at 350° for 30 minutes, stirring at 10 minute intervals.

Continued

Add chicken and white fish. Poke mussels into top of rice. Bake 10 minutes. Add steamed clams in their shells and crab legs and cook 5 minutes longer or until rice is tender and mussels have opened. Garnish with red pepper and remaining green pepper.

CALAMARI

1½	pounds squid
1	cup white wine
2	cloves garlic
¾	pound linguine, cooked
2	tablespoons safflower oil
⅓	cup olive oil
	juice of 1 lemon
½	teaspoon or less salt
¼	teaspoon pepper
2	tablespoons chopped fresh parsley

Thoroughly wash squid; split and remove cartilage, eyes and ink sacks.

Heat wine and garlic in wok or heavy skillet. Sauté squid 3-5 minutes — just until color changes and squid become tender; do not overcook or squid will become rubbery. Drain off liquid.

Arrange squid over pasta; sprinkle with safflower oil, olive oil, lemon juice, salt, pepper and parsley. Toss until squid and linguine are well-coated.

Note: If you are not familiar with the proper method to clean squid, ask the personnel at your fish market to show you.

BOUILLABAISSE

2 pounds clams
2 pounds mussels
2 cups dry white wine
4 cups chicken broth* (page 295)
½ cup safflower oil
¼ cup olive oil
1 onion, chopped
1 leek with green top, chopped
4 cloves garlic
4 large ripe tomatoes, chopped
1 28-oz. can plum tomatoes
2 sprigs fresh basil
3 drops Tabasco sauce
½ teaspoon salt
1 bay leaf
  dash each cayenne, thyme and fennel
2 green peppers, chopped
¾ pound red snapper, cut into 3-inch cubes
¾ pound cod, cut into 3-inch cubes
¼ pound scallops
¾ pound crab legs
6 red potatoes, sliced and steamed in their jackets until just tender

Wash and soak clams and mussels*(see page 416).
Continued

Bring wine, chicken broth, safflower oil and olive oil to a boil in a large stock pot. Add onion, leek and garlic; simmer 20 minutes. Add fresh and canned tomatoes, basil, Tabasco sauce and seasonings; heat just to boiling, but do not allow to boil. Add clams and mussels. Cover. Steam just until shells begin to open; add green pepper and remaining seafood. Cook 5 minutes. Add potatoes; simmer 2-3 minutes or until most clams and mussels have opened and red snapper and cod are cooked. Do not overcook seafood. Serves 8-10.

LINGUINE WITH TUNA SAUCE

3	large ripe tomatoes, chopped
2	tablespoons olive oil
½	cup chopped fresh parsley
1	bunch green onions with tops, chopped
½	teaspoon chopped fresh basil or ¼ teaspoon dried basil
1	lemon
1	6½-oz. can water pack tuna, drained
1	teaspoon pepper
¾	pound linguine, cooked

Combine tomatoes, oil, parsley, green onion and basil; cook 5-7 minutes. Squeeze lemon over tuna. Grate rind of lemon; sprinkle over tuna and toss with pepper. Add to tomatoes and onion; cook 5-7 minutes. Serve over linguine.

CIOPPINO

1   pound clams
1   pound mussels
1   cup dry white wine
2   cups chicken broth* (page 295)
1   8-oz. can tomato sauce
3   tablespoons tomato paste
3   tablespoons safflower oil
3   tablespoons olive oil
1   onion, chopped
1   leek with green top, chopped
2   cloves garlic
3   fresh ripe tomatoes, chopped
1   1-lb. can plum tomatoes
2   sprigs fresh basil or ½ teaspoon
     dried
1   bay leaf
     dash each fennel, thyme and
      cayenne
2   drops Tabasco sauce
¾   teaspoon salt
1   green pepper, chopped
¼   pound red snapper, cut into 3-inch
     cubes
¼   pound cod, cut into 3-inch cubes
¼   pound scallops
¼   pound crab legs
2   cups cooked seashell-shaped pasta

Wash and soak clams and mussels following procedure for steamed clams with fresh lemon* (page 416).

Bring wine, chicken broth, tomato sauce, tomato paste, safflower oil, and olive oil to a boil. Add onion, leek and garlic; simmer 20 minutes. *Continued*

Add fresh and canned tomatoes and remaining seasonings; heat just to boiling. Add clams and mussels. Cover. Steam just until shells begin to open; add green pepper and remaining seafood. Cook 5 minutes; add pasta. Simmer 2-3 minutes or until most clams and mussels have opened and red snapper and cod are cooked.

TUNA NOODLE CASSEROLE

1   8-oz. package salad macaroni, cooked
1   6½-oz. can water pack tuna, drained
1   8-oz. can sliced waterchestnuts, drained
3   cups cream of chicken soup* (page 316)

Combine all ingredients. Pour into a 2-quart casserole. Bake at 375° for 25-30 minutes.

CHAPTER SEVENTEEN

POULTRY

ROAST TURKEY

---

       1   turkey
           sage
           pepper
           garlic powder
     2-3   stalks celery, cut into 2-inch pieces
     1-2   onions, quartered

Wipe inside of turkey with a damp paper towel; wash outside with cold water. Rub inside cavity with sage, pepper and garlic powder. Place celery and onions inside cavity. Skewer neck skin to back; tuck wing tips behind shoulder joints.

Place breast side up on rack in shallow roasting pan; roast at 325°. Turkey is done when drum sticks move easily or twist out of joint. A meat thermometer should register 195°. If turkey browns too quickly, cover it with a cap of aluminum foil.

Roasting Chart
   6-8   pounds 2¾ to 3½ hours
  8-12   pounds 3¼ to 4   hours
 12-16   pounds 3¾ to 5   hours
 16-20   pounds 4¾ to 6½ hours
 20-24   pounds 6¼ to 8   hours

Note: For Positive Diet purposes the turkey should not be stuffed as fat from the turkey drips into the dressing. There is an excellent stuffing recipe in this book that is cooked along side the turkey.

Helpful Hint: Be sure to save the carcass for soup.

BARBECUED TURKEY

1   turkey
    sage
    pepper
    garlic powder
2   stalks celery, chopped
1   large onion, chopped
    safflower oil

Wipe inside of turkey with a damp paper towel; wash outside with cold water. Rub inside cavity with sage, pepper and garlic powder. Place celery and onions inside cavity. Skewer neck skin to back; tuck wing tips behind shoulder joints. Rub outside of turkey with safflower oil.

Place 25 briquets on each side of barbecue kettle. When coals are ready put in drip pan. Put turkey in roast holder position on grill. Every hour add 8 briquets per side.

For a 12-pound turkey allow 2½-hours cooking time; for a 20-pound turkey allow 11 minutes per pound.

Note: The roast holder and drip pan which are necessary to barbecue a turkey are available in hardware stores and discount stores.

ROAST TURKEY BREAST

turkey breasts
safflower oil
sage

Remove skin from breast; rub with safflower oil and season with sage. Roast on a rack at 350° for 1½-hours or until juices run free when pricked with a fork.

STEAMED TURKEY BREAST

turkey breast
lemon juice

Remove skin from turkey breast. Place breast in a steamer over boiling water and add a dash of lemon juice. Cover. Steam 30-35 minutes or until juices run free when pricked with a fork.

OVEN-FRIED CHICKEN

½-1   chicken breast per person
        safflower oil
        flour or bread crumbs
        dash pepper
        paprika

Remove skin from chicken. Brush each piece with safflower oil. Dredge lightly in flour or bread crumbs. Season with pepper. Sprinkle with paprika. Bake at 425° 35-40 minutes. Turn; bake 10-25 minutes longer or until tender.

EXTRA CRISPY OVEN-FRIED CHICKEN

2   chicken breasts, halved
½   cup skim milk
½   cup Grape Nuts Flakes

Remove skin from chicken; debone if desired. Dip chicken in milk, then in Grape Nuts Flakes. Bake in a teflon pan at 400° for ½ hour. Reduce heat to 350°. Cover loosely with foil. Bake 20-30 minutes longer. Do not turn chicken during baking.

BAKED' CHICKEN WITH OLIVE OIL AND FRESH LEMON

2   chicken breasts, halved
2   tablespoons safflower oil
2   tablespoons olive oil
¼   cup fresh lemon juice
1   clove garlic, minced
¼   teaspoon oregano
¼   teaspoon tarragon

Remove skin from chicken breasts; debone. Combine safflower oil, olive oil, lemon juice, garlic, oregano and tarragon; pour over chicken. Marinate 20 minutes. Bake at 350° 35-45 minutes or until done. Baste frequently during baking.

Helpful Hint: To debone chicken breasts, tear off skin. Break breast in two by splitting bone in center of breast. Cut meat free from the long rib cage bone. Then cut around upper edge of breast. Pull the rest of the meat away from bones. Loosen the tendons and remove.

To save chicken bones for soup, keep a plastic bag in the freezer just for bones reserved from boning breasts. When bag is full, add extra backs, necks and wings and make chicken soup.

MICROWAVE BAKED CHICKEN

2   chicken breasts, halved
    safflower oil

Remove skin from chicken breasts; debone. Brush with safflower oil. Place in glass pie plate — place larger pieces to the outside of dish. Cover with plastic wrap; prick for steam to escape. Cook 8 minutes; turn. Rearrange pieces in dish; cook 6 minutes longer or until done.

ROAST CHICKEN

1   3-4 pound broiler-fryer chicken
    sage
    pepper
    garlic powder
2   stalks chopped celery with leaves
1   onion, quartered

Wipe inside of chicken with a damp paper towel; wash outside with cold water. Rub inside cavity with sage, pepper and garlic powder. Place celery and onions inside cavity. Skewer neck skin to back; tuck wing tips behind shoulder joints. Place breast side up in shallow roasting pan. Roast 60-75 minutes at 350°. Let stand 10 minutes before slicing.

Serve with oven-roasted vegetables.

Note: Be sure to save the carcass for soup.

ROAST CHICKEN ORIENTAL STYLE

1   bunch leaf lettuce
1   roast chicken, thinly sliced* (page 452)
1   bunch green onions with tops
12 spring roll (lumpia) wrappers
     hot Chinese mustard
     toasted sesame seeds

Tear lettuce into bite-size pieces; arrange on a platter or tray. Layer chicken over lettuce. Slice green onions lengthwise into 2-inch strips; arrange around edge of lettuce.

Place spring roll wrappers in a vegetable steamer rack over boiling water; steam 3-5 minutes or until hot or wrap spring roll wrappers in a damp dish towel and steam 1-2 minutes in the microwave. Remove to a napkin-lined basket.

Everyone prepares their own meal as follows: Lay spring roll wrapper flat. Place a slice of chicken, some lettuce and green onion lengthwise in center of wrapper. Fold bottom edge up, left and right sides over and roll as for crêpes.

Dip in hot Chinese mustard and sesame seeds* (page 247).

Note: Won Ton Soup* (page 298) and new variety rice* (page 410) are especially good accompaniments.

POACHED CHICKEN

      tub safflower margarine
   4 chicken breasts
  ½ fresh lemon
  ¼ cup dry white wine
  ¼ cup chicken broth* (page 295)
      dash pepper
      dash salt

Grease a baking dish with tub safflower margarine. Remove skin from chicken breast; debone. Arrange chicken breasts in baking dish; drizzle with lemon juice. Season. Add wine and broth. Cover dish tightly. Bake at 400° 10-15 minutes or until tender and no sign of pink remains.

BOILED CHICKEN

      chicken breasts
      celery with leaves
      onion
      carrot
      piece of fresh ginger

Remove skin from chicken breast; debone if desired. Place chicken in small stock pot; add some celery, onion and carrot and a piece of fresh ginger. Add enough cold water to cover by 2-inches; bring to a boil. Cook 10-20 minutes or until chicken is tender and no sign of pink remains; do not overcook.

STEAMED CHICKEN

chicken breasts
fresh lemon juice

Remove skin from chicken breast; debone if desired. Place breast in a vegetable steamer basket over boiling water; add a dash of lemon juice. Cover. Steam 15-25 minutes or until chicken is tender and no sign of pink remains; do not overcook.

Serve with fresh lemon wedges; sprinkle with ground pepper.

Note: Fresh raw spinach with a dressing of fresh lemon and ground pepper* (page 363) and sliced tomatoes with fresh basil* (page 338) are nice accompaniments.

BARBECUED CHICKEN BREASTS

½-1   chicken breast per person, skin
        removed
      barbecue sauce

Place chicken breasts over hot coals; cook 10 minutes. Turn; cook 10 minutes. Turn; baste with barbecue sauce. Cook 5 minutes. Turn; baste. Cook 5 minutes longer. Chicken is done when it can easily be pulled away from bone.

Note: Be sure to read labels when selecting a barbecue sauce to insure it contains only heart-healthy ingredients.

BARBECUED CHICKEN WITH FRESH LIME

3   chicken breasts, halved
⅔   cup fresh lime juice
    juice of 2 lemons
⅔   cup safflower oil
2   teaspoons rosemary
¼   teaspoon pepper

Remove skin from chicken; debone if desired. Combine all ingredients, except chicken in a covered jar; shake. Pour over chicken. Marinate several hours or overnight. Grill chicken over medium coals about 50 minutes. Baste with marinade and turn frequently during cooking.

BARBECUED CHICKEN ITALIAN STYLE

1   recipe oil and vinegar dressing*
    (page 362)
2   tablespoons Dijon mustard
¼   cup dry white wine
1   broiler-fryer chicken, cut up
½   pound fresh mushrooms
2   onions quartered
2   tomatoes, halved

Combine dressing, Dijon and wine; pour over chicken and vegetables. Marinate 2 hours. When coals are ready, arrange chicken on barbecue; grill 20 minutes. Turn; grill 20 minutes longer. Turn; add vegetables. Grill 10 minutes or until chicken is tender and vegetables are hot. Baste frequently during cooking.

BARBECUED CHICKEN WITH SKEWERED VEGETABLES

3	chicken breasts
3	tablespoons safflower oil
1	tablespoon olive oil
¼	cup fresh lemon juice
1	teaspoon honey
	dash tarragon
	dash oregano
12	cherry tomatoes
12	fresh mushrooms
2	onions, cut into 2-inch cubes
2	green peppers, quartered
½	fresh pineapple, cut into chunks

Skin and debone chicken; cut into 2-inch cubes. Combine safflower oil, olive oil, lemon juice, honey and seasonings; pour over chicken and vegetables. Marinate 30-60 minutes.

Alternate chicken, vegetables and fruit on skewers. Broil 4-6 inches from heat, turning frequently and basting often about 20-30 minutes or until chicken is done.

Variation: Instead of chicken parts, roast a whole chicken. Skewer vegetables separately.

DIJON CHICKEN

1   chicken breast per person
1   recipe Dijon vinaigrette* (page 361)

Broil, grill, bake, steam, roast or poach chicken. Accompany with Dijon vinaigrette for dipping.

Note: Fresh spinach salad with sesame seeds* (page 337) and sliced tomatoes drizzled with Dijon vinaigrette are nice accompaniments.

CHICKEN-STUFFED PEPPERS

4   medium green peppers
⅓   cup chopped onion
1   1-lb. can stewed tomatoes
2   cups cooked barley or rice
¼   teaspoon Tabasco sauce
    dash pepper
3   cooked chicken breasts, deboned
    and cubed
¾   cup grated low-fat Mozzarella or
    Cheddar cheese

Cut tops of green peppers; remove seeds and membrane. Sauté onion in small amount of tomato liquid; add tomatoes, rice or barley, Tabasco, pepper, chicken and ½ of the cheese. Stand peppers upright in an 8-inch square baking dish; stuff with tomato-barley filling. Bake uncovered at 350° 25-30 minutes or until hot; sprinkle with remaining cheese. Return to oven until cheese melts.

Variation: In place of chicken, use ¾-lb. extra lean ground round, cooked and drained.

STIR-FRIED CHICKEN WITH VEGETABLES

1   tablespoon ginger juice
1   tablespoon sake
1   pound deboned chicken breasts, cut into bite-sized pieces
2   tablespoons potato starch
1   cup chicken broth* (page 295)
1   onion, sliced into 1/16ths
¼   pound bamboo shoots, cut into 2-inch lengths
3   stalks celery, sliced
1   carrot, sliced crosswise into rounds
2   green peppers, cut into 1/16ths
½   pound fresh snow peas
1   8-oz. can sliced waterchestnuts
½   pound fresh mushrooms, sliced

Grate ginger; squeeze pulp to get 1 tablespoon juice. Mix ginger juice with sake; pour over chicken. Let stand 10 minutes; sprinkle with potato starch.

Cook chicken in a pre-heated teflon skillet over medium-high heat until chicken turns white. Set aside.

Heat ½ cup of broth in wok or heavy skillet; stir-fry onions, bamboo shoots, celery and carrots until just crisp-tender. Stir in green pepper and snow peas; stir-fry 2-3 minutes. Add waterchestnuts and mushrooms; stir-fry 1-2 minutes. Add more broth as needed during cooking. Toss chicken with vegetables. Serve at once.

Note: Good with steamed rice.

STIR-FRIED CHICKEN WITH GREEN PEPPERS

1 pound deboned chicken breasts
1 tablespoon sake
2 tablespoons potato starch
½ cup chicken broth* (page 295)
4 green peppers, seeded and cut
   lengthwise into thin strips

Cut chicken into bite-size pieces; toss with sake. Let stand 10 minutes; sprinkle with potato starch. Cook in a pre-heated teflon skillet over medium high heat until chicken turns white. Set aside. Heat chicken broth in wok or heavy skillet; stir-fry green peppers 2-3 minutes or until just crisp-tender. Toss with chicken.

CHICKEN A LA KING

½ pound fresh mushrooms, sliced
½ green pepper, sliced
1½ cups cooked chicken, diced
1 recipe cream of chicken soup*
   (page 316)
   rice, biscuits or toast

Sauté mushrooms and green pepper in small amount of chicken broth, water or white wine until tender. Stir in chicken and soup. Heat to serving temperature. Serve over rice, biscuits or toast.

Note: If serving over rice, pack rice into a ring mold. Turn out at once onto a hot platter. Fill center with chicken a la king.

CHICKEN POT PIE

½   cup diced carrots
¼   cup diced celery
¼   cup chopped white onion
      chicken broth* (page 295)
1½ cups cooked chicken, diced
3   cups cream of chicken soup*
      (page 316)
½   cup fresh snow peas
½   cup thinly sliced fresh mushrooms
⅛   teaspoon pepper
1   recipe double pie crust* (page 507)

Sauté carrots, celery and onion in small amount of chicken broth, water or white wine until tender. Add chicken, soup, remaining vegetables and seasoning; set aside. Roll out pastry dough. Line one 9-inch pie pan or 3-4 individual size pans with ½ of the dough. Fill with chicken filling. Adjust top crust. Tuck edges under and flute. Cut steam holes. Bake at 400° for 20 minutes or until lightly browned and inside mixture is bubbly.

CHICKEN AND DUMPLINGS

1   3-pound chicken
1   onion, sliced
2   stalks celery, chopped
½   teaspoon or less salt
5   peppercorns
1   bay leaf
5   cups water
2   carrots, quartered lengthwise
½   pound fresh mushrooms, sliced
2   tablespoons flour plus ¼ cup water
¾   cup snow peas

Place chicken, onion, celery, salt, peppercorns, bay leaf and water in stock pot; heat to boiling. Cover, reduce heat and simmer 2-3 hours. Strain. Slice and wrap chicken. Refrigerate chicken and broth overnight. Skim fat. Shortly before serving, heat broth to boiling; add carrots and cook 10-15 minutes or until tender. Prepare dumplings.

Dumplings
1   cup flour
2   teaspoons baking powder
¼   teaspoon or less salt
½   cup skim milk
2   tablespoons safflower oil

Sift together flour, baking powder and salt. Combine milk and safflower oil and add to dry ingredients; stir just until moistened.
Continued

Add chicken and mushrooms to boiling broth; bring to a second boil. Drop dumplings by table-spoonsful on top of bubbling stew. Cover tightly; bring to a boil. Reduce heat; simmer 12-15 minutes. Caution: do not lift cover from dumplings during cooking process.

Remove dumplings from pan. Combine flour and water to make a smooth paste; quickly stir into broth to make a gravy. Add snow peas. Heat. Serve.

CANTONESE HOT POT

1½	pounds deboned chicken breasts
5	carrots, cut into thin rounds
4	cups chicken broth* (page 295)
2	bunches fresh spinach leaves
1	head Chinese cabbage
½	pound fresh mushrooms
1	8-oz. can whole waterchestnuts
1	bunch broccoli, flowerets only
1	white onion, cut into 2-inch cubes
1	cake Tofu, cubed

Skin chicken; cut into 2-inch cubes. Sauté carrots in small amount of broth until just crisp-tender. Arrange meats and vegetables on a large tray. Heat broth to boiling; pour into fondue pot. Light flame underneath to keep broth boiling.

Each person cooks his own meal by skewering meat and vegetables on fondue forks. When all vegetables and chicken are gone, ladle the broth into individual bowls and serve.

Note: New variety rice* (page 410) and Chinese buckwheat (soba) noodles are nice accompaniments.

CHICKEN DIVAN

3	chicken breasts, halved
¾	pound asparagus spears
1½	cups cream of chicken soup* (page 316)
⅔	cup safflower mayonnaise
⅓	cup low-fat evaporated milk
½	cup grated low-fat Cheddar cheese
1	teaspoon lemon juice
½	teaspoon curry powder
½	cup bread crumbs

Remove skin from chicken and debone; brown chicken lightly on both sides in a teflon skillet. Steam asparagus in vegetable steamer basket over boiling water 2-3 minutes; arrange in an 8-inch square baking dish and top with chicken. Combine soup, mayonnaise, milk, cheese, lemon juice and curry; pour over chicken. Sprinkle with bread crumbs. Bake at 350° 25-30 minutes.

Note: Serve with steamed red potatoes.

Variation: Substitute broccoli for asparagus.

CHICKEN CURRY

½   cup chopped onion
2   cups chicken broth* (page 295)
2   cups skim milk
½   cup flour
½   teaspoon or less salt
1   tablespoon curry powder
¼   teaspoon ground ginger
1   tablespoon lemon juice
4   cups cooked chicken, diced
1   8-oz. can sliced waterchestnuts
    steamed rice
    unsalted peanuts for garnish
       (optional)
    raisins for garnish (optional)
    pineapple chunks for garnish
       (optional)
    homemade chutney (optional)

Sauté onion in small amount of chicken broth until tender; add remaining broth. Bring to a boil. Shake milk and flour in a covered jar to form a smooth paste; gradually add to boiling broth, stirring constantly until thick. Add seasonings. Pour lemon juice over chicken; add to sauce. Stir in waterchestnuts. Heat. Serve over steamed rice. If desired, garnish with unsalted peanuts, raisins, pineapple chunks and chutney.

Note: Frozen bananas* (page 502) make a perfect dessert.

CHICKEN CREOLE

1 medium onion, chopped
1 clove garlic, minced
½ cup celery, finely chopped
1 8-oz. can tomato sauce
½ cup water
1 bay leaf
¼ teaspoon salt
⅛ teaspoon cayenne
2 tablespoons safflower oil
1 green pepper, finely chopped
1 cup cooked chicken, cubed
1 teaspoon fresh parsley, chopped
steamed rice

Combine onion, garlic, celery, tomato sauce, water, bay leaf, salt, cayenne and safflower oil in a 4-quart saucepan; bring to a boil. Cover, reduce heat and simmer 45-60 minutes. Add green pepper and chicken. Cover; simmer 10-15 minutes. Sprinkle with parsley. Serve over steamed rice.

CHICKEN CACCIATORE

1 28-oz. can plum tomatoes
1 tablespoon safflower oil
1 onion, chopped
3 carrots, peeled and thinly sliced
3 stalks celery, thinly sliced
2 tablespoons red wine vinegar
¼ teaspoon pepper
¾ teaspoon sage
½ teaspoon or less salt
¼ teaspoon sugar
2 chicken breasts, halved
¾ pound shell-shaped macaroni

Combine all ingredients, except chicken and pasta in a stew pot or Dutch oven; bring to a boil. Reduce heat; cover and simmer 25-30 minutes. Skin and debone chicken; add to sauce and cook 25-30 minutes or until tender. Serve over cooked pasta.

Note: Crusty French bread and a tossed green salad with oil and vinegar dressing are nice accompaniments.

CHILI CON POLLO

1	28-oz. can plum tomatoes
½	teaspoon or less salt
1½	teaspoons dry mustard
1½	teaspoons chili powder
2	small cloves garlic, minced
1	pound deboned, cooked chicken breast, diced
4	cups cooked red kidney beans
2	cups cooked salad macaroni

Combine tomatoes, salt, dry mustard, chili powder and garlic; simmer uncovered for 1½-2 hours. Add chicken and kidney beans; heat to boiling. Stir in pasta. Heat to serving temperature.

Variation: Two 15-oz. cans kidney beans with liquid may be used in place of the fresh.

CHICKEN TOSTADOS

corn tortillas
cooked chicken, cubed
lettuce, diced
ripe tomatoes, diced
white onion, diced
chopped green chilies (optional)
low-fat Cheddar or Mozzarella cheese,
    grated
tomato salsa* (page 361)
plain non-fat yogurt (optional)
    (page 202)

Place tortillas on a teflon baking sheet. Heat in a 350° oven 3 minutes; turn. Heat 3 more minutes or until warm. Spread tortillas with chicken; top with lettuce, tomato, onion, green chilies, cheese, salsa and yogurt.

Variation: Substitute extra-lean ground round for chicken.

CHICKEN ENCHILADAS

    2 cups cooked chicken, shredded
    1 small ripe tomato, chopped
    1 onion, chopped
    1 8-oz. can chopped green chilies
 1¼ cups grated low-fat Cheddar cheese
    1 recipe tomato salsa* (page 361)
    8 corn tortillas
    1 8-oz. can tomato puree
    3 cloves garlic
    3 drops Tabasco sauce

Combine chicken, tomato, ¼ cup chopped onion, 1 tablespoon chopped green chilies, 1 tablespoon cheese and 1 tablespoon salsa. Set aside. Heat tortillas on a teflon baking sheet in a 350° oven about 3 minutes on each side to soften. Put 3 tablespoons chicken filling in center of each tortilla and roll; arrange seam side down in a shallow oven-proof baking dish. Set aside. Place tomato puree, garlic and remaining onion in blender; purée until smooth. Stir in remaining green chilies and Tabasco sauce; pour over enchiladas. Bake at 375° 15 minutes. Sprinkle with remaining cheese. Bake 10 minutes longer.

CHICKEN CHALUPAS

2 cups chicken broth* (page 295)
2 large ripe tomatoes, chopped
1 large onion, chopped
1 clove garlic
3 cooked chicken breasts, cubed
⅛ teaspoon cayenne pepper
⅛ teaspoon black pepper
⅛ teaspoon salt
  corn tortillas

Topping
  chopped ripe tomatoes
  chopped white onion
  low-fat Cheddar cheese, grated
  tomato salsa* (page 361)
  plain non-fat yogurt* (page 202)
    (optional)

Bring chicken broth to a boil; add tomatoes, onion and garlic. Bring to a second boil; cook about 1 hour or until liquid is nearly absorbed. Stir in chicken, cayenne pepper, black pepper and salt; simmer 45-60 minutes or until all liquid is absorbed.

Place tortillas on a teflon baking sheet. Heat in a 350° oven 3 minutes; turn. Heat 3 more minutes or until warm. Top each with chicken filling, then with tomato, onion and cheese. Sprinkle with salsa; top with yogurt, if desired.

Variation: Just before serving, stir 1-2 cups baked beans* (page 408) into chicken filling; heat to serving temperature.

471

LEMON CHICKEN WITH FRESH SPINACH

        3   chicken breasts
        1   tablespoon ginger juice
        1   tablespoon sake
       ½   cup fresh lemon juice
        2   cups chicken broth* (page 295)
       ¼   cup flour
       ½   cup water
        2   tablespoons potato starch
        1   bunch fresh spinach

Remove skin from chicken; debone and cut into cubes. Sprinkle with ginger juice and sake. Let stand 10 minutes.

Combine lemon juice and broth in medium saucepan; reserve ⅓ cup and set aside. Heat remainder to boiling. Shake flour and water in a covered jar to form a smooth paste; gradually add to boiling broth, stirring constantly until thick. Reduce heat and let simmer 5-10 minutes.

Sprinkle chicken with potato starch. Heat reserved broth in wok or heavy skillet; stir-fry chicken. Tear spinach into bite-size pieces; toss with chicken. Serve onto plates. Pour sauce over.

LEMON CHICKEN WITH MAYONNAISE AND FRESH TOMATOES

3 chicken breasts, halved
⅛ teaspoon safflower oil
¼ cup dry vermouth
¼ teaspoon white pepper
½ cup lemon juice
½ cup safflower mayonnaise
1 teaspoon grated onion
watercress
fresh tomato slices
fresh parsley

Remove skin from chicken; debone. Brush with safflower oil. Lightly brown chicken on both sides in a teflon skillet; remove to baking dish.

Pour vermouth into skillet; bring to a boil and reduce by ⅓. Remove from heat; add white pepper and 6 tablespoons of the lemon juice; pour over chicken. Bake covered in a 350° oven for 20 minutes or until chicken is done. Baste frequently during cooking. Cool to room temperature. Refrigerate several hours.

Mix remaining lemon juice with mayonnaise and grated onion. Let chicken come to room temperature (about 1 hour) before serving; place on a bed of watercress that has been topped with sliced tomatoes. Garnish with parsley. Serve with lemon mayonnaise.

Note: Homemade safflower mayonnaise* (page 360) is especially good with this

CHAPTER EIGHTEEN

RED MEATS

BROILED LAMB CHOPS

4   extra lean lamb chops

Score fat edges of chops; place on rack in broiling pan. Broil 3 inches from heat 8-10 minutes; turn. Broil 5-8 minutes.

Variation: Place canned pear or peach halves beside chops the last 3 minutes of cooking. If desired, fill with mint jelly the last 2 minutes of cooking.

SHISH KEBOB

3	tablespoons safflower oil
1	tablespoon olive oil
½	cup dry white wine or vermouth
1	teaspoon lemon juice
¼	teaspoon or less salt
1-2	pounds lamb, cut into 1-inch cubes
2	green peppers, quartered lengthwise
10-12	cherry tomatoes
8-10	artichoke hearts
10-12	fresh mushrooms
1	onion, cut into wedges
2	cups fresh pineapple, cut into chunks

Combine oils, wine, lemon juice and salt; pour over lamb and vegetables. Marinate several hours. Arrange lamb, vegetables and pineapple alternately on skewers. Grill over hot coals or broil basting frequently and turning often until lamb is done.

477

ROAST LEG OF LAMB

1   leg of lamb
    pepper
    rosemary
    garlic powder

Season lamb with pepper, rosemary and garlic powder. Place fat side up on rack in roasting pan. Insert meat thermometer. Roast at 325° 30-35 minutes per pound. Meat thermometer should read 175° for medium or 182° for well done.

Variation: Use a crown roast; fill the center with barley and mushroom pilaf* (page 410) just before serving.

LAMB BURGERS

1   pound extra lean ground lamb
    pita bread
½   pound low-fat Mozzarella cheese,
        sliced
    red lettuce leaves
    sliced tomato
    sliced white onion

Press ground lamb into patties. Grill over hot coals or broil on rack 3-inches from heat, 4-6 minutes on each side. Turn when juices begin to form on top of meat. Serve into pita bread. Top with cheese, lettuce, tomato and onion.

BARBECUED LAMB ROAST

3-4   pounds leg of lamb, butterflied
      thyme
      garlic powder
      rosemary
      pepper
3   tablespoons safflower oil
1   tablespoon olive oil
½   cup dry white wine
1   tablespoon fresh lemon juice
      fresh parsley for garnish
      fresh lemon wedges for garnish
      cherry tomatoes
      mushroom caps, steamed 2-3 minutes
      asparagus spears, steamed 3-5 minutes

Have butcher remove bone from leg of lamb and open roast; season with thyme, garlic powder, rosemary and pepper. Combine safflower oil, olive oil, wine and lemon juice; pour over meat. Marinate in refrigerator, turning several times, 4 hours or overnight. Allow to stand at room temperature at least 1 hour before grilling.

Build a medium fire in barbecue. Grill 4-inches from heat, turning and basting with marinade every 10 minutes, 30-40 minutes for rare, 40-50 minutes for medium and 50-60 minutes for well-done. Place on carving platter and let set 10 minutes. Carve into diagonal slices. Garnish with parsley, lemon wedges, cherry tomatoes, mushroom caps and fresh asparagus spears.

Variation: To oven roast, place lamb on rack in roasting pan. Cook 15 minutes at 450°; reduce heat to 350° and roast approximately 1¼ hours or until lamb reaches desired doneness. Baste frequently while roasting.

ROAST VEAL

1   veal shoulder, loin, saddle or rack of
      veal roast
2   teaspoons olive oil
      juice of ½ lemon
      pinch of thyme
      garlic powder to taste
      black pepper to taste

Remove meat from refrigerator and let stand at room temperature for 1 hour; rub with olive oil. Sprinkle with lemon juice; season with thyme, garlic powder and black pepper. Place fat side up on rack in roasting pan. Insert a meat thermometer through outside fat into thickest part of meat. Bake uncovered at 425°. Cover loosely with foil. Roast 15-20 minutes per pound; meat thermometer should register 170°.

VEAL BURGERS

1   pound extra lean ground veal
      French bread
      sliced white onion
      red lettuce leaves
      sliced tomato
      safflower mayonnaise

Press veal into patties. Grill over hot coals or broil on rack 3-inches from heat, 4-6 minutes on each side. Turn when juices begin to form on top of meat. Serve on French bread. Top with onion, lettuce, tomato and mayonnaise.

VEAL ITALIAN STYLE

¼   teaspoon safflower oil
¼   teaspoon olive oil
2   small cloves garlic, minced
3   tomatoes, chopped, peeled and
      seeded
    dash oregano
    dash pepper
1   pound veal, sliced very thin and
      pounded extra-thin
4   slices low-fat Mozzarella cheese

Heat oils, garlic, tomatoes, oregano and pepper just to boiling. Remove from heat; cover to keep warm. Place veal on rack in broiler pan; broil 3-inches from heat 2-3 minutes. Turn when juices begin to form on top of meat; broil 1-2 minutes. Cover with cheese. Return to broiler until cheese melts. Serve with sauce.

ROAST PORK

1   very lean pork roast
    pepper
    sage
    garlic powder

Heat oven to 350°. Season meat. Place fat side up on rack in roasting pan. Insert a meat thermometer through outside fat into thickest part of meat. Roast 40 minutes per pound; meat thermometer should register 185°.

Note: Warm applesauce and homemade dumplings are nice accompaniments.

GRILLED VEAL STEAKS WITH FRESH LEMON AND MUSHROOMS

1¼	pound veal round steaks, pounded very thin
3	tablespoons safflower oil
1	tablespoon olive oil
½	cup dry white wine
1	tablespoon fresh lemon juice
1	pound fresh mushrooms, thinly sliced
1	15-oz. can quartered artichoke hearts
2	lemons, cut into quarters

Grill veal over hot coals or broil on rack 3-inches from heat. Turn when juices begin to form on top of meat; cook 3-4 minutes longer or to desired doneness. While meat is cooking, combine safflower oil, olive oil, wine and lemon juice; pour ½ of mixture into a skillet and heat. Add mushrooms and sauté, add artichokes during the last few minutes of cooking. Remove mushrooms and artichokes to a platter; cover to keep warm. Quickly heat remaining sauce. Garnish veal with mushrooms and artichokes, squeeze lemon over; drizzle with wine sauce.

ROAST BEEF

1 beef roast
2 cloves of garlic
 salt
 pepper

Heat oven to 325°. Season meat with salt and pepper; insert garlic. Place fat side up on rack in roasting pan. Insert a meat thermometer through outside fat into thickest part of meat. Roast 20-26 minutes per pound for rare; meat thermometer should register 140°. Roast 27-30 minutes per pound for medium; meat thermometer should register 160°. Roast 31-35 minutes per pound for well done; meat thermometer should register 170°. Add 10 extra minutes per pound for rolled roasts. For very rare meat, roast at 200° for 1 hour per pound.

Note: Remember for Positive Diet purposes, meat should be roasted to medium or to well done.

SWISS STEAK

1 pound extra-lean flank or round
 steak
¼ cup flour
 dash pepper
1 onion, cut into rings
¼ cup red wine
1 1-lb. can plum tomatoes

Shake meat in paper bag with flour and pepper. Brown onion and meat on both sides in wine. Drain, if necessary to remove any excess fat. Stir in tomatoes. Cover tightly. Cook slowly 1½-2 hours or until tender.

SKEWERED BEEF

¼	cup safflower oil
¼	cup red wine vinegar
½	cup dry red wine
1	clove garlic, minced
¼	teaspoon black pepper
1-2	pounds round or chuck steak, cut into 1-inch cubes
¾	pound fresh mushrooms
12	cherry tomatoes
12	artichoke hearts
1	white onion, cut into 2-inch cubes
2	green peppers, quartered lengthwise

Combine oil, vinegar, wine, garlic and pepper; pour over meat and vegetables. Cover. Chill 1-4 hours. Drain. Alternate meat and vegetables on skewers. Grill over medium hot coals or broil 4-6 inches from heat, basting frequently and turning often.

Variation: Marinate a rump roast or a chuck roast; barbecue or bake. Skewer vegetables separately; barbecue or broil.

HAMBURGERS

extra lean ground round
French rolls, French bread or
   hamburger buns
tomato slices
lettuce
white onion slices
safflower mayonnaise

Press ground round into patties. Grill or broil on rack 3-inches from heat 4-6 minutes on each side. Turn when juices begin to form on top of meat. Serve immediately on warm buns, French bread or French rolls. Garnish with tomato slices, lettuce and onion.

GRILLED STEAK

extra-lean steaks

Score steak by cutting through outside fat every inch or so to prevent meat from curling during cooking. Grill or broil on rack 3 inches from heat. Turn when juices begin to form on top of meat. For 1-inch thick steaks grill 5 minutes on each side for rare; 6 minutes on each side for medium; and 8 minutes on each side for well done. For 2-inch thick steaks grill 16 minutes on each side for rare; 18 minutes on each side for medium; and 20 minutes on each side for well done.

Note: For Positive Diet purposes, meat should be roasted to medium or to well done.

COUNTRY POT ROAST

2-3 pound chuck, blade, rump or pot
     roast
  1 2-pound can plum tomatoes
  2 teaspoons caraway seeds
  ½ teaspoon or less salt
2-3 drops Tabasco sauce (optional)
  1 bay leaf
  ¼ teaspoon black pepper
  4 potatoes, peeled and quartered
  6 carrots, peeled and quartered
  6 stalks celery, peeled and quartered
  4 small onions
 12 fresh mushrooms

Brown meat in a small amount of tomato liquid; drain, if necessary to remove any excess fat. Add tomatoes and seasonings. Cover and simmer 1½ hours; add potatoes, carrots, celery and onions. Cover and simmer about 1 hour — until vegetables are crisp-tender. Add mushrooms and simmer 15 minutes.

BEEF STEW

2	pounds chuck roast
1	2-pound can plum tomatoes
¼	teaspoon black pepper
¼	cup red wine (optional)
4	stalks celery, sliced on the diagonal into quarters
1	onion, cut into eighths
5	carrots, peeled and quartered
½	pound fresh mushrooms, sliced
½	pound fresh green beans, cooked
1	15-oz. can artichoke hearts
½	teaspoon safflower oil
3-4	drops hot chili oil (La Yu)
2	cups cooked macaroni

Brown chuck roast in small amount of tomato liquid; drain if necessary, to remove any excess fat. Add tomatoes, pepper and wine; bring to a boil. Add celery, onion and carrots; simmer 45 minutes. Add mushrooms, beans and artichoke hearts; simmer 15 minutes. Add safflower oil, chili oil and pasta. Heat.

Note: Hot chili oil (La Yu) is available in oriental markets.

OLD FASHIONED HASH

1½	cups coarsely ground left over roast or steak
3	coarsely ground cooked potatoes
½	onion, coarsely ground
¼	pound fresh mushrooms, coarsely ground
1	green pepper, coarsely ground
¼	cup chopped fresh parsley
½	teaspoon or less salt
¼-½	teaspoon black pepper
⅔	cup low-fat evaporated milk
⅓	cup crushed corn flakes plus 1 tablespoon olive oil for topping (optional)

Combine all ingredients except corn flakes and olive oil. Grease a loaf pan with tub safflower margarine. Mold hash into pan. Sprinkle with corn flake topping, if desired. Bake at 350° 30 minutes or until hot. Serve with ketchup and mustard.

DUTCH MEAT LOAF

1   15-oz. can tomato sauce
¼   cup water
2   tablespoons prepared mustard
1   tablespoon vinegar
1   pound extra-lean ground round
1   cup bread crumbs
¼   cup egg substitute
1   medium onion, chopped
¼   teaspoon pepper

Combine tomato sauce, water, mustard and vinegar. Mix beef with bread crumbs, egg, onion, pepper and ¼ of the tomato sauce mixture. Shape into a loaf pan. Pour enough sauce over top of meat loaf to coat. Bake at 350° for 1 hour, basting often. Warm remaining sauce; serve over sliced meat loaf.

TOSTADOS

8   corn tortillas
1   pound extra-lean ground round,
      cooked and drained
½   head of lettuce, chopped
2   ripe tomatoes, chopped
1   white onion, chopped
1   cup low-fat Mozzarella or Cheddar
      cheese, grated
1   recipe tomato salsa* (page 361)

Place tortillas on a teflon baking sheet. Heat in a 350° oven 3 minutes on each side or until warm. Spread with ground round. Top with lettuce, tomato, onion, cheese and salsa. Serve.

OVEN TACOS

4   corn tortillas
1   pound extra-lean ground round,
        cooked and drained
1   cup grated low-fat Cheddar cheese
1   white onion, chopped
1   green pepper, chopped
    chopped green chilies (optional)
2   ripe tomatoes, chopped
½   head of lettuce, chopped
    sprouts
1   recipe tomato salsa* (page 361)
    plain non-fat yogurt* (page 202)
        (optional)

Spread tortillas on a teflon baking sheet. Place ground round lengthwise in the center of each tortilla. Cover meat with cheese. Top cheese with onions, green pepper, green chilies and tomatoes. Bake at 400° for 10-15 minutes or until cheese melts. Remove from oven. Top with lettuce, sprouts and salsa. Fold left and right edges of tortilla over center to cover filling. Top with yogurt.

CHILI CON CARNE

1 pound extra-lean ground round
1 onion, chopped
2 cloves garlic, minced
1 28-oz. can tomatoes
½ teaspoon ground cumin
1 teaspoon cayenne pepper
1 tablespoon chili powder
4 cups cooked kidney beans or two
  15-oz. cans red kidney beans
  with liquid
2 cups salad macaroni, cooked
1 7-oz. can chopped green chilies
  (optional)

Brown ground beef with onions and garlic; drain off any excess fat. Add tomatoes and seasonings; simmer uncovered 1½-2 hours. Add kidney beans; heat to boiling. Add macaroni; heat to serving temperature. Sprinkle with green chilies.

Note: This recipe is very hot. For a milder flavor, reduce the cumin and the cayenne.

SPAGHETTI SAUCE

  1   28-oz. can plum tomatoes
  1   28-oz. can tomato puree
  1   12-oz. can tomato paste
  1   8-oz. can tomato sauce
  3   cups water
1½ teaspoons or less salt
1½ teaspoons basil
 ¾ teaspoon oregano
  5   extra-lean pork chops
  2   pounds pasta
      crushed red pepper (optional)

Purée tomatoes in blender; pour into stock pot. Add remaining ingredients; except for meat, pasta and red pepper. Stir and bring to a boil; reduce heat.
Remove all visible fat from pork chops; brown chops on both sides using a teflon skillet. Add to sauce. Cover and simmer ½ hour. Add meat balls. Cover and simmer over low heat for 2-2½ hours. Serves 8-10.

     Meat Balls
  2   lbs. extra-lean ground round or veal
      ground black pepper to taste
      garlic powder to taste
  1   cup dry bread crumbs
 ½ cup egg substitute
 ½ cup skim milk
 ½ cup chopped fresh parsley
Continued

Sprinkle ground meat with black pepper and garlic powder; add bread crumbs, egg, milk and parsley. Knead; add additional milk if needed for moisture. Form meat into 32 very firm meat balls.

Note: If you have a source for extra-lean Italian sausage, add 4-8 sausages to the sauce.

Sauce and meat balls may be frozen.

BEEF STROGANOFF

1	pound extra-lean ground round
¾	cup onion, finely chopped
1	clove garlic, minced
½	pound fresh mushrooms, sliced
¼	teaspoon or less salt
⅛	teaspoon pepper
⅛	teaspoon rosemary
2	tablespoons flour
1½	cups cream of chicken soup* (page 316)
1	cup plain non-fat yogurt* (page 202)
1	1-pound package bowtie-shaped pasta, cooked
	poppy seeds
	fresh parsley for garnish

Sauté ground beef, onion and garlic; drain off any excess fat. Add mushrooms; cook 3-5 minutes. Stir in salt, pepper, rosemary and flour; simmer uncovered 10 minutes. Add soup and heat. Stir in yogurt; heat, but do not boil. Arrange pasta around edges of large platter; spoon stroganoff into center. Sprinkle pasta with poppy seeds. Garnish with fresh parsley.

LASAGNA

1½-2	pounds extra-lean ground round
1	clove garlic
1	small onion
3	pounds canned plum tomatoes
3½	teaspoons safflower oil
3½	teaspoons olive oil
1	24-oz. can tomato sauce
½	teaspoon or less salt
½	teaspoon oregano
1	teaspoon basil
¼	teaspoon pepper
2	bunches fresh spinach
2	cups skim ricotta cheese
1	package lasagna, cooked and drained crushed red pepper
½-¾	lbs. thinly sliced Mozzarella cheese

Brown ground round with garlic and onion in a teflon skillet; drain excess fat. Set aside. Purée tomatoes in blender; add oils, tomato sauce and spices. Whirl 2-3 minutes. Set aside. Wash spinach; shake dry and remove any tough lower stems. Steam in a covered skillet 2-3 minutes or until wilted. Squeeze dry; chop. Combine spinach, ground round and ricotta.

Cover bottom of a 13"x9"x2" pan with tomato sauce. Add a layer of noodles. Spread with spinach mixture. Sprinkle with red pepper. Add a layer of Mozzarella. Cover with sauce. Repeat layers 2-3 more times. Pour remaining sauce over final layer. Top with additional cheese. Bake covered at 350° for 45-60 minutes. Serves 8-10.
Continued

Note: For a smaller group use two 8-inch square pans and put one in the freezer.

Variations: If you have a source for extra-lean Italian sausage, use that in place of ground round. Boil the sausage 10-15 minutes; remove and discard casings. Chop sausage.

Extra-lean ground pork or ground veal or chicken may also be used in place of ground round.

BARBECUED ROUND STEAK

⅓ cup safflower oil
2 tablespoons olive oil
3 tablespoons lemon juice
1 tablespoon red wine vinegar
2 cloves garlic
   pinch thyme
½ teaspoon chili powder
   pinch oregano
2 pounds extra-lean round steak
1 large onion, sliced

Combine safflower oil, olive oil, lemon juice, vinegar and seasonings; pour over steak. Top with onion. Cover. Marinate in refrigerator 24 hours, turning several times to coat. Drain. Grill steaks over hot coals 7-8 minutes on each side or to desired doneness. Sprinkle with pepper.

PIZZA

Crust

1	package active dry yeast
¾	cup warm water
4	cups flour
½	teaspoon sugar
½	teaspoon salt
2	tablespoons olive oil
1	egg or ¼ cup egg substitute, beaten

Dissolve yeast in ¾ cup warm water. Mix flour with sugar and salt; add to yeast along with oil and egg and stir until mixed. Knead on a heavily floured board until smooth and elastic. (Add additional water if needed for moisture.) Put dough in a bowl greased with tub safflower margarine; cover and let rise in a warm place for 1 hour. Punch down. Knead slightly. Let rise 1 more hour. Divide dough in half. Roll into two 9-inch crusts. Dough may be frozen.

Sauce per Crust

1	1-lb. can plum tomatoes
1	tablespoon tomato paste
1	tablespoon olive oil
¼	teaspoon oregano
¼	teaspoon basil
¼	teaspoon pepper
½	lb. grated low-fat Mozzarella cheese

Drain tomatoes; dice. Reserve ½ cup of the juice; mix juice with tomato paste, diced tomatoes, and olive oil. Spread over crust; sprinkle with oregano, basil and pepper. Add choice of toppings.
Continued

Toppings:
>fresh ripe tomatoes
>sauteed onions
>fresh mushrooms, sliced and
>>steamed 2-3 minutes
>green onions
>green chili peppers
>extra-lean ground round,
>>cooked and drained
>cooked chicken
>chopped clams
>fresh pineapple
>sprouts

Sprinkle with cheese. Bake at 450° for 20 minutes or until crust is done and cheese is melted.

MEXICAN STYLE STEAK

1   recipe barbecued round steak*
    (page 495)
8   corn tortillas
½   head of lettuce, chopped
2   ripe tomatoes, chopped
1   white onion, chopped
1   recipe tomato salsa* (page 361)

Prepare steak according to recipe (page 495). Wrap tortillas in a damp kitchen towel. Heat in a 350° oven for 15 minutes. Slice steak into very thin strips. Place several strips on each tortilla. Top with lettuce, tomato and onion. Roll. Serve with salsa.

CHAPTER NINETEEN

DESSERTS

Note: Because sugar reduction is essential to good cardiac health, desserts should be used sparingly, and only for very special occasions.

Remember, the premier dessert is fresh fruit.

APPLESAUCE

8-10 large cooking apples, peeled, cored and
cut into chunks
½ cup water
½ cup or less sugar
1 teaspoon cinnamon

Put apples and water in saucepan; cover and simmer, stirring frequently, until apples are barely tender. Add sugar and continue cooking about 30 minutes or until sugar dissolves. Stir in cinnamon.

Note: For a smooth, rather than a chunk type sauce, purée apples in the blender or food processor before adding sugar. Proceed as for chunk style.

If using a crock pot, combine all ingredients. Cover. Cook on low 8 hours or overnight.

BAKED APPLES

¼ cup or less brown sugar
1 teaspoon cinnamon
1 tablespoon safflower oil
⅓ cup raisins
6-8 medium baking apples

Mix sugar, cinnamon, oil and raisins. Fill center of apples. Place upright in baking dish. Pour 1 cup water around apples. Bake at 375° 45-60 minutes, basting frequently.

Note: If using a crock pot, reduce water to ½ cup. Cook on low 8 hours or overnight.

FRESH STRAWBERRIES WITH YOGURT AND BROWN SUGAR

fresh strawberries with stems
plain non-fat yogurt* (page 202)
fresh mint leaves
brown sugar

Arrange berries in a basket or serving bowl. Place yogurt in a chilled bowl; garnish with mint. Pass with brown sugar. To eat, dip berries first in yogurt, then in brown sugar.

STRAWBERRY SHORTCAKE

angel food cake
fresh strawberries
whipped cream substitute* (page 202)

Slice cake; top with crushed or sliced berries. Garnish with whipped cream substitute and fresh whole berries.

Note: Most angel food cake mixes are acceptable on the Positive Diet. Be sure to read the label to verify heart-healthy ingredients.

FROZEN BANANAS

Peel bananas. Wrap in plastic wrap. Freeze.

BAKED APRICOTS

fresh apricots, halved and pitted
2   teaspoons water per apricot
vanilla sugar (instructions follow)
plain non-fat yogurt* (page 202)

Place apricots and water in a baking dish; sprinkle with vanilla sugar. Bake in a 375° oven for 30-35 minutes. Garnish with a dollop of non-fat yogurt.

Vanilla Sugar: Store 2 vanilla beans with 2 cups sugar in a covered jar for several weeks. The longer it is stored, the better the flavor.

GLAZED FRUITS

fresh fruits in season—strawberries, cherries, blueberries, raspberries, grapes, apples, oranges, bananas
1   egg white per 2-3 persons
2   tablespoons water per egg white
2   tablespoons granulated sugar per egg white

Arrange fruit in a basket. Beat egg whites and water until fluffy; pour into a serving bowl. Pass with granulated sugar. To eat, dip fruits first in the beaten egg white, then in sugar.

FROSTED GRAPES

Put grapes in the freezer. Freeze until firm.

BROILED PAPAYA HALVES

1-2 fresh papayas
fresh lime juice
wedges of fresh lime

Cut papayas in half lengthwise. Remove seeds. Brush with lime juice. Place skin side down on broiler rack; cook 2-3 minutes. Serve with lime wedges.

Note: To barbecue, place split papayas on edge of barbecue, grill 5-6 minutes — just until hot.

BAKED BANANAS

1½ teaspoons fresh lemon juice
1 teaspoon grated lemon rind
1 tablespoon brown sugar
4 bananas, peeled and sliced
lengthwise

Combine lemon juice, lemon rind and brown sugar; brush over bananas. Bake at 375° for 15 minutes. Serve at once.

BANANAS WITH HONEY AND BROWN SUGAR

Peel bananas and place in baking dish. Drizzle with honey; sprinkle with brown sugar. Top with nuts, if desired. Bake at 375° for 15 minutes.

POACHED PEARS

  1   cup white wine
  1   vanilla bean, split open
4-6   firm, ripe pears
  ¼   cup lemon juice
  2   tablespoons orange juice
      fresh mint for garnish
      fresh fruits for garnish

Place wine and vanilla bean in medium saucepan; bring to a boil. Peel and quarter pears; dip in lemon juice. Place pears in vegetable steamer over boiling wine; cover and steam 8-10 minutes or until tender. Remove from pan. Boil poaching liquid 2-3 minutes to reduce. Remove and discard vanilla bean. Combine 2 tablespoons poaching liquid with 2 tablespoons lemon juice and 2 tablespoons orange juice.

Serve pears at room temperature on individual dessert plates with a small amount of sauce. Garnish with fresh mint and fresh fruits in season, such as sliced fresh peaches (dip in lemon juice to preserve color), grapes, kiwi, bananas, cantaloupe, watermelon, plums, peeled orange segments or mandarin oranges.

FROZEN WATERMELON

Layer slices of watermelon in a 13"x9"x2" pan; cover with plastic wrap and freeze 30 minutes. Turn. Return to freezer until ready to serve. Garnish with sherbets, sorbets or ices, or fresh fruits and sprigs of mint.

RHUBARB SAUCE

4 cups rhubarb, cut into 1-inch slices
½ cup sugar or 4 tablespoons honey
1-2 tablespoons water

Combine all ingredients in a saucepan; cover. Cook slowly about 10 minutes or until fruit is tender.

Variations: Warm, serve over sliced bananas. Or serve with Yogurt Topping — combine 1 cup plain non-fat yogurt* (page 202) with the juice and rind of ½ lemon; add a dash of honey.

APPLE CRISP

6-7 tart cooking apples
1 tablespoon lemon juice
⅓ cup granulated sugar
1 teaspoon cinnamon
¾ cup rolled oats
½ cup flour
1 cup brown sugar
3 tablespoons safflower oil

Place apples in a deep baking dish; sprinkle with lemon juice, sugar and cinnamon. Combine remaining ingredients; pour over apples. Bake at 375° for 30 minutes or until apples are tender.

SINGLE PASTRY CRUST

1½ cups all-purpose flour
1½ teaspoons sugar
¾ teaspoon salt
½ cup safflower oil
2 tablespoons skim milk

Combine flour, sugar and salt. Mix together oil
and milk; add to flour. Using a pastry blender or
fork, work mixture into a soft dough. Add additional milk if needed. Form into a ball. Roll out on
a well-floured pastry cloth. Place in a 9" pie plate.
Adjust crust. Flute edges.

Note: If a baked shell is needed, prick bottom and
sides of crust with a fork. Bake at 450° 10-12 minutes or until golden. If filling and crust are to be
baked together, do not prick crust.

DOUBLE PASTRY CRUST

2 cups all-purpose flour
½ teaspoon salt
4 tablespoons ice water
⅔ cup safflower mayonnaise
1½ tablespoons skim milk

Combine flour and salt. Mix ice water with
mayonnaise; add to flour. Using a pastry blender
or fork, work mixture together; add milk. Form
into a ball. Divide dough in half. Roll out on a
well-floured pastry cloth. Place in a 9" pie plate;
adjust crust. Fill. Add top crust; flute edges.

Note: It is very important that the ice water be ice
cold.

STRAWBERRY-RHUBARB PIE

½	cup sugar
¼	cup flour
¼	teaspoon salt
¼	teaspoon nutmeg
3	cups rhubarb, cut into ½-inch pieces
1	cup strawberries, sliced
1	9-inch double pastry crust* (page 507)

Combine sugar, flour, salt and nutmeg. Add fruit. Toss to coat. Let stand 20 minutes. Spoon into pastry-lined pie plate. Adjust top crust. Flute edges. Prick. Bake at 400° 40-45 minutes.

FRESH BERRY PIE

1	9-inch double pastry crust* (page 507)
2	tablespoons flour
½	cup sugar
⅛	teaspoon salt
4	cups fresh raspberries, strawberries, or blackberries
1	teaspoon lemon juice

Line a 9-inch pie plate with pastry. Mix together flour, sugar and salt; sprinkle ¼ of the mixture on uncooked bottom crust. Coat berries with lemon juice and toss with remaining sugar mixture. Spoon into pie plate. Adjust top crust; flute edges. Prick. Bake at 450° for 15 minutes. Reduce heat to 350° and continue baking 25-30 minutes.

APPLE PIE

6 cups apples, pared and sliced
1¼ tablespoons lemon juice
¼ cup sugar
½ teaspoon cinnamon
⅛ teaspoon salt
2 tablespoons flour
1 9-inch double pastry crust* (page 507)

Toss apples with lemon juice. Combine sugar, salt, cinnamon and flour; mix with apples. Spoon into pastry-lined pie plate. Adjust top crust. Flute edges. Prick. Bake at 450° for 10 minutes. Reduce heat to 375° and continue baking 40-50 minutes.

PUMPKIN PIE

1 1-lb. can pumpkin
¾ cup firmly packed brown sugar
¾ cup egg substitute
¼ teaspoon salt
1 teaspoon cinnamon
½ teaspoon ginger
½ teaspoon nutmeg
¼ teaspoon cloves
1 13-oz. can skim evaporated milk
1 9-inch single pastry crust* (page 507)

Combine pumpkin, brown sugar, egg substitute, salt and spices; add milk and blend. Pour into pie shell. Adjust top crust; flute edges. Prick. Bake at 400° for 50 minutes or until done.

Note: To test for doneness, insert a knife into center of pie. When pie is done, the knife will come out clean.

TOPPING FOR FRUIT COBBLER

1   cup all-purpose flour, sifted
½   teaspoon salt
1½   teaspoons baking powder
⅓   cup skim milk
3 .   tablespoons safflower oil

Combine flour, salt and baking powder. Mix milk with oil; add to flour. Using a fork or pastry blender, work dough into a ball. Drop by spoonfuls onto fruit cobbler. (Recipes follow.)

BERRY COBBLER

¾   cup water
2   tablespoons cornstarch
½   cup sugar
3   cups strawberries, raspberries,
      blueberries or blackberries
1   recipe cobbler topping* (recipe above)

In medium saucepan, combine water, cornstarch, and sugar; bring to a boil. Cook for 1 minute, stirring constantly. Add berries and remove from heat. Pour into a 9-inch or a 10-inch pie plate. Top with cobbler topping. Bake at 425° 25-30 minutes or until topping is lightly browned.

CHERRY COBBLER

1 20-oz. can pitted, tart pie cherries
    with liquid
½ cup sugar
1 tablespoon minute tapioca
1 recipe cobbler topping* (page 510)

Combine cherries, sugar and tapioca in medium saucepan; cook, stirring constantly until sugar is dissolved and syrup is clear. Pour into a 9-inch or a 10-inch pie plate. Dot with cobbler topping. Bake at 425° 25-30 minutes or until topping is lightly browned.

RHUBARB COBBLER

4 cups rhubarb, cut into 1-inch slices
½ cup sugar
1-2 tablespoons water
2 tablespoons cornstarch
1 recipe cobbler topping* (page 510)

In medium saucepan, combine rhubarb, sugar, water and cornstarch. Bring to a boil; cook for 1 minute, stirring constantly. Pour into a 9-inch or a 10-inch pie plate. Dot with cobbler topping. Bake at 425° 25-30 minutes or until topping is lightly browned.

FREEZING AND BEATING ICES

Pour mixture into large mixing bowl suitable for freezing. Cover. Freeze 1-2 hours or until solid around edges, but still slightly slushy in center. Remove from freezer. Beat with electric mixer on medium speed until mixture is smooth and no large crystals remain. Cover. Refreeze for 1 hour. Serve at once or refreeze. If refrozen, allow mixture to soften 5-10 minutes at room temperature or for 30 minutes at refrigerator temperature before serving.

Note: It is important that the bowl used for freezing be large because the mixture must not be too deep if it is to freeze properly. When doubling a recipe, use 2 bowls, rather than one.

Serve ices in chilled, stemmed glasses, in fresh lemon or orange shells, in cantaloupe or other melon boats. Garnish with whole fresh fruits and a sprig of mint.

FRESH STRAWBERRY ICE

4 cups hulled strawberries
1½ teaspoons lemon juice
2 teaspoons sugar

Purée berries in blender; add lemon juice and sugar and whirl 2-3 minutes. Pour into large bowl. Follow preceding instructions for freezing and beating ices.

LEMON ICE

2   cups water
2½ tablespoons sugar
½   cup fresh lemon juice
    grated rinds of 2 lemons

Combine water and sugar in saucepan; boil without stirring for 5 minutes. Cool. Add lemon juice and rind; stir. Pour into large bowl suitable for freezing. Follow instructions for freezing and beating ices (page 512).

To Serve: Cut tops from whole lemons; squeeze out juice (reserve for lemon ice or for lemonade). Remove pulp. Fill shells with lemon ice. Garnish with violets or with blueberries and a sprig of mint.

LIME ICE

2   cups water
½   cup sugar
1   cup fresh lime juice
    juice of 1 orange

Combine water and sugar in medium saucepan; boil without stirring for 5 minutes. Cool. Add lime juice and orange juice. Pour into a large mixing bowl suitable for freezing. Follow instructions for freezing and beating ices (page 512).

To Serve: Cut tops from whole limes; squeeze out juice (reserve for limeade). Remove pulp. Fill shells with lime ice. Garnish with sliced papaya or peeled orange segments and a sprig of fresh mint.

WATERMELON ICE

---

3   cups watermelon pulp
⅓   cup sugar
    juice of 1 large orange

Purée watermelon pulp in blender; add remaining ingredients and whirl 3-4 minutes. Pour into large mixing bowl suitable for freezing. Follow instructions for freezing and beating ices* (page 512).

To Serve: Spoon over cantaloupe or honeydew boats. Garnish with fresh mint.

PAPAYA ICE

---

2   ripe papayas, peeled
2   tablespoons sugar
⅓   cup water
2   tablespoons fresh lime juice

Purée papaya in blender. Combine sugar and water in saucepan; boil 5 minutes without stirring. Cool to room temperature. Pour lime juice over papaya. Add cooled syrup. Whirl in blender 3-4 minutes. Pour into large mixing bowl suitable for freezing. Follow instructions for freezing and beating ices* (page 512).

PINEAPPLE ICE

3   cups unsweetened pineapple juice

Pour juice into blender; whirl 3-4 minutes. Pour into large mixing bowl suitable for freezing. Follow instructions for freezing and beating ices* (page 512).

KIWI ICE

2   cups peeled kiwi
½   teaspoon lemon juice
¼   cup water
¼   cup sugar

Purée kiwi in blender; add remaining ingredients and whirl 2-3 minutes. Pour into large mixing bowl suitable for freezing. Follow instructions for freezing and beating ices* (page 512).

GRANITA DE CAFÈ CON PANE

2   cups decaffeinated espresso coffee
3   teaspoons sugar or lightly to taste
1   recipe whipped cream substitute*
     (page 202).

Combine brewed coffee and sugar. Pour into large mixing bowl suitable for freezing. Follow instructions for freezing and beating ices* (page 512).

To Serve: Spoon into stemmed glasses. Garnish with whipped cream substitute.

FREEZING AND BEATING SORBETS

Pour mixture into large mixing bowl suitable for freezing. Cover. Freeze 1-2 hours or until solid around edges but still slightly slushy in center; remove from freezer. Beat until smooth and no large crystals remain. Set aside. In small mixing bowl, beat egg whites. Fold into sorbets. Return to freezer. Freeze without stirring 1-2 hours.

*Note: It is important that the bowl used for freezing be large because the mixture must not be too deep if it is to freeze properly. When doubling a recipe, use 2 bowls, rather than one.

The amount of sugar may be varied depending on the sweetness of the fruit. If additional sugar is necessary, add it to the egg whites before beating.

For creamier sorbet, add an additional egg white.

These sorbets have a good texture and will keep a long while in the freezer.

WATERMELON SORBET

3 cups watermelon pulp, puréed in blender
⅓ cup sugar or lightly to taste
juice of 1 large orange
2 egg whites, beaten until stiff

Combine watermelon purée, sugar and orange juice. Pour into large bowl. Follow preceding instructions for freezing and beating sorbets.

LEMON SORBET

1   cup fresh lemon juice
    grated rind of 3 lemons
2   cups water
½   cup sugar
3   egg whites, beaten until frothy

Combine water and sugar in medium saucepan; boil without stirring for 5 minutes. Cool. Add lemon juice. Pour into blender; whirl 3 minutes. Pour into large mixing bowl. Follow instructions for freezing and beating sorbets* (page 516).

Note: To make Lime Sorbet, substitute lime juice for lemon juice and add the juice of 1 orange. Omit the grated rind of 3 lemons.

PAPAYA SORBET

2   ripe papayas, peeled
3   tablespoons sugar
⅓   cup water
2   tablespoons fresh lime juice
2   egg whites, beaten until frothy

Purée papaya in blender. Combine sugar and water in medium saucepan; boil 5 minutes without stirring. Cool to room temperature. Pour lime juice over papaya. Add cooled syrup. Pour into blender; whirl 3 minutes. Pour into large mixing bowl. Follow instructions for freezing and beating sorbets* (page 516).

VANILLA ICE CREAM

2 cups skim milk
1 envelope Knox gelatin
1¼ cups sugar
2 cups skim evaporated milk
1½ teaspoons vanilla

Heat skim milk just to scalding; do not boil. Remove from heat; stir in gelatin and sugar. Stir until dissolved. Pour into blender. Whirl 3-5 minutes. Add evaporated milk; whirl 2 minutes. Chill 5 hours or overnight. Process in ice cream freezer according to manufacturer's directions. Stir in vanilla. Chill 30-60 minutes.

Variations: Just before serving, top with fresh berries or with blueberry* or raspberry sauce* (page 287).

CHOCOLATE ICE CREAM: Add 6 tablespoons unsweetened cocoa powder and ¼-½ teaspoon cinnamon to vanilla recipe.

ROCKY ROAD ICE CREAM: Prepare chocolate ice cream. After processing add ¾ cup miniature marshmallows.

COFFEE ICE CREAM: Prepare vanilla ice cream. Add 2 tablespoons decaffeinated instant coffee powder when stirring in the gelatin and sugar. Process as directed. Then add 1½ tablespoons finely ground, decaffeinated espresso coffee.

PECAN ICE CREAM: Prepare vanilla ice cream. After processing add 1 cup whole pecans.
Continued

FRESH PEACH ICE CREAM: Prepare vanilla ice cream, substituting ¼ teaspoon almond extract for vanilla. Purée 3 ripe, peeled peaches in blender. Peel and slice 2 additional peaches. Stir into processed recipe. Chill.

FRESH STRAWBERRY, RASPBERRY, BLUEBERRY OR BLACKBERRY ICE CREAM: Prepare vanilla ice cream. Process. Purée 2 cups fresh berries in blender. Slice an additional 1 cup of berries. Fold into processed recipe. Chill.

FRESH CHERRY ICE CREAM: Prepare strawberry ice cream. Substitute pitted cherries for berries.

FRESH APRICOT OR PLUM ICE CREAM: Prepare strawberry ice cream. Substitute plums or apricots for berries.

FRUITSICLES

Use fruit juice, such as apple, orange, grape, grapefruit, or lemonade. Or use canned fruit, such as peaches, pears, plums or apricots — purée in blender. Or use fresh or frozen berries — purée in blender with a small amount of water.

Pour into popsicle molds. Freeze until firm. Or pour into ice cube trays with separators; place a tongue depressor or toothpick in each square and freeze until firm.

Note: If using canned fruits, use only those packed in their own juice. Avoid those with heavy syrup.

FROZEN YOGURT POPS

Prepare nonfat fruit-flavored yogurt* (page 203), using either method 1 or method 2. Chill. Pour into popsicle molds. Freeze until firm.

TAPIOCA PUDDING

1   egg, separated
2   cups skim milk
3   tablespoons minute tapioca
⅛   teaspoon salt
4   tablespoons sugar
¾   teaspoon vanilla

In medium saucepan combine egg yolk, milk, tapioca, salt and 3 tablespoons of the sugar; let stand 5 minutes. Beat egg white until foamy; gradually beat in remaining sugar. Beat until egg whites form stiff peaks. Set aside. Cook tapioca over medium heat, stirring constantly, until mixture comes to a full boil — about 6-8 minutes. Gradually fold into beaten egg whites. Add vanilla. Stir only enough to mix. Let cool for 20 minutes. Chill.

Note: For chocolate tapioca, add cocoa powder to completed recipe.

PEANUT BUTTER COOKIES

4   egg whites
2   cups non-hydrogenated peanut
     butter
1⅔ cups granulated sugar

Beat egg whites until stiff. Set aside. Combine peanut butter and sugar; fold in egg whites. Drop by teaspoonfuls onto teflon baking sheets. Flatten slightly with prongs of fork. Bake at 325° for 20 minutes. Remove to wire racks to cool.

RICE KRISPIE COOKIES

3   tablespoons safflower oil
40 regular size marshmallows
½   teaspoon vanilla
4   cups Rice Krispie cereal

Warm oil. Add marshmallows; cook over medium heat until marshmallows are melted, stirring constantly. Add vanilla. Pour in cereal. Mix well. Drop by teaspoonfuls onto a sheet of waxed paper.

MOLASSES COOKIES

2 cups all-purpose flour
¼ teaspoon salt
1 teaspoon baking powder
1 teaspoon baking soda
½ teaspoon ground cloves
1¼ teaspoon ground ginger
1¼ teaspoon cinnamon
⅔ cup safflower oil
¼ cup molasses
1 egg or ¼ cup egg substitute
1 cup firmly packed brown sugar
granulated sugar

Sift together flour, salt, baking powder, baking soda, cloves, ginger and cinnamon. Set aside. Using lowest speed of electric mixer, blend oil, molasses and egg; add sugar. Blend. Gradually add flour and dry ingredients; mix well.

Chill dough 2 hours. Form into 1-inch balls. Roll each ball in granulated sugar. Place on teflon baking sheets. Sprinkle each cookie with 2-3 drops of water. Bake at 375° 8-10 minutes.

RAISIN-OATMEAL COOKIES

1	orange with rind
6	tablespoons safflower oil
¾	cup honey
½	cup skim milk
2	teaspoons vanilla
1	cup whole wheat pastry flour
1½	cups rolled oats
½	teaspoon baking soda
½	teaspoon salt
½	teaspoon baking powder
1	teaspoon cinnamon
1	teaspoon nutmeg
1½	cups raisins

Grind orange with rind in grinder or blender; add oil, honey, milk and vanilla; blend. Combine remaining ingredients; add to orange mixture. Stir to blend. Drop by large serving-spoonfuls onto teflon baking sheets. Bake at 300° for 25-30 minutes. Remove to wire racks to cool.

Note: If less orange flavor is desired, use less orange rind.

For smaller cookies, drop by teaspoonfuls.

GINGERBREAD MUFFINS

1	cup molasses
½	cup firmly packed brown sugar
½	cup safflower oil
1¼	teaspoon cinnamon
½	teaspoon ground cloves
½	teaspoon nutmeg
1½	teaspoon ground ginger
1	cup boiling water
2	cups all-purpose flour, sifted
1	teaspoon baking soda

Using low speed of electric mixer, blend molasses, brown sugar, oil, cinnamon, ground cloves, nutmeg and ginger. Add boiling water; blend. Gradually add flour; beat 2 minutes or until smooth. Dissolve baking soda in 2 tablespoons hot water; add to batter. Blend. Pour into an 8-inch square teflon baking pan or into paper-lined muffin tins. Bake at 350° for 25-30 minutes.

Variation: Just before serving, top with sliced bananas and whipped cream substitute* (page 202).

YELLOW CHIFFON CAKE

  2   eggs, separated
1¼ cups sugar
2¼ cups flour
  3   teaspoons baking powder
 ¾ teaspoon salt
 ⅓ cup safflower oil
  1   cup skim milk
1½ teaspoons vanilla

Beat egg whites until frothy. Gradually add ½ cup sugar; beat until egg whites are stiff. Set aside. In large bowl, sift together remaining sugar, flour, baking powder and salt; add oil, ½ of the milk and vanilla. Beat 1 minute on medium speed; add remaining milk and egg yolks. Beat 1 minute longer. Gently fold in egg whites. Bake in teflon cake pans at 350° for 30-35 minutes.

SEVEN MINUTE ICING

  2   egg whites
1¼ cups sugar
     dash salt
 ½ cup water
 ¼ teaspoon cream of tartar
  1   teaspoon vanilla

Bring 2 cups water to a boil in bottom of double boiler. In top of double boiler, combine egg whites, sugar, salt, water and cream of tartar; beat 1 minute. Place over boiling water. Using highest speed of electric mixer, beat constantly 5-7 minutes or until frosting stands in stiff peaks. Remove from heat. Stir in vanilla.

CHOCOLATE CAKE

2 eggs, separated
1¼ cups sugar
1¾ cups flour
¾ teaspoon baking soda
¾ teaspoon salt
½ cup safflower oil
1 cup skim milk plus 1 tablespoon vinegar
¼ cup unsweetened cocoa powder
½ teaspoon vanilla

Beat egg whites until frothy. Gradually beat in ½ cup sugar; beat until egg whites are stiff. Set aside. In large mixing bowl, sift together remaining sugar, flour, baking soda and salt; add oil, ½ of the milk and vanilla. Beat 1 minute on medium speed; add remaining milk, egg yolks and cocoa powder. Beat 1 minute longer. Fold in egg whites. Bake in teflon cake pans or in paper-lined muffin cups at 350° for 30-35 minutes. Cool on wire racks.

CHOCOLATE-FUDGE CAKE

———————————————————————

    2   cups flour
1¼   cups sugar
   ½   cup unsweetened cocoa powder
   ½   teaspoon salt
   1   tablespoon baking soda
  ⅔   cup safflower oil
   1   cup skim milk
   1   cup strong decaffeinated coffee

Combine flour, sugar, cocoa, salt and baking soda; add oil and milk and blend with a spoon. Stir in boiling coffee. Pour into an 8-inch square teflon baking pan, into paper-lined muffin cups or into a 9-inch round teflon baking pan. Bake at 350° for 35-40 minutes. Cool on wire racks. Frost with chocolate fudge frosting* (recipe below).

CHOCOLATE-FUDGE FROSTING

———————————————————————

   3   tablespoons unsweetened cocoa
           powder
   1   cup sugar
  ⅓   cup evaporated skim milk
   3   tablespoons safflower oil
  ¼   teaspoon salt
   1   teaspoon vanilla

In medium saucepan, combine all ingredients, except vanilla. Bring to a boil, reduce heat and simmer 1 minute. Remove from heat. Add vanilla; beat 5 minutes. Spread over cake.

Note: Add additional milk or water if needed for a creamier spreading consistency.

SOURCE NOTES

The chart on the sugar content of breakfast cereals is from the *Journal of Dentistry for Children* (September/October, 1974) and is reproduced with permission from the American Society of Dentistry for Children.

The chart on the amount of sugar found in common foods is reproduced with permission from Kurt W. Donsbach, Ph.D., copyright 1975.

The chart on the sodium content of common spices is reproduced with permission of the American Spice Trade Association.

The recipe for Herb Seasoning is reproduced with permission from the American Heart Association, copyright 1978.

The chart on the fat content of fast foods is based upon information from "On the Fast Food Trail," by Wendy Midgley, R.D. (*Diabetes Forecast* July/August 1979), and is used with permission of the American Diabetes Association, copyright 1979; and from "How Good Are Fast Foods," by Jane E. Brody (*New York Times*, Sept. 19, 1979) and is used with permission of The New York Times Company, copyright 1979.

Information on body fat percentages is from *Fit or Fat?* by Covert Bailey, copyright 1977, and is used with permission.

Information on diet foods is from "The Good — And Bad — Of Diet Foods," by Francis Sheridan Goulart (*Consumer Digest*, September/October 1979) and is used with permission of Consumer Digest, Inc., copyright 1979.

The information concerning the size, shape and location of the heart, and the reference to the former Mayor of Chicago, are from *Learning How To Live With Heart Trouble* by Arthur J. Snider and is used with permission of Budlong Press Company, copyright 1973.

The quote from John W. Farquhar, M.D., is from a speech given in Honolulu, Hawaii, in December, 1979, and is used with permission.

The quote from Mark Hegsted, M.D., is from *Jane Brody's Nutrition Book* (W.W. Norton & Company), copyright 1981, and is used with permission.

The quotes from Congressman Albert Gore and Craig Claiborne are from the March 15, 1982, cover story of *Time* and are used with permission.

BIBLIOGRAPHY

American Heart Association. *Cooking Without Your Salt Shaker.* Cleveland, Ohio: American Heart Association Northeast Ohio Affiliate, Inc., 1978.

American Heart Association. "Dietary Fat And Its Relation to Heart Attack and Strokes." *Circulation 23,* 1961.

American Heart Association. *Heartbook.* New York: E.P. Dutton, 1980.

American Heart Association. *The American Heart Association Cookbook.* New York: Ballantine, 1977.

Armstrong, M.L. et. al. "Regression of Coronary Arthermomatosis in Rhesus Monkeys." *Circulatory Research,* 1959.

Aykroyd, W.R. *The Story of Sugar.* Chicago: Quadrangle, 1967.

Bailey, Covert. *Fit or Fat?* Pleasant Hills, California: Covert Bailey, 1977.

Blackburn, Henry. "Progress in the Epidemiology and Prevention of Coronary Heart Disease." *Progress in Cardiology, Vol. 3,* edited by Paul N. Yu and John F. Goodwin, 1974.

Blumenfeld, Arthur. *Heart Attack: Are You A Candidate?* New York: Pyramid Books, 1971.

Benditt, E.P. "The Origin of Atherosclerosis." *Scientific American,* February, 1977.

Bond, C.Y. et al. *The Low Fat Low Cholesterol Diet.* Garden City, N.Y.: Doubleday & Co., Inc., 1971.

Bowen, Angela. *The Diabetic Gourmet.* New York: Harper & Row Publishers, Inc., 1970.

Brody, Jane E. "How Good Are Fast Foods." *The New York Times,* Sept. 19, 1979.

Brody, Jane E. *Jane Brody's Nutrition Book.* New York: W.W. Norton & Co., 1981.

"Cardiovascular Surgery." *Public Health Service, Publication No. 1701,* 1969.

"Composition of Foods in the United States — 1909 to 1948." *U.S. Department of Agriculture,* 1949.

"Composition of Foods: Dairy and Egg Products, Raw, Processed, Prepared." *U.S. Department of Agriculture,* 1976.

"Composition of Foods: Fats and Oils, Raw, Processed, Prepared." *U.S. Department of Agriculture,* 1979.

"Composition of Foods: Poultry Products, Raw Processed, Prepared." *U.S. Department of Agriculture,* 1979.

"Composition of Foods: Soups, Sauces and Gravies, Raw, Processed, Prepared." *U.S. Department of Agriculture,* 1979.

"Composition of Foods: Spices and Herbs, Raw, Processed, Prepared." *U.S. Department of Agriculture,* 1977.

"Composition of Foods: Raw, Processed, Prepared." *U.S. Department of Agriculture,* 1975.

Cooper, Kenneth H. *Aerobics.* New York: M. Evans and Co., 1968.

Cooper, Kenneth H. *The New Aerobics.* New York: Evans and Co., Inc., 1970.

Clarke, N.E. Sr. "Atherosclerosis, Occlusive Vascular Disease and EDTA." *American Journal of Cardiology, Vol. VI,* 1960.

Daubar, R.R., and Kannel, W.B. "Some Factors Associated With the Development of Coronary Heart Disease. Six Years Follow Up Experience In The Framingham Study." *American Journal of Public Health 49,* 1959.

Enos, W.F., et. al. "Pathogenesis of Coronary Disease in American Soldiers Killed in Korea." *Journal of the American Medical Association,* 1955.

Ewald, Ellen B. *Recipes for a Small Planet.* New York: Random House, 1973.

Farquhar, John W. *The American Way Of Life Need Not Be Hazardous To Your Health.* New York: W.W. Norton & Co., 1978.

Ferguson, J.M. *Habits, Not Diets: The Real Way To Weight Control.* Palo Alto, Calif.: Bull Publishing, 1976.

Friedman, Meyer, and Rosenman, Ray H. *Type A Behavior and the Heart.* New York: Alfred A. Knopf, 1974.

Goulart, Francis Sheridan. "The Good — And Bad — of Diet Foods." *Consumer Digest,* September/October, 1979.

Guthrie, Helen A. *Introductory Nutrition.* St. Louis: C.V. Mosby Co., 1971.

Hanssen, Maurice. *Everything You Wanted To Know About Salt.* New York: Pyramid Books, 1968.

"Heart Facts."*American Heart Association,* 1980.

Hur, Robin. *Food Reform: Our Desperate Need.* Austin, Texas: Heidelberg Publishers, 1975.

Jones, Jerome. *Diet For a Happy Heart.* San Francisco: 101 Publications, 1978.

Keys, A. "Coronary Heart Disease Among Minnesota Business and Professional Men Followed After Fifteen Years." *Circulation 27,* 1963.

Keys. A. "Coronary Heart Disease in Seven Countries." *Circulation 41, Supplement 1,* 1970.

Keys, A. "The Diet and the Development of Coronary Heart Disease." *Journal of Chronic Diseases, 4,* 1956.

Keys, A. and Keys, M. *Eat Well and Stay Well.* Garden City, New York: Doubleday & Co., Inc., 1959.

Kullman, Donald A. *ABC Milligram Cholesterol Diet Guide.* North Miami Beach, Florida: Merit Publications, Inc., 1977.

Kraus, Barbara. *Calories and Carbohydrates.* New York: The New American Library, Inc., 1981.

Kraus, Barbara. *The Dictionary of Sodium, Fats and Cholesterol.* New York: Grosset & Dunlap, 1974.

Lappe, Francis Moore. *Diet For A Small Planet.* New York: Ballantine, 1975.

Linde, S.M., and Finnerty, F., Jr. *High Blood Pressure.* New York: David McKay Co., Inc., 1975.

Luna, David. *The Lean Machine.* Culver City, California: Peace Press, 1980.

Mayer, Jean. *A Diet For Living.* New York: Pocket Books, 1976.

Mayer, Jean. *Obesity: Causes, Cost and Control.* Englewood Cliffs, N.J.: Prentice-Hall, 1968.

McNamara, J.J., et. al. "Coronary Artery Disease In Viet Nam Casualties." *Journal of the American Medical Association,* 1971.

Midgley, W. "On The Fast Food Trail. . ." *Diabetes Forecast,* 1979.

"Nutritive Value of American Foods in Common Units." *U.S. Department of Agriculture,* 1979.

Page, H., and Schroeder, J. *The Whole Family Low Cholesterol Cookbook.* New York: Grosset & Dunlap, 1976.

Page, I.H., et. al. "Prediction of Coronary Heart Disease Based on Clinical Suspicion, Age, Total Cholesterol, and Triglyceride." *Circulation 42,* 1970.

Pritikin, N., Leonard, J., Hofer, J., *Live Longer Now.* New York: Grosset and Dunlap, 1974

Pritikin, N., and McGrady, P.M., Jr. *The Pritikin Program for Diet and Exercise.* New York: Grosset and Dunlap, 1979.

Rinse, J. "Atherosclerosis, Chemistry and Nutritions, Some Observations, Experiences and an Hypothesis." *American Laboratory,* 1973.

Robinson, C.H. *Basic Nutrition and Diet Therapy.* New York: Macmillan Co., 1970.

Simonton, O. Carl, et. al. *Getting Well Again.* Los Angeles: J.P. Tucker, Inc., 1978.

Shekelle, R.B. "Western Electric Study." *New England Journal of Medicine,* 1981.

Sipple, H.L., and McNutt, K. *Sugars In Nutrition.* New York: Academic Press, 1974.

Snider, Arthur J., and Oparil, Suzanne. *Hypertension.* Chicago: Budlong Press Co., 1976.

Snider, Arthur J. *Learning How to Live With Heart Trouble.* Chicago: Budlong Press Co., 1973.

Stunkard, Albert J. *The Pain Of Obesity.* Palo Alto, Calif.: Bull Publishing Co., 1976.

Swank, Roy L., and Pullen, Mary-Ellen. *The Multiple Sclerosis Diet Book.* Garden City, New York: Doubleday & Co., Inc., 1977.

Toufexis, Anastasia. "Taming The No. 1 Killer." *Time,* June 1, 1981.

Waldo, Myra. *The Low Salt, Low Cholesterol Cookbook.* New York: G.P. Putnam's Sons, 1974.

Wallis, Claudia. "Salt: A New Villain?" *Time,* March 15, 1982.

Wright, I.S. "Correct Levels of Serum Cholesterol." *Journal of the American Medical Association,* 1976.

Wisser, R.W. et. al. "Atherosclerosis and The Influence of Diet: An Experimental Mode." *Journal of the American Medical Association,* 1965.

Yudkin, John. "Sugar and Coronary Heart Disease." *Food and Nutrition News, 36, No. 6,* 1965.

Yudkin, John. *Sweet and Dangerous.* New York: Bantam Books, 1972.

A

Adams, Dr. Forest H., 48

Alcohol, 10, 32, 59, 60
    sugar in, 143

American diet, myths of, 82–89
    fast foods as nutritious,
        86–87
    gaining weight (as you get
        older), 89
    high protein breakfast, 85
    processed foods as
        nutritious, 87
    red meat consumption,
        83–84
    refined sugar as energy,
        87–88
    salt as a needed
        preservative, 88–89
    whole milk dairy products,
        84–85

American Heart Association,
    19, 27, 30, 32, 60, 105, 208,
    230

American Restaurant
    Association, 171

Angina pectoris, 13, 18
    meaning of, 53
    physical activity and, 54
    results of, 53–54

Aorta, 43

Appetizers, tips for ordering
    (in a restaurant), 174

Aquinas, St. Thomas, 89–90

Armstrong, Dr. M. L., 90, 91

Arteriogram. See Coronary
    arteriogram

Arteriosclerosis, 14

Artery blockages, 45

Atherosclerosis, 57–58, 74
    development of, 52
    meaning of, 47
    reversibility of, 90–91

    See also Coronary heart
        disease

Atrium, 41–42

Attitude, weight control, 168

B

Bailey, Dr. Covert, 160

Bakery products, commercially
    prepared, 191–92

Baking, cooking by, 189

Barbecuing, 189

Belgium, 65

Beverages, 82
    meal planning, 229
    sugar content in, 148
    tips for ordering (in a
        restaurant), 177

Blockage (plaque), 51–53

Blood
    coronary arteries and, 42–45
    high in oxygen, 41
    low in oxygen, 41
    resistance to flow, 41–42

Blood cholesterol. See
    Cholesterol

Blood clot, 53

Blood vessel system, heart
    and, 40–41

Brazil, 74

Bread, tips for ordering (in a
    restaurant), 175

Breakfast
    low-fat, 120–24
    Positive Diet suggestions,
        209–11
    tips for ordering (in a
        restaurant), 176

Breakfast cereals, sugar in,
    144–47

British Isles, 65

Broiling, cooking by, 189

Bureau of Foods (Food and

Drug Administration), 164
Burger King's French fries, 86
Burton, Sir Richard, 9
Butterfat, sources of, 125–26
Butterfat reduction, 97, 124–129
  how to begin, 126–29
  identification of sources,
    125–26
  planning and practice
    stages, 155
  refinement stage, 155
  timing sequence chart, 158

C

Cakes, sugar content, 148
Calcium, 84
Calories, 31, 59, 60, 77, 79, 89,
  96
  compared to fat content,
    184–85
  control of, 165–66
  density of foods, 79
  fat consumption, 70
Candy, sugar content, 149
Canned foods, 27
  sugar content of fruit and
    juices, 149
Carbohydrates, 70, 79, 86
Cheese, low-fat, 128–29
Chest pain. *See* Angina pectoris
Cholesterol, 10, 18, 26, 27, 29,
  30, 31, 32, 33, 51, 53, 58, 59,
  60, 85, 96, 166, 186
  average American
    consumption, 105
  diet pattern and cardiac
    disease, 61–69
  distinction between
    body-produced and
    dietary, 66
  one-for-one substitutions,
    110–11
  production of, 66
  in red meat, 106
  role of, 65–68

sources of, 66, 106–8
studies and field tests, 61–65
testing cardiac risk potential,
  68–69
two-week meal plan, 108–14
in vegetarians, 69
Cholesterol reduction, 97,
  105–24, 130
  buttermilk, 97, 124–29, 155
  first basic principle, 105–6
  how to begin, 108–11
  identification of sources,
    106–8
  refinement stage, 154
  planning and practice
    stages, 154
  summing up, 130
  timing sequence chart, 158
  two-week dinner plan,
    112–24
Cigarette smoking, 10, 26, 27
Claiborne, Craig, 72
Coca Cola, 28
Concentrated sugar, 78
  foods high in, 78–79
  foods rich in, 80
Congestive heart failure, 56–57
Consumer Digest, 164
Convenience foods, 27, 70, 186
Cookies, sugar content, 148
Cooking equipment and
  staples, 231
Cooking terms and procedures,
  232–33
Cooking Without Your Salt Shaker
  (American Heart
  Association), 208
Cooley, Dr. Denton A., 9–11
Copeland, Dr. Jack G., 13–15
Coronary arteries, 42–45
  diagram, 44
  heart and, 42–45
  location of, 43–45
  tears, 45

Coronary arteriogram, 18, 25

Coronary artery bypass surgery, 13–15

Coronary artery disease, diet and, 14–15

Coronary heart disease, 47–58, 90
  blockage (or plaque), 51–53
  cardiac conditions, 53–57
  development of, 26–27, 50–53
  EKG examination, 49–50
  fatalities, 21, 47
  in females, 48–49
  focusing on the problem, 57–58
  introduction to, 17–35
  in the middle-aged and elderly, 48
  risk factors, 23, 25–29, 160–63
  surgery, 23–24
  in young people, 48

Creative substitution, Positive Diet, 101–3

D

Dairy products
  fat in, 125
  myth of consumption, 84–85
  sugar content, 149

Death, leading causes of (1979), 20

Desserts
  sugar content, 150
  tips for ordering (in a restaurant), 176

Diet pattern, cardiac disease and, 27–35, 59–91
  control, 32
  coronary fatalities, 31–32
  epidemiologic studies, 31
  fat and cholesterol, 61–71
  myths of American diet, 82–89
  responsibility for change, 32
  reversibility of athersclerosis, 90–91

salt, 72–77
sugar, 77–82

Dinner, Positive Diet suggestions, 218–25

E

Early, Dr. James, 17

East Africa, 80

Edema, 56, 72

Egg substitute, 102

El Cordobes (matador), 21

Electrocardiogram (EKG), 17–18, 49–50

Entrees, tips for ordering (in a restaurant), 175

Estrogen (hormone), 49

Exercise, 10, 26, 27, 89

F

Farquhar, Dr. John W., 59, 77

Fast foods, 27
  fat content, 115
  nutritious and healthful myth, 86–87

Fat reduction, 97, 105–24, 130
  buttermilk, 97, 124–29, 155
  first basic principle, 105–6
  how to begin, 108–11
  identification of sources, 106–8
  planning and practice stages, 154
  refinement stage, 154
  summing up, 130
  timing sequence chart, 158
  two-week dinner plan, 111–24

Fats, 18, 26, 27, 28, 31, 51, 53, 58, 59, 60, 79, 85, 96, 166
  average American consumption, 105
  caloric consumption, 70
  daily nutritional needs, 230
  diet pattern and cardiac disease, 69–71

in fast foods, 115
foods with high fat values, 70
how to calculate food
   content, 184–85
one-for-one substitutions,
   110–11
in red meat, 106
role of, 69–71
sources of, 106–8
two-week meal plan, 108–14
types of, 71
whole milk products, 125

Fatty streak, 51

Fibrillation, 57

Finland, 64, 161

Fish oil, 101–2

Food and Drug Administration
   (FDA), 135, 164

Framingham Study, 63

French fries, 102–3

Frozen foods, 27

Fruits, daily nutritional needs,
   230

G

Genetics, 26

Gluttony, 9

Gore, Albert, 136–37

Grain, daily nutritional needs,
   230

Greece, 64, 65, 160, 161

Greene, Graham, 96

Guleck, Dr. Charles J., 48

H

Harvard University, 74–75

Health food stores, 192

Heart, 37–42
   how it works, 40–42
   location of, 39
   meanings of, 37–38
   misconceptions, 39
   pumping action, 38–39, 41–42
   shape of, 39

Heart attack, 32, 54–56, 90
   cholesterol level and, 62–63,
      64, 69
   death rate, 21, 28, 56
   diagram, 55
   number per year, 47
   odds of having, 56
   "sudden," 49
   See also Coronary heart disease

Heartbeat, 38, 50, 57

Heart disease. *See* Coronary
   heart disease

Heart-lung machine, 23, 25

Hegsted, Dr. Mark, 60–61

Herbs and seasonings, 205–8

High blood pressure
   (hypertension) 26, 31–32, 72,
      74–75, 90
   causes of, 74
   genetic predisposition to, 75

High-density lipoprotein (HDL), 66, 68

High protein breakfast myth, 85

Human Nutrition Center
   (Department of Agriculture), 60–61

Hydrogenation, 186–87

Hypertension. *See* High blood
   pressure

I, J

India, 69

Intima (tissue), 50

Italy, 64, 65, 69, 160, 161

Jams and jellies, sugar content,
   150

Japan, 64, 69, 74, 80, 160, 161

Junk foods, 27

K

Kennedy, John F., 22

Keys, Dr. Ancel, 62, 63, 64, 159

Kidney disease, 72

Korean War, 48, 65

Kraus, Barbara, 137

L

Labels, reading, 143, 184
Left coronary arteries, 43
Life expectancy rate, 28
Lipoprotein, 66
London University, 78
Long John Silver's fish, 86
Lunch
   low-fat, 118–20
   Positive Diet suggestions,
     213–17

M

McDonald's (restaurant chain),
   28, 86
Malnutrition, 27–28
Mars candy, 28
Meal planning, 98–100, 195–233
   breakfast suggestions, 209–12
   cooking terms and
     procedures, 232–33
   dinner suggestions, 218–25
   egg substitute, 201
   fruit yogurt, 202
   guide to basic foods, 195–97
   list of staples, 231
   lunch suggestions, 213–17
   plain nonfat yogurt, 202
   skim milk, 201
   snack suggestions, 226–29
   table of substitutions,
     198–200
   tips on herbs, 204–8
   whipped cream substitute, 203
   See also Index of Recipes;
     Positive Diet
Monosaturated fats, 186
Myocardial infarction (MI). *See*
   Heart attack

N

Nagle, Dr. John, 17–19, 21, 22,
   23, 25–26, 27–29, 30, 33–34,
   61, 95

National Center for Health
   Statistics, 80
National Heart, Lung and
   Blood Institute, 74
National Research Council, 75
Natural sugar, 78
   foods containing, 79
Netherlands, 64, 65, 160, 161
New Guinea, 74

O

Obesity, 26, 31, 70, 80, 159–60
   as cardiac risk factor, 160–63
Oils, daily nutritional needs, 230
Overweight males (ages 40–49),
   161

P

Page, Dr. Lot, 74–75
Pediatric Atherosclerosis
   (University of California at
   Los Angeles), 48
Peru, 69
Portion control, 167
Positive Diet, 33–35, 93–150
   applying basic principles
     and tools, 103–4
   basic principles, 96–97
   basic tools, 98–103
   butterfat reduction, 97,
     124–29
   creative substitution, 101–3
   eating in restaurants, 171–77
   elements of, 94
   fat and cholesterol
     reduction, 97, 105–24, 130
   lifestyle and, 93–96
   salt reduction, 97, 131–39
   sugar reduction, 97, 140–50
   timing, as key to success,
     151–58
   weight control, 159–69
   See also Meal planning
Processed food, 60, 82, 185–86

nutritious as natural foods myth, 87
salt in, 76, 77, 135–36

Protein, 70, 78, 79
animal food, 84
daily nutritional needs, 230

Public Health Service, 63

Pulmonary edema, 56

Q

Quick weight loss approach, 163–64

R

Recreation, importance of, 10

Red meat
calories from fat, 106
myth of consumerism, 83–84
two-week meal plan, 108–14

Refined sugar, 140
energy food myth, 87–88

Rest, importance of, 10

Restaurants, eating in (how to handle), 171–77
"doom and gloom" approach, 174
guidelines, 172
tips for ordering, 174–77

Roasting, cooking by, 189

S

Safflower oil, 102

Salad, tips for ordering (in a restaurant), 175–76

Salt, 26, 27, 28, 31, 59, 60, 72–77, 82, 96, 166
"adequate and safe" level of intake, 75
intake (U.S.), 75–77
positive and negative characteristics, 72–75
preservative myth, 88–89
in processed foods, 76, 77 135–36
sodium content of spices, 139

Salt reduction, 97, 105–24, 130, 193–94
how to begin, 132–37
identification of sources, 121–32
planning and practice stages, 156
refinement stage, 156
summing up, 137–38
timing sequence chart, 158

Sandwiches
Positive Diet suggestions, 215–16
tips for ordering (in a restaurant), 176

Saturated fat, 71, 85, 185, 186

Sauces, sugar content, 150

Schauss, Dr. Alexander G., 82

Seven Country study, 64

Skim milk, 126–27

Sleep, importance of, 10

Snack foods, 27

Snack suggestions, 226–29

Sodium chloride. *See* Salt

Sodium, Fats, and Cholesterol (Kraus), 137

Solomon Islands, 74–75

Sorbitol, 164

Soup, tips for ordering (in a restaurant), 174–75

South Africa, 80

Spain, 65

Spices, sodium content of, 139

Stanford Heart Disease Prevention Program, 59

Stewing, cooking by, 189

Stress, 10, 26

Stroke, 28, 32, 72

Sucrose, 78

Substitution, diet, 101–3

Sugar, 10, 26, 27, 28, 31, 32,

59, 60, 77–82, 96, 166
in alcohol, 143
average U.S. consumption, 82
in breakfast cereals, 144–47
in common foods, 148–50
diet high in, 80
label reading, 143
in processed foods, 77–78
sweet tooth syndrome,
    81–82
types of, 78–79
Sugar reduction, 140–50, 194
how to begin, 141–43
identification of concentrated
    sources, 140–41
planning and practice
    stages, 157
refinement stage, 157
summing up, 144
timing sequence chart, 158
Sweet tooth syndrome, 81–82
snack suggestions, 228
Switzerland, 65

T

Tachycardia, 57
Taco Bell Taco, 86
Tacoma General Hospital, 23
Thyroid disease, 72
Time (magazine), 136–37
Triglycerides, 10, 80

U

U.S. Census Bureau, 108
U.S. Department of
    Agriculture, 32, 60–61, 106,
    134, 142
U.S. Department of Agriculture
    Composition of Food
    Analysis, 124
U.S. Department of Health and
    Human Services, 32
U.S. Senate Select Committee
    on Nutrition, 27, 32, 72, 105
    diet recommendations, 60

U.S. Surgeon General, 32, 72
University of California at Los
    Angeles (UCLA), 48
University of Cincinnati, 48
University of Minnesota, 62
Unsaturated fat, 71, 185, 186

V

Vegetable oil, 185–86
Vegetables
    daily nutritional needs, 230
    tips for ordering (in a
        restaurant), 175
Vegetarians, 69
Ventricle, 41–42
Viet Nam War, 22, 48, 65
Vitikainen, Dr. Kari, 23

W

Washington State University, 142
Weight control, 159–69
    attitude, 168
    calories, 165–66
    eating in restaurants, 171–77
    obesity as a cardiac risk
        factor, 160–63
    overweight males, 163
    portion control, 167
    positive approach to, 164–69
    quick weight loss approach,
        163–64
    tips, 168–69
Weight gain myth (as you get
    older), 89
Whole milk products, fat in,
    125; *See also* Dairy products
World War II, 32

Y

Yemen, 80
Yogurt, low-fat, 129
Yudkin, Dr. John, 78, 82
Yugoslavia, 64, 160, 161

A

Almond Peas, 387

Antipasto, 331
　Eggplant, 248
　Fruit, 251
　Salad, 332
　Tuna, 248
　Vegetable, 249

Appetizers, 237–59
　Artichoke Dip, 258
　Artichokes with Fresh
　　Lemon, 243
　Cheese Burritos, 255
　Cheese Pie, 245
　Cheese Tortilla Chips, 256
　Cheese Tostados, 256
　Crab and Artichokes with
　　Dijon, 242
　Crab Cocktail, 241
　Cracked Crab, 241
　Dijon Cucumber Sticks, 244
　Eggplant Antipasto, 248
　Eggplant Rounds, 252
　Fruit Antipasto, 251
　Hot Mustard and Sesame
　　Seeds, 247
　Ketchup and Horseradish
　　Sauce, 247
　Marinated Mushrooms, 244
　Marinated Salmon, 239
　Munchies, 254
　Nachos, 255
　Oysters on the Half Shell,
　　238
　Oysters Rockefeller, 238
　Pizza, 253
　Popcorn, 259
　Potato Skins, 254
　Seviche, 240
　Skewered Fruit, 250
　Spanish Dip, 257
　Spinach and Crab Coquette,
　　242
　Spinach Dip, 258
　Spring Rolls, 246–47
　Steamed Clams Bordelaise, 237
　Steamed Mussels with Wine
　　and Garlic, 237
　Stuffed Mushrooms, 245
　Toasted Pumpkin Seeds, 259
　Tomato Salsa, 257
　Tortilla Chips, 256
　Tuna Antipasto, 248
　Vegetable Antipasto, 249

Apple(s)
　Baked, 501
　Crisp, 506
　Pie, 509

Applesauce, 501

Apricot(s)
　Baked, 503
　Ice Cream, 519

Artichoke(s)
　Breaded Hearts of, 371
　and Crab with Dijon, 242
　Dip, 258
　Fresh, 370
　with Fresh Lemon, 243
　Hearts with Lemon, Garlic
　　and Olive Oil, 371
　Soup, Cream of, 315
　Stuffed, 346
　Tomato, Mushroom, and
　　Green Bean Salad, 342

Asparagus
　Fresh, with Lemon, 372
　Soup, Cream of, 315

B

Bagels, 274

Baked Apples, 501

Baked Apricots, 503

Baked Bananas, 504

Baked Beans, 408

Baked Chicken with Olive Oil
　and Fresh Lemon, 451

Baked Eggplant, 379
　Provencale, 380

Baked Fillets with Lemon and
　Fennel, 425

Baked Onions, 386

Baked Potatoes, 390

Baked Squash, 398

Banana(s)
Baked, 504
Frozen, 502
with Honey and Brown
Sugar, 504
-Raisin Bread, 280

Barbecued Beef Sandwich, 323

Barbecued Chicken Breasts, 455

Barbecued Chicken with Fresh
Lime, 456

Barbecued Chicken Italian
Style, 456

Barbecued Chicken with
Skewered Vegetables, 457

Barbecued Eggplant, 378

Barbecued Fillets, 426

Barbecued Lamb Roast, 479

Barbecued Round Steak, 495

Barbecued Turkey, 448

Barbecued Zucchini, 399

Barley
and Mushroom Pilaf, 410
-Mushroom Soup, 303

Basil
Tomatoes, and Cheese,
Pasta with, 403
and Tomatoes, Fettuccini
with, 404
Tomatoes, and Mozzarella
Salad, 338

Beans
Baked, 408
Dried, 407
Three Bean Salad, 356
See also Green Beans

Beef, 483–97
Barbecued Round Steak, 495
Barbecued Sandwich, 323
Broth, 302
Broth Parisian, 303
Chili con Carne, 491

Country Pot Roast, 486

Cube Steak Sandwich, 323

Dutch Meat Loaf, 489

Grilled Steak, 485

Hamburgers, 485

Lasagna, 494–95

Mexican Style Steak, 497

Old Fashioned Hash, 488

Oven Tacos, 490

Roast, 483

Skewered, 484

Spaghetti Sauce, 492–93

Stew, 487

Stroganoff, 493

Swiss Steak, 483

Tostados, 489

Berry
Cobbler, 510
Ice Cream, 519
Pie, Fresh, 508
See also names of berries

Beverages, 260–64
Cappuccino, 264
Chocolate Whip with
Cinnamon, 264
Fresh Lemonade, 260
Fruit Shake, 260
Hot Cider, 263
Iced Tea, 263
Orange Cooler, 261
Sangria, 262
Strawberry Frost, 261

Blackberry Ice Cream, 519

Black Pepper and Lemon,
Green Beans with, 374

Blueberry Ice Cream, 519

Bouillabaisse, 440–41

Boiled Chicken, 454

Bouillon, Court, 423
Easy, 423

Bread Crumbs, 270

Breaded Artichoke Hearts, 371

Breads, 265–86
Bagels, 274
Banana-Raisin, 280
Bread Crumbs, 270

Challah, 272–73
Cheese, 276
Cinnamon, 279
Coffee Cake, 278
Corn, 277
Crêpes, 285
Croutons, 270
Energy Bars, 282
Enriched White, 267
French, 269
French Toast, 286
Garlic, 270
Granola, 283
Health, 271
Honey Wheat, 268
Muffins, 277
Pancakes, 284
Soft Pretzels, 276
Sticks, 275
Stuffing, 411
Waffles, 286
Yogurt Pancakes, 284
Zucchini, 281

Breakfast Quiche, 290

Breast of Chicken Sandwich, 321

Broccoli
Fresh, with Safflower
  Mayonnaise, 376
Stir-fried, 375

Broiled Fillets with Fresh
  Lemon, 424

Broiled Lamb Chops, 477

Broiled Papaya Halves, 504

Broiled Scallops, 418

Broiled Tomato Halves, 396

Broth
Beef, 302
Beef Parisian, 303
Chicken, 295
Turkey, 301

Brown Sugar
and Honey, Bananas with, 504
and Yogurt, Stawberries
  with, 502

Buckwheat Noodles, Chicken
Soup with, 300

Burritos, Cheese, 255

C
Caesar Salad a la Positive Diet, 333

Cakes, 526–28
Chocolate, 527
Chocolate-Fudge, 528
Coffee Cake, 278
Yellow Chiffon, 526

Calamari, 439

Canned Tomatoes, 395

Cantonese Hot Pot, 463

Cappuccino, 264

Carrots
Nippy, 377
and Zucchini Julienne, 400

Casseroles
Tuna Noodle, 443
Zucchini-Mozzarella, 401

Celery
Remoulade, 372
Soup, Cream of, 317

Challah, 272–73

Cheese
Bread, 276
Burritos, 255
and Crab Sandwich, Hot, 325
and Egg Muffins, 291
Macaroni and, 405
Pie, 245
-stuffed Zucchini, 400
Toasted Sandwich, 327
Tomatoes, and Basil, Pasta
  with, 403
Tortilla Chips, 256
Tostados, 256
and Vegetables, Fillets with, 429
and Yogurt, Fresh Sole
  with, 433

Chef's Salad, 350

Cherry
Cobbler, 511
Ice Cream, 519

Chicken, 450–73

Baked with Olive Oil and
  Fresh Lemon, 451
Barbecued Breasts, 455
Barbecued with Fresh Lime,
  456
Barbecued with Skewered
  Vegetables, 457
Boiled, 454
Breast Sandwich, 321
Broth, 295
Cacciatore, 467
Cantonese Hot Pot, 463
Chalupas, 471
Chili con Pollo, 468
Creole, 466
Curry, 465
Dijon, 458
Divan, 464
and Dumplings, 462–63
Enchiladas, 470
Extra Crispy Oven-fried, 450
and Green Peppers,
  Stir-fried, 460
Hearty Cream Soup, 316
Italian Style Barbecued, 456
a la King, 460
Lemon with Fresh Spinach,
  472
Lemon, with Mayonnaise
  and Fresh Tomatoes, 473
Microwave Baked, 452
Noodle Soup, 300
Oven-fried, 450
Poached, 454
Pot Pie, 461
Roast, 452
Roast, Oriental Style, 453
Salad, 349
Sandwich Filling, 321
Soup with Buckwheat
  Noodles, 300
Soup with Chinese
  Vegetables, 296
Soup, Cream of, 316
Soup with Lemon, 297
Soup with Spinach and
  Saifun, 297
Soup with Tomato and
  Green Onion, 296

Steamed, 455
Stir-fried with Vegetables, 459
-stuffed Peppers, 458
Tomatoes, and Spinach
  Salad, 340
Tostados, 469
Vegetable Soup, 299

Chili
  con Carne, 491
  con Pollo, 468
  Soup, Mexican, 308

Chilled Pea Soup, 308

Chocolate
  Cake, 527
  -Fudge Cake, 528
  -Fudge Frosting, 528
  Ice Cream, 518
  Whip with Cinnamon, 264

Chowder
  Manhattan Clam, 312
  New England Clam, 313
  Seafood, 311

Cider, Hot, 263

Cinnamon
  Bread, 279
  Chocolate Whip with, 264

Cioppino, 442–43

Clam(s)
  Bordelaise Steamed, 237
  Italian Style, 417
  Manhattan Chowder, 312
  Nectar, Hearty, 314
  New England Chowder, 313
  Sauce, Linguine with, 437
  Steamed, with Fresh
    Lemon, 416
  -stuffed Sole, 431

Club House Sandwich, 322

Cobbler, 510–11
  Berry, 510
  Cherry, 511
  Rhubarb, 511
  Topping for, 510

Coffee
  Granita de Cafè con Pane, 515

Ice Cream, 518
Coffee Cake, 278

Coleslaw, 356

Cookies, 522–24
Molasses, 523
Peanut Butter, 522
Raisin-Oatmeal, 524
Rice Krispie, 522

Corn
Bread, 277
on the Cob, 378

Cottage Fries, 388

Country Pot Roast, 486

Court Bouillon, 423
Easy, 423

Crab
and Artichokes with Dijon, 242
and Cheese Sandwich, Hot, 325
Cocktail, 241
Cracked, 241
Louis (Salad), 347
Papaya, and Cucumber
Salad, 344
Sandwich Filling, 325
and Spinach Coquette, 242
Stuffed Peppers, 345
-stuffed Sole, 432
-stuffed Trout, 422
Zucchini Stuffed with, 343

Cranberry Relish, 358

Cream Soups, 315–19
Artichoke, 315
Asparagus, 315
Celery, 317
Chicken, 316
Cucumber, 317
Hearty Chicken, 316
Mushroom, 319
Pea, 318
Zucchini, 320

Creamy French Dressing, 364

Crêpes, 285

Croutons, 270

Crunchy Peanut Butter
Sandwich, 326

Cube Steak Sandwich, 323

Cucumber
Crab, and Papaya Salad, 344
and Onion Salad, 340
Soup, Cream of, 317
Sticks with Dijon, 244
and Tomato Salad, 338

Curry
Potato Salad, 353
Chicken, 465

D

Desserts, 501–28
Apple Crisp, 506
Apple Pie, 509
Applesauce, 501
Baked Apples, 501
Baked Apricots, 503
Baked Bananas, 504
Bananas with Honey and
Brown Sugar, 504
Berry Cobbler, 510
Broiled Papaya Halves, 504
Cherry Cobbler, 511
Chocolate Cake, 527
Chocolate-Fudge Cake, 528
Chocolate-Fudge Frosting, 528
Double Pastry Crust, 507
freezing and beating ices, 512
freezing and beating
sorbets, 516
Fresh Berry Pie, 508
Fresh Strawberries with
Yogurt and Brown Sugar, 502
Fresh Strawberry Ice, 512
Frosted Grapes, 503
Frozen Bananas, 502
Frozen Watermelon, 505
Frozen Yogurt Pops, 520
Fruitsicles, 520
Gingerbread Muffins, 525
Glazed Fruits, 503
Granita de Cafè con Pane, 515
Ice Creams, 518–19
Kiwi Ice, 515
Lemon Ice, 513
Lemon Sorbet, 517
Lime Ice, 513

Molasses Cookies, 523
Papaya Ice, 514
Papaya Sorbet, 517
Peanut Butter Cookies, 522
Pineapple Ice, 515
Poached Pears, 505
Pumpkin Pie, 509
Raisin-Oatmeal Cookies, 524
Rhubarb Cobbler, 511
Rhubarb Sauce, 506
Rice Krispie Cookies, 522
Seven Minute Icing, 526
Single Pastry Crust, 507
Strawberry-Rhubarb Pie, 508
Strawberry Shortcake, 502
Tapioca Pudding, 521
Topping for Fruit Cobbler, 510
Watermelon Ice, 514
Watermelon Sorbet, 516
Yellow Chiffon Cake, 526
Dijon Mustard
    Chicken with, 458
    Crab and Artichokes with, 242
    and Cucumber Sticks, 244
    Pasta Primavera with, 403
    Vegetables with, 376
    and Vegetables, Fillet of
        Sole with, 430
    Vinaigrette, 361
Dill and Onion, Potatoes with, 391
Dips
    Artichoke, 258
    Spanish, 257
    Spinach, 258
Double Pastry Crust, 507
Dumplings, Chicken and, 462–63
Dutch Meat Loaf, 489

E

Easy Court Bouillon, 423
Egg/Egg Substitute, 201, 288–91
    Breakfast Quiche, 290
    Cheese and Egg Muffins, 291
    Egg Drop Soup, 299
    French Omelet, 288
    Huevos Rancheros, 289
    Scrambled, 290

Eggplant, 378–81
    Antipasto, 248
    Baked, 379
    Barbecued, 378
    Provencale, Baked, 380
    Rounds, 252
Enchiladas, Chicken, 470
Energy Bars, 282
Enriched White Bread, 267
Extra Crispy Oven-fried
    Chicken, 450

F

Fat-free Gravy, 394
Fennel and Lemon, Baked
    Fillets with, 425
Fettuccini
    with Fresh Basil and
        Tomatoes, 404
    Napoli, 404
    Seafood, 436
Fillet of Sole with Fresh
    Vegetables and Dijon, 430
Fillets with Fresh Vegetables
    and Cheese, 429
Fillets with Vermouth and
    Orange Sauce, 427
Fillets with Wine and Tomato
    Sauce, 428
Fish. *See* Seafood
Freezing and beating ices, 512
Freezing and beating sorbets, 516
French Bread, 269
French Dip Sandwich, 322
French Dressing
    Creamy, 364
    Garlic, 364
French Fried Potatoes, 388
French Omelet, 288
French Toast, 286
Fresh Artichokes, 370
Fresh Asparagus with Lemon,
    372

Fresh Berry Pie, 508

Fresh Broccoli with Safflower Mayonnaise, 376

Fresh Lemonade, 260

Fresh Mushroom Salad, 341

Fresh Mushroom Soup with Mozzarella Cheese, 304

Fresh Sole with Yogurt and Cheese, 433

Fresh Spinach Salad with Sesame Seeds, 337

Fresh Strawberries with Yogurt and Brown Sugar, 502

Fresh Strawberry Ice, 512

Fresh Tomatoes with Roast Peppers, 339

Fresh Tomato Soup, 306

Fried Onions, 386

Frosted Grapes, 503

Frosting
   Chocolate-Fudge, 528
   Seven Minute Icing, 526

Frozen Bananas, 502

Frozen Watermelon, 505

Frozen Yogurt Pops, 520

Fruit(s)
   Antipasto, 251
   Glazed, 503
   Shake, 260
   Skewered, 250
   Syrup, 287
   Yogurt, 203
   See also names of fruit

Fruitsicles, 520

Fudge-Chocolate Cake and Frosting, 528

G

Garlic
   Bread, 270
   French Dressing, 364
   Lemon, and Olive, Artichoke Hearts with, 371

and Wine, Steamed Mussels with, 237

Gazpacho, 307

Gingerbread Muffins, 525

Glazed Fruits, 503

Granita de Cafè con Pane, 515

Granola, 283

Grapes, Frosted, 503

Gravy, Fat-free, 394

Green Beans, 373–75
   with Fresh Lemon and Tarragon, 373
   Italian Style, 373
   with Lemon and Black Pepper, 374
   with Mushrooms and Pecans, 374
   with Mushrooms and Waterchestnuts, 375
   Tomato, Artichoke, and Mushroom Salad, 342

Green Goddess Salad, 345

Green Onion and Tomato, Chicken Soup with, 296

Green Peppers, Stir-fried Chicken with, 460

Grilled Steak, 485

Grilled Veal Steaks with Fresh Lemon and Mushrooms, 482

Grilled Vegetables, 382

H

Hamburgers, 485

Hash, Old Fashioned, 488

Hash Brown Potatoes, 389

Health Bread, 271

Hearty Clam Nectar, 314

Hearty Cream of Chicken Soup, 316

Hearty Turkey Soup, 301

Herb Seasoning, 208

Herbed Tomatoes, 397

Herbs, tips on, 204–8

Holiday Yams with
Marshmallows, 398

Honey
and Brown Sugar, Bananas
with, 504
Wheat Bread, 268

Horseradish and Ketchup
Sauce, 247

Hot Cider, 263

Hot Crab and Cheese
Sandwich, 325

Hot Mustard and Sesame
Seeds, 247

Hot Potato Salad, 354

Hot Tuna Salad, 349

Hot Tuna Sandwich, 324

Huevos Rancheros, 289

Hungry Joe Special, 406

I, J

Ice Cream, 518–19

Iced Tea, 263

Ices, 512–15
freezing and beating, 512
Fresh Strawberry, 512
Kiwi, 515
Lemon, 513
Lime, 513
Papaya, 514
Pineapple, 515
Watermelon, 514

Icing. *See* Frosting

Japanese New Variety Rice, 410

K

Ketchup and Horseradish
Sauce, 247

Kiwi Ice, 515

L

Lamb, 477–79
Barbecued Roast, 479
Broiled Chops, 477
Burgers, 478
Roast Leg of, 478
Shish Kebob, 477

Lasagna, 494–95

Layered Salad, 335

Lemon
Artichokes with, 243
and Black Pepper, Green
Beans with, 374
Broiled Fillets with, 424
Chicken with Fresh
Spinach, 472
Chicken with Mayonnaise
and Fresh Tomatoes, 473
Chicken Soup with, 297
Dressing, Fresh, 363
and Dry Mustard Dressing, 363
and Fennel, Baked Fillets
with, 425
Fresh Asparagus with, 372
Garlic, and Olive Oil,
Artichoke Hearts with, 371
Ice, 513
and Mushrooms, Grilled
Veal Steaks with, 482
and Olive Oil, Baked
Chicken with, 451
and Olive Oil Dressing, 363
Potatoes, 391
Sorbet, 517
Steamed Clams with, 416
and Tarragon, Green Beans
with, 373
Vinegar and Oil Dressing
with, 362

Lemonade, Fresh, 260

Lentils, Dried, 407

Lettuce
Stuffed, 336
and Tomato Sandwich, 328
Wilted, 336

Lime
Barbecued Chicken with, 456
Ice, 513

Linguine
with Clam Sauce, 437
with Tuna Sauce, 441

Lobster
  Sandwich Filling, 326
  Tails, 419

M

Macaroni
  and Cheese, 405
  Salad, 355
  Tuna Casserole, 443
Manhattan Clam Chowder, 312
Maple Syrup, 287
Marinated Fish, 420
Marinated Mushrooms, 244
Marinated Salmon, 239
Marshmallows, Yams with, 398
Mashed Potatoes, 393
Mayonnaise, Safflower, 360
  Fresh Broccoli with, 376
  and Tomatoes, Lemon
    Chicken with, 473
Meat Loaf, Dutch, 489
Meats. *See* Beef; Lamb; Pork;
  Veal
Mexican Chili Soup, 308
Mexican Salad, 342
Mexican Style Steak, 497
Microwave Baked Chicken, 452
Milk, Skim, 201
Milkshake, Fruit, 260
Minestrone Soup, 305
Minted Peas, 387
Molasses Cookies, 523
Monte Cristo Sandwich, 327
Mozzarella Cheese
  Fresh Mushroom Soup with, 304
  Tomato, and Basil Salad, 338
  -Zucchini Casserole, 401
Muffins, 277
  Cheese and Egg, 291
  Gingerbread, 525
Munchies, 254
Mushroom(s)

and Barley Pilaf, 410
-Barley Soup, 303
and Lemon, Grilled Veal
  Steaks with, 482
Marinated, 244
and Pecans, Green Beans
  with, 374
Salad, 341
Sautèed, 384
Soup, Cream of, 319
Soup with Mozzarella
  Cheese, 304
Stuffed, 245
Tomato, Artichoke, and
  Green Bean Salad, 342
and Waterchestnuts, 341
and Waterchestnuts, Green
  Beans with, 375
Mussels
  Italian Style, 415
  Steamed, with Wine and
    Garlic, 237
Mustard
  Hot, with Sesame Seeds, 247
  and Lemon Dressing, 363
  See also Dijon Mustard

N

Nachos, 255
New England Clam Chowder,
  313
New Potatoes and Fresh
  Vegetables, 392
Niçoise Salad, 348
Nippy Carrots, 377
Noodle(s)
  Buckwheat, Chicken Soup
    with, 300
  Chicken Soup with, 300
  Saifun, Chicken Soup with
    Spinach and, 297
  Tuna Casserole, 443

O

Oatmeal-Raisin Cookies, 524
Oil and Vinegar Dressing, 362
  with Lemon, 362

Old Fashioned Hash, 488

Olive Oil
    and Lemon, Baked Chicken
      with, 51
    and Lemon Dressing, 363
    Lemon, and Garlic,
      Artichoke Hearts with, 371

Omelet, French, 288

Onion(s)
    Baked, 386
    and Cucumber Salad, 340
    and Dill, Potatoes with, 391
    Fried, 386
    Rings, 385
    and Tomato, Chicken Soup
      with, 296
    Vinaigrette, 385

Orange
    Cooler, 261
    and Vermouth Sauce, Fillets
      with, 427

Oven-fried Chicken, 450

Oven Tacos, 490

Overnight Salad, 334

Oyster(s)
    on the Half Shell, 238
    Rockefeller, 238
    Stew, 310

P

Paella, 428–29

Pancakes, 284
    Yogurt, 284

Papaya
    Crab, and Cucumber Salad, 344
    Halves, Broiled, 504
    Ice, 514
    Sorbet, 517

Parsleyed Potatoes, 392

Pasta, 402–5
    Calamari, 439
    Fettuccini with Fresh Basil
      and Tomatoes, 404
    Fettuccini Napoli, 404
    with Fresh Tomatoes, Basil,
      and Cheese, 403
    Lasagna, 494–95
    Linguine with Clam Sauce, 437
    Linguine with Tuna Sauce, 441
    Macaroni and Cheese, 405
    Macaroni Salad, 355
    Primavera with Dijon, 403
    Primavera with Tomatoes, 402
    Seafood Fettuccini, 436
    Spaghetti Sauce, 492–93
    Tuna Noodle Casserole, 443

Pastry Crust, Single or Double, 507

Pea(s)
    Almond, 387
    Dried, 407
    Minted, 387
    Soup, Cream of, 318
    Soup, Chilled, 308

Peach Ice Cream, 519

Peanut Butter
    Cookies, 522
    Crunchy Sandwich, 326

Pears, Poached, 505

Pecan(s)
    Ice Cream, 518
    and Mushrooms, Green
      Beans with, 374

Peppers
    Chicken-stuffed, 458
    Crab stuffed, 345
    Roast, 399
    Roasted, with Tomatoes in
      Salad, 339
    Stir-fried Chicken with, 460

Pies, 508–9
    Apple, 509
    Cheese, 245
    Chicken Pot Pie, 461
    Fresh Berry, 508
    Pumpkin, 509
    Strawberry-Rhubarb, 508

Pineapple Ice, 515

Pizza, 496–97
    Appetizer, 253

Plain Nonfat Yogurt, 202

Plum Ice Cream, 519

Poached Chicken, 454

Poached Fish, 424

Poached Pears, 505

Popcorn, 259

Pork Roast, 481

Potato(es), 388–94
  Baked, 390
  Chips, 389
  Cottage Fries, 388
  Epicure, 393
  Fat-free Gravy, 394
  French Fried, 388
  and Fresh Vegetables, 392
  Hash Brown, 389
  Lemon, 391
  Mashed, 393
  with Onion and Dill, 391
  Parsleyed, 392
  Skins, 254
  Twice-baked, 390

Potato Salad, 353
  Curried, 353
  Hot, 354

Pot Roast, Country, 486

Poultry. *See* Chicken; Turkey

Pretzels, Soft, 276

Primavera Dressing, 360

Pudding, Tapioca, 521

Pumpkin
  Pie, 509
  Seeds, Toasted, 259

Q

Quiche, Breakfast, 290

R

Raisin
  -Banana Bread, 280
  -Oatmeal Cookies, 524

Raspberry Ice Cream, 519

Ratatouille, 381

Relish, Cranberry, 358

Rhubarb

Cobbler, 511
  Sauce, 506
  -Strawberry Pie, 508

Rice, 408–10
  Barley and Mushroom Pilaf, 410
  Japanese New Variety, 410
  Paella, 428–29
  Pilaf, 409
  Tabbouli Pilaf, 409
  Wild, 408

Rice Krispie Cookies, 522

Roast Beef, 483

Roast Chicken, 452
  Oriental Style, 453

Roast Leg of Lamb, 478

Roast Peppers, 399

Roast Pork, 481

Roast Turkey, 447
  Breast, 449

Roast Veal, 480

Rocky Road Ice Cream, 518

Russian Dressing, 365

S

Safflower Mayonnaise, 360
  Fresh Broccoli with, 376
  and Tomatoes, Lemon Chicken with, 473

Saifun Noodles and Spinach, Chicken Soup with, 297

Salad Dressings, 360–65
  Creamy French, 364
  Dijon Vinaigrette, 361
  Fresh Lemon, 363
  Fresh Lemon and Dry Mustard, 363
  Fresh Lemon and Olive Oil, 363
  Garlic French, 364
  Oil and Vinegar, 362
  Oil and Vinegar with Lemon, 362
  Primavera, 360
  Russian, 365
  Safflower Mayonnaise, 360

Thousand Island, 365
Tomato Salsa, 361
Yogurt, 365
Salads, 331–59
    Antipasto, 331, 332
    Caesar, a la Positive Diet, 333
    Chef's, 350
    Chicken, 349
    Coleslaw, 356
    Crab Louis, 347
    Crab Stuffed Peppers, 345
    Cranberry Relish, 358
    Cucumber and Onion, 340
    Curried Potato, 353
    Fresh Mushroom, 341
    Fresh Mushrooms and
        Waterchestnuts, 341
    Fresh Spinach with Sesame
        Seeds, 337
    Fresh Tomatoes with Roast
        Peppers, 339
    Green Beans, Tomatoes,
        Artichokes and
        Mushrooms, 342
    Green Goddess, 345
    Hot Potato, 354
    Hot Tuna, 349
    Layered, 335
    Macaroni, 355
    Mexican, 342
    Niçoise, 348
    Overnight, 334
    Papaya, Crab and
        Cucumber, 344
    Potato, 353
    Seviche, 333
    Spinach, 337
    Stuffed Artichoke, 346
    Stuffed Lettuce, 336
    Summer, 358
    Super Taco, 352
    Sweet and Sour, 332
    Taco, 351
    Three Bean, 356
    Tomato and Cucumber, 338
    Tomatoes, Mozzarella and
        Basil, 338
    Tomatoes, Spinach and
        Chicken, 340

Tomatoes Vinaigrette, 339
Watermelon, 357
Wilted Lettuce, 336
Winter, 359
Zucchini, 343
Zucchini Stuffed with Crab, 343
Salmon, Marinated, 239
Salsa, Tomato, 257, 361
Sandwiches, 320–28
    Barbecued Beef, 323
    Breast of Chicken, 321
    Chicken Filling, 321
    Club House, 322
    Crab Filling, 325
    Crunchy Peanut Butter, 326
    Cube Steak, 323
    French Dip, 322
    Hot Crab and Cheese, 325
    Hot Tuna, 324
    Lettuce and Tomato, 328
    Lobster Filling, 326
    Monte Cristo, 327
    Toasted Cheese, 327
    Tuna Filling, 324
    Vegie, 328
Sangria, 262
Sauces
    Clam, Linguine with, 437
    Ketchup and Horseradish, 247
    Orange and Vermouth,
        Fillets with, 427
    Rhubarb, 506
    Spaghetti, 492–93
    Tuna, Linguine with, 441
    Wine and Tomato, Fillets
        with, 428
Sautèed Mushrooms, 384
Sautèed Vegetables, 384
Scallops, Broiled, 418
Scrambled Eggs, 290
Seafood, 414–43
    Baked Fillets with Lemon
        and Fennel, 425
    Barbecued Fillets, 426
    Bouillabaisse, 440–41
    Broiled Fillets with Fresh

Lemon, 424
Broiled Scallops, 418
Calamari, 439
Chowder, 311
Cioppino, 442–43
Clams Italian Style, 417
Clam-stuffed Sole, 431
Court Bouillon, 423
Crab-stuffed Sole, 432
Crab-stuffed Trout, 422
Easy Court Bouillon, 423
Fettuccini, 436
Fillet of Sole with Fresh
    Vegetables and Dijon, 430
Fillets with Fresh Vegetables
    and Cheese, 429
Fillets with Vermouth and
    Orange Sauce, 427
Fillets with Wine and
    Tomato Sauce, 428
Fish Oriental Style, 435
Fresh Sole with Yogurt and
    Cheese, 433
Linguine with Clam Sauce, 437
Linguine with Tuna Sauce, 441
Lobster Tails, 419
Marinated Fish, 420
Mussels Italian Style, 415
Paella, 428–29
Poached Fish, 424
Steamed Clams with Fresh
    Lemon, 416
Stuffed Whole Fish, 421
Szechwan Fish Rolls, 434–35
Tuna Burgers, 433
Tuna Noodle Casserole, 443
See also names of seafood
Sesame Seeds
    Fresh Spinach with, 337, 397
    Hot Mustard and, 247
Seven Minute Icing, 526
Seviche, 240
    Salad, 333
    Soup, 309
Shish Kebob, 477
Single Pastry Crust, 507
Skewered Beef, 484

Skewered Fruit, 250
Skim Milk, 201
Soft Pretzels, 276
Sole
    Clam-stuffed, 431
    Crab-stuffed, 432
    with Fresh Vegetables and
        Dijon, 430
    with Yogurt and Cheese, 433
Sorbets, 516–17
    freezing and beating, 516
    Lemon, 517
    Papaya, 517
    Watermelon, 516
Soups, 295–319
    Beef Broth, 302
    Beef Broth Parisian, 303
    Chicken Broth, 295
    Chicken with Buckwheat
        Noodles, 300
    Chicken with Chinese
        Vegetables, 296
    Chicken with Lemon, 297
    Chicken Noodle, 300
    Chicken with Spinach and
        Saifun, 297
    Chicken with Tomato and
        Green Onion, 296
    Chicken Vegetable, 299
    Chilled Pea, 308
    Cream of Artichoke, 315
    Cream of Asparagus, 315
    Cream of Celery, 317
    Cream of Chicken, 316
    Cream of Cucumber, 317
    Cream of Mushroom, 319
    Cream of Pea, 318
    Cream of Zucchini, 319
    Egg Drop, 299
    Fresh Mushroom with
        Mozzarella Cheese, 304
    Fresh Tomato, 306
    Gazpacho, 307
    Hearty Clam Nectar, 314
    Hearty Cream of Chicken, 316
    Hearty Turkey, 301
    Manhattan Clam Chowder, 312
    Mexican Chili, 308

Minestrone, 305
Mushroom-Barley, 303
New England Clam
 Chowder, 313
Oyster Stew, 310
Seafood Chowder, 311
Seviche, 309
Turkey Broth, 301
Won Ton, 298
Spaghetti Sauce, 492–93
Spanish Dip, 257
Spinach
 and Crab Coquette, 242
 Dip, 258
 Lemon Chicken with, 472
 and Saifun, Chicken Soup
  with, 297
 Salad, 337
 with Sesame Seeds, 337, 397
 Tomato, and Chicken Salad, 340
Spring Rolls, 246–47
Squash, Baked, 398
Steamed Chicken, 455
Steamed Clams
 Bordelaise, 237
 with Fresh Lemon, 416
Steamed Mussels with Wine
 and Garlic, 237
Steamed Turkey Breast, 449
Stews
 Beef, 487
 Bouillabaisse, 440–41
 Cioppino, 442–43
 Oyster, 310
Stir-fried Broccoli, 375
Stir-fried Chicken
 with Green Peppers, 460
 with Vegetables, 459
Stir-fried Vegetables, 383
Strawberry(ies)
 Frost, 261
 Ice, 512
 Ice Cream, 519
 -Rhubarb Pie, 508

Shortcake, 502
 with Yogurt and Brown
  Sugar, 502
Stroganoff, Beef, 493
Stuffed Artichoke Salad, 346
Stuffed Lettuce, 336
Stuffed Mushrooms, 245
Stuffed Whole Fish, 421
Stuffing, Bread, 411
Summer Salad, 358
Super Taco Salad, 352
Sweet and Sour Salad, 332
Swiss Steak, 483
Syrup
 Fruit, 287
 Maple, 287
Szechwan Fish Rolls, 434–35

T
Tabbouli Pilaf, 409
Taco(s)
 Oven, 490
 Salad, 351
 Super Salad, 352
Tapioca Pudding, 521
Tarragon and Lemon, Green
 Beans with, 373
Tea, Iced, 263
Thousand Island Dressing, 365
Three Bean Salad, 356
Toasted Cheese Sandwich, 327
Toasted Pumpkin Seeds, 259
Tomato(es), 395–97
 Artichoke, Mushroom, and
  Green Bean Salad, 342
 Basil, and Cheese, Pasta
  with, 403
 and Basil, Fettuccini with, 404
 Canned, 395
 and Cucumber Salad, 338
 and Green Onion, Chicken
  Soup with, 296

Halves, Broiled, 396
Herbed, 397
and Lettuce Sandwich, 328
and Mayonnaise, Lemon
Chicken with, 473
Mozzarella, and Basil Salad,
338
Pasta Primavera with, 402
and Roast Peppers Salad,
339
Salsa, 257, 361
Soup, Fresh, 306
Spinach, and Chicken
Salad, 340
Vera Cruz, 396
Vinaigrette, 339
and Wine Sauce, Fillets
with, 428
Topping for Fruit Cobbler, 510
Tortilla Chips, 256
Cheese, 256
Tostados, 489
Cheese, 256
Chicken, 469
Trout, Crab-stuffed, 422
Tuna
Antipasto, 248
Burgers, 433
Hot Sandwich, 324
Noodle Casserole, 443
Salad, Hot, 349
Sandwich Filling, 324
Sauce, Linguine with, 441
Turkey, 447–49
Barbecued, 448
Broth, 301
Roast, 447
Roast Breast, 449
Soup, Hearty, 301
Steamed Breast, 449
Twice-baked Potatoes, 390

V

Veal, 480–82
Burgers, 480
Grilled Steaks with Fresh
Lemon and Mushrooms, 482

Italian Style, 481
Roast, 480
Vegetable(s), 368–401
Almond Peas, 387
Antipasto, 249
Artichoke Hearts with
Lemon, Garlic and Olive
Oil, 371
Baked Eggplant, 379
Baked Eggplant Provencale, 380
Baked Onions, 386
Baked Potatoes, 390
Baked Squash, 398
Barbecued Eggplant, 378
Barbecued Zucchini, 399
Breaded Artichoke Hearts, 371
Broiled Tomato Halves, 396
Canned Tomatoes, 395
Celery Remoulade, 372
and Cheese, Fillets with, 429
Cheese-stuffed Zucchini, 400
Chicken Soup, 299
Chinese, Chicken Soup
with, 296
Corn on the Cob, 378
Cottage Fries, 388
Dijon, 376
and Dijon, Fillet of Sole
with, 430
French Fried Potatoes, 388
Fresh Artichokes, 370
Fresh Asparagus with
Lemon, 372
Fresh Broccoli with
Safflower Mayonnaise, 376
Fried Onions, 386
Green Beans with Fresh
Lemon and Tarragon, 373
Green Beans Italian Style, 373
Green Beans with Lemon
and Black Pepper, 374
Green Beans with
Mushrooms and Pecans, 374
Green Beans with
Mushrooms and
Waterchestnuts, 375
Grilled, 382
Hash Brown Potatoes, 389

Herbed Tomatoes, 397
Holiday Yams with
    Marshmallows, 398
Lemon Potatoes, 391
Mashed Potatoes, 393
Minted Peas, 387
New Potatoes and Fresh
    Vegetables, 392
Nippy Carrots, 377
notes on cooking, 368–69
Onion Rings, 385
Onions Vinaigrette, 385
Oriental, 382
Parsleyed Potatoes, 392
Potato Chips, 389
Potatoes Epicure, 393
Potatoes with Onion and
    Dill, 391
Ratatouille, 381
Roast Peppers, 399
Sautèed, 384
Sautèed Mushrooms, 384
Sesame Spinach, 397
Skewered, Barbecued
    Chicken with, 457
Stir-fried, 383
Stir-fried Broccoli, 375
Stir-fried Chicken with, 459
Twice-baked Potatoes, 390
Vera Cruz Tomatoes, 396
Zucchini and Carrots
    Julienne, 400
Zucchini-Mozzarella
    Casserole, 401

Vegie Sandwich, 328

Vera Cruz Tomatoes, 396

Vermouth and Orange Sauce,
    Fillets with, 427

Vinaigrette
    Dijon, 361
    Onions with, 385
    Tomatoes with, 339

Vinegar and Oil Dressing, 362
    with Lemon, 362

W

Waffles, 286

Waterchestnuts and Fresh
    Mushrooms, 341
    Green Beans with, 375

Watermelon
    Frozen, 505
    Ice, 514
    Salad, 357
    Sorbet, 516

Wheat Bread, Honey, 268

Whipped Cream Substitute, 202

White Bread, Enriched, 267

Wild Rice, 408

Wilted Lettuce, 336

Wine
    and Garlic, Steamed
        Mussels with, 237
    and Tomato Sauce, Fillets
        with, 428

Winter Salad, 359

Won Ton Soup, 298

Y

Yams with Marshmallows, 398

Yellow Chiffon Cake, 526

Yogurt
    and Brown Sugar,
        Strawberries with, 502
    and Cheese, Fresh Sole
        with, 433
    Dressing, 365
    Frozen Pops, 520
    Fruit, 203
    Pancakes, 284
    Plain Nonfat, 202

Z

Zucchini, 399–401
    Barbecued, 399
    Bread, 281
    and Carrots Julienne, 400
    Cheese-stuffed, 400
    -Mozzarella Casserole, 401
    Salad, 343
    Soup, Cream of, 319
    Stuffed with Crab, 343